MW01245831

From Bob Knight

to Bobby Wampler

Stories from the Heartland

by Lynn Houser

This book is dedicated to my wife, Pat, who knew a good story idea when she heard one, who wasn't afraid to tell me of a bad story idea when she heard one, and who, in the end, was the best editor, proof-reader and spell-checker a writer ever had.

M. T. Publishing Company, Inc.™

P.O. Box 6802
Evansville, Indiana 47719-6802
www.mtpublishing.com

Copyright © 2014
Lynn Houser

Graphic Designer: Amanda Reyher

Library of Congress Control Number: 2014941728
ISBN: 978-1-938730-35-1

Printed in the United States of America.

Thanks, reader, for taking an interest in this book. I lived it, and I hope you can relive it — the laughter, the tears, the thrills.

Lynn Houser

Contents

Chapter 3
Adventures and Misadventures

Chapter 4
Closer to Home

Chapter 5
On the Beaten Path

Chapter 6
The General's Last Stand

Chapter 7
Old Generals Never Die

Chapter 8
Out of the Blues Comes 2002

Chapter 9
Gamers

Chapter 10
The Long Haul

Chapter 11
Going Pro

Chapter 12
Characters

Chapter 13
Good-Bye, So Long, Farewell

Index

Acknowledgements

This project would never have taken flight had it not been for the cooperation of two publishers, Mayer Maloney of the *Bloomington Herald-Times* and Terry Housholder of the *Kendallville News-Sun*. Without their blessing to reprint all the articles, there would have been no book.

I should also credit *Sports Illustrated* for letting me reprint the article on pencil baseball; *Indianapolis Monthly*, for allowing me to reprint "*Hoosiers*, Ten Years After" and "Fallen Hoosier;" *Indiana Alumni Magazine*, for allowing me to reprint the article on the resurgence of IU athletics and also the article on George William Thompson.

A lot of others deserve some thanks. Bob Hammel, the retired *Herald-Times* Sports Editor, is the best mentor a writer could ever have -- the ultimate professional.

I also would like to thank John Peirce, the former *News-Sun* editor who gave me a chance to learn and grow as a sports writer.

Above all I would like to thank my wife, Pat, the best editor a reporter could ever have. Her input and feedback over the years has steered many an article on the right path.

Foreword

Did I Mention Bob Knight?

There, I did it. I shamelessly worked Bob Knight into my book title.

Bob Knight probably would rather I left him out of it, but how else is a rather obscure writer like me going to lure a reader into these pages? What other title could I come up with -- "The Greatest Hits of a Writer You Never Heard Of?"

Bob Knight sells, folks, and now that I am retired, I need to supplement my fixed income. Drawing a sportswriter's salary for 36 years is not going to take you very far, but before Coach Knight excommunicates me, I hope he will take the time to read the chapters devoted to him.

My intent is to not pile up on Knight like a lot of writers have done over the years. I was fortunate to get a closer look at the man thanks to my position as a sports writer for the *Bloomington Herald-Times*. I was able to see the man's genius and also his flaws.

I was courtside in Bloomington when he threw "The Chair" in 1985. I was courtside in

New Orleans when he won his last NCAA title in 1987. I was in Indianapolis in 2000 when Indiana University President Myles Brand announced that Knight no longer would be coaching the IU basketball team. And I was there in Lubbock in 2001 when Knight began a new chapter at Texas Tech.

Four of the 13 chapters in this book pertain to Knight, so the title isn't misleading at all. By the thread of the written word, Bob Knight has been woven into the life of this Indiana writer.

Keep in mind that the *Bloomington Herald-Times*, the home-town newspaper, tended to take Knight's side over the years. The H-T's long-time sports editor, Bob Hammel, my mentor, had a strong, personal friendship with Knight that filtered down to the rest of the staff. Today, that would be frowned upon, but in the 1970s, '80s and early '90s it was not at all viewed as a lack of professionalism. The H-T realized early on that Knight sold newspapers, and it was in our best interests to cultivate that relationship.

So when I followed as Hammel as IU basketball beat writer in 1998, I took the same approach with Knight. Although I never reached the level of friendship Hammel did, I believe I did earn the man's trust and respect.

That's not to say we didn't have our differences. There was an occasion where Knight was so upset with one of my columns that he called me to his office and demanded an apology. Before I could explain my position, he asked me to leave his office in no uncertain terms. It was if he were exercising his authority as "The General," and I was the duty-bound soldier to oblige. However, he eventually cooled down and actually became more tolerant of me from that point on.

It helped open a door when he was hired by Texas Tech in 2001. The H-T sent me out to Lubbock to cover the event, and I was surprised to find Knight welcoming me with open arms. There is an entire chapter of this book devoted to his resurfacing in Texas, along with chapters covering his last season at IU, his controversial dismissal and his early years. And don't miss the feature on the 1976 Hoosiers, "The Spirit of '76," in Chapter 10, "The Long Haul.'

I do want to emphasize that this book encompasses a lot more than Knight. It is a collection of pieces on a multitude of topics.

You will read about the IU basketball player who carried a bullet in his side while he played for Knight.

You will read about a Hoosier player who lost his mother to a tornado.

You will discover how another Hoosier had to confront his lack of confidence.

You will see baseball player Mickey Mantle golfer John Daly like you have never seen them before.

You will follow me on a look back into the early 1900s, when Jim Thorpe roamed IU's Jordan Field and when a rather obscure black athlete went on to become a civil rights leader in a distant Midwestern town.

These pages span a wide range of eras, topics and personalities, taking you from the simplicity of the high school stage to the vastness of the college and professional sports arena, from Bob Knight to, well, Bobby Wampler.

Of all the personalities I came across in 36 years, Bobby Wampler is one of the most loveable. If nothing else, please read the two stories about this inspirational young man in Chapter 12.

Also, don't miss the stories on the movie, *Hoosiers*, especially "The Fallen Hoosier," the tragic account of the final days of Kent Poole, the young man who played "Merle." Look for those stories in Chapter 10.

I hope you will find something entertaining in all the stories and see how the writing evolved over 30-plus years. You will note a number of clichés, I must confess. However, most of them were still fresh at the time they were written. To put each story in its proper historical perspective, I have included the publication dates. Each piece also is prefaced with a brief editor's note explaining the origin or background.

The articles selected were either award-winners, reader favorites or personal favorites. Some of them date back to the 1970s, when I was sports writer for the *Kendallville News-Sun*, a small daily in northeastern Indiana. I started there in 1976 and remained in that position for eight years. In 1984 I took a sports position at the *Bloomington Herald-Telephone*, which was renamed the *Herald-Times* in 1989. I remained there until my retirement in 2012.

So, ripped from the headlines, I give you 36 years of newspaper writing. Turn the page and dive in. As you will see, there is a story behind the story, including mine.

Lynn Houser

Chapter 1
Close Encounters of the First Kind

Any Indiana sportswriter who worked his craft during the 1970s, '80s and '90s can thank Bob Knight for being a steady source of copy. This chapter covers Knight's early years, including his 1979 run-in with the Puerto Rican authorities, the 1985 chair-throwing incident and the 1987 national championship season. It ends with Knight contemplating a move to New Mexico.

Your Basic Bob Knight

The first article in this book is actually the last one thrown into the mix. As I was about to wrap up this project, I came upon this manuscript in an old scrapbook. It details my very first encounter with Bob Knight, going back to my student days at Indiana University. In the fall of 1971 I was taking a magazine writing class. One of our assignments was to focus on a public figure. I chose the new head basketball coach, and he made time to meet with me one-on-one and allow me to attend some pre-season practices. Although the writing wasn't good enough to interest a magazine, I think it does give the reader an insight into what the young coach was all about. And little did I know at the time, it was the very first thread in a fabric that helped shape my career.

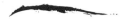

December 1971
(unpublished)

An Indiana University basketball practice: Two squads of players are performing rigorous basketball drills at opposite ends of the court. Standing on the big, red "I" encircled at center court is a tall and muscular figure who is watching the action with an absorbing intensity. Except for his short, frosty-black hair, the man's youthful face radiates a boyishness which makes him look almost as young as the players.

Sometimes this man will shout with authority at the players. At other times he will address them in a conversational manner. And then occasionally he will just shake his head and say nothing at all. No matter how he communicates to the players, they watch and listen because he is the boss. He is Bob Knight, the new head basketball coach of Indiana University.

As a new coach he brings new methods, new philosophies and new approaches to Hoosier basketball. This change has been long overdue, according to some followers of IU.

After two last place finishes in the Big Ten prior to the 1970-71 season, the fans began to question the coaching of Lou Watson. But the skepticism of Watson's earlier years was replaced by hope as one of the most heralded crops of sophomores in IU history became eligible for the 1970-71 season. (It wasn't until the 1972-73 season that freshmen were allowed to suit up immediately).

With names like George McGinnis, Steve Downing, Ed Daniels, John Ritter, Bootsy White, Frank Wilson, Kim Pemberton and Jerry Memering added to the Hoosier roster, many expected to see Indiana in the Houston Astrodome for the NCAA finals.

But Indiana had to win the Big Ten first (only conference champs qualified), and it failed to do that when Wisconsin eliminated the Hoosiers from the race in a stunning overtime defeat. At the next home game, the chants of "We're No. 1" heard earlier in the season were replaced by boos and jeers aimed particularly at Watson.

While the fans were disappointed with Watson because of Indiana's failure to win the Big Ten, they weren't the only ones who were displeased. Some of the players also were discontented with the head coach because they felt he was partial to certain members of the team (mainly McGinnis). At a secret meeting, they aired their views their views and considered boycotting the upcoming Ohio State game. Although the boycott never materialized, the knowledge of the meeting and the players' dissent was enough to make Watson resign less than 48 hours after the Ohio State contest.

Upon Watson's resignation, many of his supporters such as trustee Robert H. Menke lashed out at both the players and fans.

Said Menke, "In the future, players should understand that they must go the season, and that applies to the coach, too – no matter what pressure is exerted by irate or chauvinistic fans."

Even some of the players themselves condemned the treatment of Watson. Ritter, who had voted against the proposed boycott, was so upset he pondered quitting basketball altogether.

"I love basketball," he said, "but after this year, considering my relationship with the other players are not the best, I'm not sure if I could play."

Thus, the year that was supposed to be IU's ended dismally. There was no NCAA, no championship, no celebration and, furthermore, no coach.

Speculation as to who would fill the coaching vacancy ranged from such notables as Bill Russell and Elgin Baylor to assistant coach Jerry Oliver. It wasn't very easy trying to recruit a coach when his mission would be, should he decide to accept, to bring a basketball program back from the dead.

But on March 27, 17 days after the departure of Watson, Indiana hired the head coach of the United States Military Academy, Bob Knight.

A "disciplinarian" by label, the university could hardly have hired a man with a more impressive record. After six years at Army, Knight's teams compiled a record of 102 wins and 50 losses – almost a .700 clip. Consistently in those years his teams ranked high in the nation in defense, and in four of those years Army was invited to the National Invitational Tournament.

His best year was in 1968 when his team established an Army record of 22 wins in a single season and finished 16th in the final polls. And Knight did all that without ever having a player over 6-foot-6.

The selection of Knight undoubtedly raised a few eyebrows among IU followers.

"What kind of coach was this who could mold a basketball also-ran like Army into a top contender?" they asked. "Could he do the same with a broken and torn IU"

The fans waited eagerly for the first public appearance of Knight.

They didn't have to wait long. On March 31, Knight called his first press conference. At that meeting the new coach did not talk about Watson and the boycott, as expected. He refused to do so on the grounds that he didn't have all the facts. Instead, he talked about things like "discipline, "defense" and a "new season."

Although a comment on the past would not have been out of order, it appeared Knight couldn't care less about what had preceded him. In a strange way, his reluctance to talk about those events was reassuring because Knight seemed to be issuing an official signal to forget the past and welcome the future. As far as he was concerned, the "new season" had already begun.

It has been almost eight months since that first press conference, and Knight still is determined to forget the past. With season opening this month, he continues to talk about the future, whether he has all the facts about last year or not.

"I don't have any feeling whatsoever as to what transpired in the past," Knight says. "If the players are going to worry about last year, then we are not going to make any headway this year. I don't really know what happened, and I don't really care. This is a new year."

So rather than dwelling on yesterday, Knight is requiring his players to concentrate on what he wants them to do tomorrow. This is where the discipline comes in.

By "discipline" Knight means doing the right thing at the right time – in all phases of the game.

"When a guy drives towards the basket, fakes, and the defenseman does not leave his feet, that's discipline," Knight says. "Of if a guy is on a fast break and passes the ball off, that's discipline, too."

But discipline does not come easy, especially in the Knight tradition. His definition requires "repetition, repetition and more repetition" of practice drills. This means a lot of free throw shooting, passing and plain running. It's hard work, but even though Knight is a former Army man, his practices are not like boot camp.

Knight does not try to wear out his players, nor does he consistently find fault with them. On the other hand, he does not hesitate to compliment them when they do the right things. When he does correct them, he attacks the mistake and not the player personally. Sometimes his corrections can even make a player laugh at himself.

In one instance, Knight had just corrected senior forward Joby Wright for a defensive mistake when he added, "You're going to make mistakes once in a while – maybe one every three games."

Such tactics in practice create a kind of looseness which makes the hard work less strenuous and seemingly more worthwhile. As Wilson says, "This is the only way to go. If you want to win you have to practice hard."

After discipline comes Knights stock and trade, defense. Knight's brand of defense is a vicious man-to-man which constantly goes for the ball, the rebound and the open offensive player. In a day of zone defenses, "box" zones and "sagging" zones, the stingy man-to-man defense is almost a work of art.

A man-to-man requires an enormous amount of individual effort and teamwork, particularly if the other team has an Austin Carr (the Notre Dame star) or a Sydney Wicks (UCLA). When it is up to one man to stop the likes of one of those, he has a monumental responsibility. But you can't stop a Carr or Wicks every time, so what do you do?

That's where the teamwork comes in, according to Knight. If one defensive player has his hands full, the others take up the slack when the situation calls for it. If the primary defensive player is "burned," the nearest defenseman leaves his player long enough to fill the vacancy. Meanwhile, the other defensive players are covering the remaining opponents until the original defenseman recovers.

Complicated? Now you can see what a good man-to-man is sort of a rarity. Things could get rather frantic if the opposing team has more than one superstar.

You can also see why discipline is necessary to play such a defense. It takes discipline to cover one and sometimes two players at the same time.

Despite the difficulty, Knight still is sold on his kind of defense because "the more you put into defense, the less mistakes are going to hurt you. A score often results from defensive mistakes than offensive effort."

On Knight's word, defense is the basis of winning, and winning is the goal of all sports. He agrees with the philosophy that "winning isn't everything; it's the only thing." To Knight, winning is the ultimate objective.

"Winning is important. Period," he says. "After all, why are we working so hard? Why? It's like war. Who wants to finish second?"

Knight adds that he does not believe in unethical practices just to build a winner, but when winning itself is concerned, he doesn't believe it can be over-emphasized. And when it comes to pressure situations, he states that each player should be assessed individually to "see who can get the job done."

At the same time, Knight tries to take a realistic approach to winning. He knows that losing is almost inevitable, so he cautions against "getting down" on a team for losing.

"Losing can be as much an experience as winning, because you can learn by your mistakes," Knight says. "When a team loses, look at how much effort was put out, and then make your judgment."

Before a team can consider winning, it must have what Knight calls the "proper mental approach." The kind of mental attitude Knight is looking for in his players consists of the desire to learn, obey and sacrifice for the sake of the team. These characteristics are important to Knight because he feels that the mental approach is just as important as the physical. In fact, he says, "Without the proper mental attitude, it is difficult to develop the abilities you have."

Without the right mental attitude, all the work put into discipline and defense is wasted, in Knight's eyes. It is all a part of his formula for winning:

VICTORY = DISCIPLINE + DEFENSE + DESIRE.

It is with this formula that Knight hopes to put the pieces back together at IU. Whether he succeeds remains to be seen through the course of the new season.

Perhaps some clue to things to come is contained in this observation by Wright: "In high school we had a disciplinarian coach, and at the end of my senior year we won the state championship. If everyone works hard, we can win the Big Ten this year."

Editor's Note: Knight's first team finished fourth in the Big Ten and lost in the first round of the NIT. He second team won the Big Ten and went to the Final Four.

Mission Improbable

I did not have the opportunity to cover Bob Knight's early Final Four runs because I was in the Navy from 1972-76. But once I got back into my chosen field, I discovered that Knight was a constant provider of column material. His run-in with a Puerto Rican policeman at the 1979 Pan Am Games offered all sorts of possible angles. I chose a slightly different approach, a gimmick that took first place in the annual Hoosier State Press Association contest, my first award in sports writing. The gags and clichés are stale now, but, hey, Mission Possible *still was a popular TV show in 1979. Today, the piece smacks of political incorrectness.*

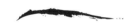

Kendallville News-Sun
July 29, 1979

In an isolated washroom in Puerto Rico, a man dressed in a business suit deposits a coin into a pay toilet. Once inside the stall, the man lifts up the toilet bowl cover and discovers a waterproof container. Inside the container are a tape recorder and 8-x-10 glossy. Pressing the switch on the recorder, he hears this message: "Buenas dias, Señor Sanchez.

"The hombre you see in the enclosed photograph is Public Enemy No. 1, the infamous Roberto Knight. On July 8, 1979, this hombre committed a heinous crime against the Republic of Puerto Rico by engaging in a shoving match with one of Puerto Rico's finest, a policeman by the name of Juan deSilva.

"The incident evolved when Knight commented on the sexual habits of Brazilian women in the presence of the Brazilian women's basketball team.

"DeSilva took issue with Knight's insult, and reminded him that he was in a Latin country. Besides, deSilva pointed out, Brazilian women are not dirty.

"Like Dr. Jekyll and Mr. Hyde, the American coach instantly turned into a raging maniac, verbally assaulting the kindly policeman about his racial background. Moments later, the Yankee swine attacked deSilva's finger with his eye, a typical dirty tactic. After that, Knight sucker-punched the bewildered policeman.

"Being the good law enforcer that he is, deSilva immediately arrested the Yankee dog on charges of assault with a deadly eye. Although his fellow policemen and our own government refused to stand behind deSilva, the noble policeman wisely made a federal case out of it. Taking up the crusade himself, the gallant deSilva shocked civilization (as we know it) by standing fast. In a heroic move, deSilva filed suit against the imperialist from the North.

"The Yankee pig cried "foul" and tried to squirm out of it, but deSilva had him by the seat of his Yankee pants.

"The charlatan pleaded for time to make his case, and Judge Rugrico Rivera, out of the kindness of his heart, granted that much-needed time. In reality, though, the tyrannical Knight was stalling so he could humiliate our beloved basketball team.

"On the evening of July 13, the boorish coach took out his anger on the basketball court, unleashing his shock troopers with a brutal vengeance. After rolling up the score against Puerto Rico's noble defenders of freedom, Knight shook his fist and gave the warm crowd the proverbial finger. What gall!

"Well, he got his in the end, Señor Sanchez. Judge Rivera, who is coming up for election this year, gave Señor Knight what he had coming to him -- the shaft.

"That was justice, amigo, especially since the coward refused to honor us with his presence. Now the gringo must "face the music," as the Yankees say.

"However, instead of serving his sentence like a man, Knight has told us to come and get him. Well, muchacho, we will.

"Your mission, Señor Sanchez, should you decide to accept, is to bring this desperado back to face justice. Extradite the bandito by whatever means necessary, just do it!

"You will find that your associates, Señor Gordon Liddy and Señor Howard Hunt, are more than capable helpers. Believe me, they are experienced in these matters.

"You will have all the supplies you need for this mission, including an amphibious assault vehicle, a Phantom jet, a militia of mercenaries and a season ticket to Indiana University basketball games.

"Good luck, Señor Sanchez. As usual, the secretary will disavow any knowledge of this conversation. This message will self-destruct in 10 seconds."

The Chair Man Has the Floor

Fast-forwarding to the incident that now is simply known as "The Chair." In the heat of the Purdue game on February 23, 1985, Bob Knight picked up a chair and hurled it across the floor of IU's Assembly Hall. From my courtside seat I knew I had a side bar that would be as well read as the game story. Purdue won, 72-63, but who really remembers the score? "The Chair" is all anybody talked about that day, and it remains one of the most talked about moments of Knight's career.

Bloomington *Herald -Telephone*
February 24, 1985

Five minutes before Saturday's game at Indiana, Purdue guard Steve Reid received a friendly cuff on the back of the head by IU coach Bob Knight, the ultimate compliment Knight pays to opposing seniors the last time he faces them.

Five minutes into the game, Reid almost got another Knight greeting. He was at the free throw line when a chair came skidding past him, courtesy of Knight, who was protesting a technical foul. Aside from the fact the Purdue went on to beat the Hoosiers 72-63 to complete a season sweep for the first time since 1977, the vision of that chair sliding past him will be the most lasting impression for Reid.

"I was shocked," said the plucky 5-9 senior from Dodge City, Kansas. "I've never seen a chair come flying in front of me when shooting a free throw. I was just going up to the line to get the ball when it came winging by. It kind of startled me."

Reid was preparing to shoot the first of two technical shots when the unexpected missile delayed his mission. Two more technicals later, Reid was at the line shooting a total of six penalty shots. With the Hoosier crowd doing its best to distract him, Reid sank the first two shots. He then yielded to the crowd's will by missing the next three shots before sinking the final attempt.

"There was such a big gap between the time it started and the time it was resolved," explained Reid, who scored 13 points. "I just wanted to get the first couple down and I don't know what the heck happened to me after that."

The already famous "Chair Incident" did little to lessen Reid's appreciation for the friendly cuff on the head by Knight, however.

"I have a lot of respect for Coach Knight's knowledge of the game and I think that (pat on the head) is a great compliment. It (the chair) just surprised me. I don't know why he did it. I know he wasn't throwing it at me. I don't think he would ever do anything to intentionally hurt someone. I just think he was frustrated."

Fellow seniors James Bullock and Mark Atkinson, two other recipients of Knight's pre-game pats on the head, expressed mixed opinions. Bullock, the bullish 6-6 forward who muscled his way to 15 points and 8 rebounds, questioned the extent of Knight's anger. "When he threw the chair, first of all, I thought it hit Steve," Bullock said. "I tried to ignore it. I got the guys in a huddle and told them, "Look, don't worry about that. Just come out and Play harder because he's trying to get them fired up.' He's a tough coach, but Gene Keady's a tough coach when you get right down to it. He (Knight) gets a little frantic now and then, but throwing chairs at a college basketball game is going a little far. I'm not going to say he's not a good coach and that I wouldn't mind playing for him, but I don't know."

Atkinson, the 6-8 forward who blanketed IU's Steve Alford for the second time this year, pointed out that Knight's wrath was directed at the officials and not the players.

"Knight is a good coach and he can basically do whatever he wants to, as long as he doesn't do anything to hurt other people. Now if that chair had hit somebody, he would have been sorry and would have come out and said something about it."

Hoosiers Beat Rebs at Own Game

Two years later, Indiana fans were celebrating a national championship. I was fortunate to be included in the Herald-Telephone's *coverage of the 1987 Final Four in New Orleans. My job was to get the opposition's side of the story. It was hard to keep a straight face in the post-game lockerroom of the UNLV Runnin' Rebs, who were not the most gracious losers. The Syracuse Orangemen, on the other hand, were nothing but classy after the final two nights later.*

Bloomington *Herald-Times*
March 29, 1987

NEW ORLEANS, LOUISIANA

They have warm-ups with names on the back like "The Hammer," "El Hud" and "G-Man."

They have cheerleaders who dress up like dance hall girls. They have fans who wear more gold than Mr. T.

They are the Runnin' Rebs of the University of Nevada-Las Vegas, the Corvettes of college basketball.

They run, they gun and they are proud of it, even in defeat.

It takes more than a 97-93 defeat to Indiana in the NCAA semifinals to impress the Rebs. If anything, they found the Hoosiers underwhelming.

"They couldn't have beat us if we had come to play," said Eldridge "El Hud" Hudson. "You hear that Bobby Knight has this good defense. Bah!"

"IU gets away with a lot," said Gary "G-Man" Graham. "They use moving picks. They travel."

"It's those crazy picks the refs don't call," grumbled Hudson. "If you taped this game, you could see the things they get away with. One time Gerald Paddio got a rebound and four guys were there to push him out of bounds and they got away with it."

"It hurts, it hurts," Paddio responded.

"Their picking game is the real story," Graham concluded. "Their offense is very well run. They get the ball to Steve Alford where he can shoot. I do think the refs overprotect him. If you even come close to him they call a foul. One time after a 3-point shot they called a foul and I didn't even touch him."

The moment Graham was referring to became a 4-point play when Alford added the free throw, giving the Hoosier their biggest lead at 41-27 with six minutes left in the first half.

"Alford is a super athlete, but they have super athletes all around," Graham said. "He scored his points (33), but if Gerald Paddio and I had done more offensively, we would have won the game. It just wasn't there today. We just didn't feel it. It's unbelievable. This hurts so bad. We can't blame anybody but ourselves. We accepted the glory when we were winning, and we have to accept this now."

"We didn't rebound and we didn't make the clutch free throws," Paddio said.

For the game, the Rebs were 10-for-19 from the line and were outrebounded 42-40. Armon "The Hammer" Gilliam was the only inside threat the Rebs had with 32 points and 10 rebounds. Their outside game was mostly limited to the long-range shooting of Freddie Banks, who led all scorers with 38 points by drilling 10 of 19 from 3-point land.

"You work so hard to get to the Final Four and now it seems so far away," Hudson said. "It was close, oh so close. We played hard. We were just a step slow. Five steals is not Runnin' Reb basketball. It's over, all over."

Hudson was so unimpressed by Indiana he predicted a "lopsided" victory for Syracuse in Monday's title game.

"It won't even be close," he said. "If Rony Seikaly comes to play, they have nobody who can guard him. If Derrick Coleman comes to play, there's no one who can guard him. If Howard Triche gets his shot from outside, they won't be able to stop him. I think Syracuse is much more physical. Indiana is not very physical at all."

Even a Runnin' Reb mother was less than awed by the Hoosiers.

"You beat Indiana," she said to Hudson as he left the lockerroom. "You just couldn't whip the refs."

Putting the 'Men" Orangemen

Now see how the Orangemen of Syracuse handled defeat.

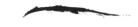

Bloomington *Herald -Telephone*
March 31, 1987

NEW ORLEANS, LOUISIANA

To win with class is easy. To lose with class takes grace.

The Syracuse Orangemen exhibited the kind of grace in defeat that proves there are no losers in championship games of the caliber played for the NCAA title Monday night.

The last-second loss to Indiana left the Orangemen in a daze and put a lot of bewildered looks on faces in the Syracuse lockerroom. But you won't see the Orangemen going off into the woods to eat berries after falling to Indiana on Keith Smart's jumper at 0:04, 74-73.

Defeats don't come any harder, especially when there is a championship on the line. However, sophomore guard Sherman Douglas spoke for the rest of his teammates when he said, "I'm not going to do nothing nasty to my life. We had a very positive season. We have a lot of young players who are going to step up in this program. We had a great team and had a great season. Just because we lost doesn't mean we're going to jump off a bridge or cut off our heads. Somebody had to lose."

Rony Seikaly, the junior center who did his part with 18 points and 10 rebounds, concurred.

"We had a great season; we were just a point short. We made a great effort to get here. To lose on a last-second shot hurts more than losing by 10, because 10 means the other team is better. The thing that's sad is that we did have control. Indiana is a great team, but when you lose on a last-second shot, there is no better team."

After rethinking his position, the native of Athens, Greece added, "As I look at it now, there is only one team in the nation better than us, and that is Indiana – and then only by a point."

Seikaly liked his chances when Howard Triche hit the front end of a one-and-one to give Syracuse a 73-70 lead with 38 seconds left. When he missed the back end, Smart promptly drove the lane and hit a jumper to make it 73-72.

The Hoosiers quickly fouled freshman Derrick Coleman, a 70 percent free throw shooter. Free throws have been hard to come by for the Orangemen at times this season, and Coleman failed on the front end of his one-and-one. Without calling time, the Hoosiers worked the clock down to 10 seconds. The Orangemen were not about to let All-American Steve Alford take the last shot. Alford was covered, so the ball ended up in Smart's hands with the seconds ticking away. Smart drove the left side and put up a 15-footer from the baseline.

"We expected Alford to get the ball," Seikaly said. "That's why it was so surprising when Smart got it. I was on the weak side and waiting for the rebound. But it hit nothing but net. The last 28 seconds we played great defense. Smart took a chance. If he misses that shot, we win."

Seikaly wasn't sure why three seconds ticked away from the time Smart's shot entered the net and the time the referees awarded a timeout with one second remaining.

"There was some confusion," Seikaly said. "As soon as the ball went through the net I went like this," he said, making a "T" with his hands. "We thought we were going to take control when we had a chance to go up four or five at the end," Seikaly said.

The Orangemen played well enough to win. They outrebounded the Hoosiers 38-35, sent them to the line only 12 times, held them to 48 percent shooting and allowed only four Hoosiers to score. They blanked starting forward Rick Calloway and four reserves.

"We played determined," Seikaly said. "We were excited about the game and ready to give it our best shot."

The Orangemen led the last eight minutes of the first half before a 3-point buzzer-beater by Alford sent them to the lockerroom down one, 34-33. The Orangemen were far from demoralized, though.

"The mood was good at halftime," Seikaly said. "We didn't want Alford to shoot that shot, but that's why he's an All-American. He can make that shot."

Alford had to work hard for his 23 points, the total leaving him one point short of Mike McGee's mark as the Big Ten's all-time leading scorer.

"Alford got some 3-point shots off screens, but most of them were off transition," said Syracuse's senior guard Greg Monroe.

After Alford's fourth 3-pointer of the first half gave Indiana its 34-33 lead, the Orangemen scored the first four points of the second half to regain the advantage. They led by as many as eight before the Hoosiers countered with a 10-0 run. That put Indiana up by two with over nine minutes to go, but the Orangemen answered with a 7-0 spurt to take a 5-point lead. It was 61-56 when Smart took over.

Playing before 64,959 Superdome fans in his home state of Louisiana, Smart scored 12 of Indiana's last 16 points to give the Hoosiers their fifth NCAA title. His heroics earned him Most Valuable Player honors for the Final Four.

"Smart played great," Seikaly said. "When we putting pressure on everybody else, he came through."

IU's 'Hoosiers' Better than Hollywood's

The night Indiana won the 1987 national championship was the same night the movie Hoosiers *was up for Academy Award honors. Indiana's last-second win over Syracuse was right out of a Hollywood script, it turned out. This column was the first of many occasions over the years in which I referenced that particular movie, as you will see.*

Bloomington Herald-Telephone
April 2, 1987

Did Indiana really win the NCAA championship Monday night, or was that another scene from the movie *Hoosiers*?

Was that Keith Smart hitting the last-second shot or Jimmy Chitwood?

Was that Bob Knight calmly sitting on the bench afterward or Norman Dale?

Was that Sharan Alford out on the floor with motherly tears or Barbara Hershey?

Naw, Sharan's prettier.

Maybe this was all a dream. Maybe it's a tasteless April Fool's joke by some jealous Purdue fans.

That's it. A bunch of Purdue fans seized control of CBS and showed some new footage from *Hoosiers* over the nation's airways Monday night. Yeah, that's the ticket.

No, it was the Boston Celtics. Yeah, the lads in green. They hijacked the IU team bus on the way to the Super Dome and demanded to play the game instead of Indiana.

Yeah, Jerry Sichting played Steve Alford because his hair never moves, either. Robert Parrish wiped the perpetual scowl off his face and played Dean Garrett. Dennis Johnson put Clearasil over his freckles to pass for Daryl Thomas. Red Auerbach stashed his cigar, put on a silver wig and rolled up a red sweater to play Bob Knight. And Larry Bird played Smart. He's the only one who could have done the things Smart did in the last 10 minutes.

This is no less harder to believe than the entire tournament trail for IU, which appropriately began at the Hoosier Dome. Whoever wrote the script for Indianapolis whetted our appetites with a come-from-behind win over Auburn, just the right kind of send-off for the regional finals in Cincinnati.

And who should shine in the Queen City but none other than the Cincinnati Kid, Rick Calloway? It was Calloway's dramatic tip against LSU that sent IU to New Orleans. A clever touch there.

Whose imagination is responsible for the championship game against Syracuse? What genius, having Smart emerge as an unexpected hero in his native state of Louisiana. Bravo!

Wonderfully, it's all so true. There it is, Smart's winning shot, again and again on TV. You can read about it in any newspaper in the land. You can listen to Don Fischer, the voice of IU, describing the final seconds on radio replays across the state. You can hear about it in any bar in Indiana, even those near West Lafayette.

For the Hoosier fans who witnessed first-hand the "Miracle on Bourbon Street," they experienced the thrill of a lifetime.

The original response was odd, though. When Smart's shot hit bottom with six seconds left – right in front of the IU cheerblock – a lot of the IU fans seemed to hesitate before letting loose with a roar. Even some of the sports writers from Indiana looked dumbfounded. Mouths were open but only air was coming out.

Did you ever want to scream for your life in a dream and couldn't? Or think back to your first attempt at speaking after having your tonsils removed.

Fans were simply stunned. The Syracuse players were so paralyzed they let precious seconds tick away before finally having the presence of mind to call a time-out.

A lot of IU heads turned quickly to the clock. Being the good basketball fans they are, they know the importance of immediately getting time called, but they were too busy coaxing the clock to cheer.

Confusion ultimately gave way to pandemonium when they realized only an absolute miracle could prevent them from winning. The only miracle was when Smart completed the script by interception the desperation pass.

It was yet another touch of Hollywood, on the very night of Hollywood's grandest event, the Academy Awards. Although *Hoosiers* did not win any Oscars, Indiana's Hoosiers won where it really counted.

One had to feel some sympathy for the Syracuse Orangemen. After Monday's bitter defeat, they sought no alibis. They took it like men and retained their self-respect.

An old funeral rite in New Orleans calls for a solemn procession to the cemetery. After sending the soul on its way to a better place, the procession turns into a joyous, musical parade. The Orangemen died a hard death in New Orleans Monday night, but their fans should celebrate a joyful passage into history. They were not losers. They were just caught up in a real-life drama called *Hoosiers*.

It Would Never Be the Same

Shortly after a disappointing 1987-88 season, Bob Knight appeared to be headed elsewhere. The University of New Mexico was making a big play for the coach, and he was listening.

Knight felt he was not appreciated in Bloomington, especially in the fury following his insensitive "rape" comment to CBS reporter Connie Chung. To paraphrase: "If rape is inevitable, you might as well enjoy it." He quickly tried to withdraw the comment, but CBS went with it.

As the firestorm grew and Knight was rumored to be leaving, Hoosier fans went into a panic, prompting this column. I didn't want him to leave without knowing how much he was appreciated. A few days later, after Knight decided to stay at IU, he told Herald-Telephone *sports editor Bob Hammel that my column helped sway his decision. It was the nicest compliment I ever received from the man.*

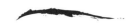

Bloomington Herald-Telephone
May 1988

Say it ain't so, Bob. Say you ain't leaving us. We're sorry if you feel betrayed, but you must believe the vast majority of Hoosiers support you.

You should have seen the switchboards light up down here at the newspaper when word got out that you were seriously thinking of leaving for New Mexico. Of the 21 calls I fielded in a 1 1/2-hour period Thursday morning, all 21 were pro-

Bob Knight. Eleven of them came from women. Apparently, a lot of women out there realize your "stress" comment had nothing to do with rape. They understand it was not the wisest choice for an analogy, but it in no way did it mean you condone such a violent act.

The gist of those phone calls was this: Indiana basketball would never be the same without you.

Bob, you are more than just a basketball coach to this state. You are an institution. Before you arrived in 1971, Indiana was just another state in the Corn Belt. Outside of the Indianapolis 500, we had nothing to show the rest of the nation.

Oh sure, high school basketball was always important to us, but it was more of a private affair. You took our limitless appetite for high school basketball and elevated it to the college level.

Then you revolutionized the college game, and us with it. You took the theories of man-to-man defense and motion offense and combined them with self discipline to create a new game. You gave college basketball a new champion in the wake of UCLA's fall to mediocrity. It is probably safe to say that the NCAA Tournament would not be the media event it is today without you.

And because of it, you gave us Hoosiers an identity. We are no longer the country bumpkins of folk lore. We are no longer the butt of crude jokes. We are no longer a state in search of a map.

You put us there, Bob. You took us and reshaped us in your own image -- proud, defiant, disciplined and uncompromisingly honest. You took our blue-collar ideals and used them to mold your basketball teams. You took our sons and made them "student athletes" -- in a time when the term is almost obsolete. You helped us forget unemployment, gas shortages and farm foreclosures. You gave us our pride back. A "Hoosier" is no longer a slang word, thanks to you.

You gave us a common bond. Wherever Hoosiers gather, your name inevitably comes up.

"You're from Indiana? Bobby Knight country? How do you put up with that guy?"

Well, I'll tell ya, partner. Just look at those three NCAA banners swaying from Assembly Hall. Look at those capacity crowds night after night. Look at the graduation rate of IU basketball players. Look at all those players who keep coming back to visit. Feel the warmth of Senior Day.

Look at all the new books in the campus library, a project supported by him. Look at the joy in the eyes of the handicapped, stationed in wheelchairs in the Hall. Look at all the charitable causes that have profited from his time.

Ask anyone confined to a hospital bed who has received an unexpected note and T-shirt from The Coach.

A typical example happened close to home this past season. During a time when he was still grieving the loss of his mother, during a time when his basketball team was flailing away, Knight took time out to autograph a basketball for a friend of mine paralyzed from an automobile accident. On his own, Knight also sent my friend a personal letter with some IU souvenirs.

Knight has been doing such things without fanfare for 17 years, but let him make one careless analogy, one misinterpreted statement, and suddenly there's a march on Showalter Fountain.

Maybe New Mexico deserves you, Bob. Maybe the fans out there will not have such short memories. You certainly don't owe us anything. You already have given of yourself in a way you ask only your players to do, completely and unequivocally.

Thank you for giving us our heyday. Thank you for teaching us about basketball and, more importantly, about life.

Those phone callers were right, Bob. It would never be the same.

Chapter 2
The Game that Transcends

What is it about baseball that makes us so nostalgic? In going through my old clips, I discovered more sentimental articles on baseball than any other subject. For whatever the reason, baseball seems to transcend time and boundaries, somehow linking us to the greats, or to greater issues.

In Search of the Proverbial Exclusive

One of the very first columns I ever wrote involved an interview with Yankee legend Mickey Mantle, who made a much-anticipated visit to little Kendallville in December, 1977. Thanks to the persistence of Bob Shook, a Kendallville restaurant owner and long-time Yankee fan, Mantle agreed to serve as the guest of honor at the grand opening of Shook's Lounge. It was a night people in Kendallville talked about for years. Mantle would return to Kendallville on a half-dozen occasions, mostly to play golf and enjoy some Hoosier hospitality. On some of those visits he brought along some pretty interesting company, Billy Martin and Whitey Ford. You will see a column pertaining to some of those visits, along with a third column written almost 20 years later when Mantle was fighting a losing battle with alcoholism.

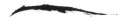

Kendallville News-Sun
December 11, 1977

"**M**ickey Mantle is coming to Kendall-ville? You're putting me on," I said when I heard the news last month. "What an exclusive that would make," I mused.

Immediately I started jotting down questions like, "What was your greatest thrill?" "Who was the toughest pitcher you ever faced?" "Who was your favorite player?" And so on.

I had all kinds of thoughtful questions ready for that one chance when I could sit down with him in some quiet booth in Shook's Lounge, the new establishment Mantle would commemorate with his appearance.

I imagined Mantle blazing into town wearing a three-piece suit, with police escorts on every side while thousands lined the streets like an old-fashioned ticker-tape parade. After all, this was no ordinary jock coming to town. This was The Mick, the legendary hero of our childhood. Yes sir, that's the way I imagined Mantle making his grand entry into Kendallville.

Now let me tell you how it really happened.

I was sitting in the Parlor Lounge watching the Indiana-Kentucky basketball game over a beer just about 90 minutes before Mantle's scheduled arrival. All of a sudden I saw Bob Shook, the owner of the new lounge and the originator of the Mantle idea. "Is he here?" I asked anxiously.

"Right there he is!" Shook roared.

And there he was, decked out in a suit all right, a Western suit -- denim jacket and Wrangler blue jeans.

Hiding my surprise at seeing Mantle dressed so informally, I watched him enter the bar and stop in front of the long mirror behind the counter. Just like the guy in the Brylcream commercial, he rubbed a hand through his perfect blonde hair while gawking spectators stood in awe.

I made my introduction by blurting some trite remark like, "Where are the girls?" referring to the same hair cream commercial.

"They're coming later," he boasted.

And then in a flash he was whisked away by Shook and a few friends. Hurriedly, I gulped down my beer and proceeded to follow them. When I arrived at Shook's Lounge, I found wall-to-wall flesh crammed into the establishment.

Trying to act inconspicuous amidst the mob, I shuffled over to the bar to watch the conclusion of the IU game and await my chance to talk with the guest of honor. It was an impossibility at first because he was smothered by well-wishers, autograph seekers and blushing females.

Many fans purchased the $2 baseballs made available for Mantle's autograph. While he was busy doing that, I decided to change my tactics and eavesdrop on some remarks made about the great slugger. This would add flavor to the article, I reasoned.

Sure enough, I heard comments like, "He's just like the rest of us," or, "He's got blue jeans on!"

One of the bartenders baited one customer by declaring that basketball superstar George McGinnis was coming next week. "Are we gonna have $2 basketballs for that?" kidded back the customer.

Other comments I picked up were, "He's the kind of guy you would want on your team … He's your kind of people, everyday people."

One woman said his wrinkles were "cute and sexy."

All the while this was going on, Mantle was signing baseballs and still unavailable for a quiet talk. I was starting to get a little impatient now and ordered another beer to pass the time. By then, I already was getting a little loose, but I wasn't too concerned because Mantle was tipping a glass or two himself.

In the meantime, I discussed the declining food prices with Roger Schermerhorn and listened to Lester Algood's explanation of why he planted a row of corn in the middle of a county road.

There were all kinds of people there I knew or recognized, among them Eldon and Sherri Ploetz and Bill and Sally Soboslay. That foursome was kind enough to help me kill some time by trading some off-beat jokes and supplying a couple more rounds of libation, which I really didn't need but couldn't refuse.

Several hours and beers later, I finally got my chance to talk to him. By that time it was midnight, and both of us were a little impatient – and none too sober, either. To top it all off, I only got five minutes with him, and that was at an open table with curious spectators nosing around.

However, that was sufficient time to find out: 1) Sandy Koufax and Don Drysdale were the toughest pitchers he faced; 2) he is content with his new role as "Mickey Mantle, executive;" 3) he doesn't get recognized in public as much as he used to; 4) he wants to be remembered by his teammates as "a guy everybody liked;" 5) his greatest thrill would be to have his No. 7 retired; and 6), to "get out of Kendallville alive."

Well, Mickey escaped the mob in Kendallville and I got my exclusive. So, on behalf of both of us, mission accomplished.

Mantle and Ford Like You and Me

How many cub reporters ever got to sit at the same table with Mickey Mantle and Whitey Ford? Color me lucky.

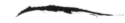

Kendallville News-Sun
July 14, 1981

When I think of a baseball Hall of Famer, I think of some old geezer sitting on his front porch whittling on a piece of wood and trying to remember "the good ol' days." Mickey Mantle and Whitey Ford shattered that image Monday night at Shook's Lounge.

There they were, the two Yankee greats, rubbing elbows with your local sportswriter and anybody else who ventured in. There were no airs, no pretenses, no half-whittled blocks of wood in that room. It was just a bunch of "good ol' boys" sharing lockerroom humor.

It was Mantle's fifth visit to Kendallville dating back to Shook's grand opening in December, 1977. I learned then there was no such thing as a serious interview with the great Yankee slugger.

I'll never forget that first attempt at what I thought was going to be my first big scoop with the *News-Sun*. By the time I finally got close enough to Mick to ask a few questions (there were too many autograph seekers in between), both of us had had our share of adult beverages. Needless to say, it was not the most coherent conversation I ever engaged in – through no fault of our own, of course.

Mantle had such a good time, though, that he has returned every year since. The welcome mat is always out at Shook's for Mantle and any other former Yankee he can con into coming with him. Two years ago, Mantle brought Billy Martin with him. This year, it was Whitey Ford's turn.

Whitey is so down-to-earth it catches you off guard. Rather than talk baseball, we talked about his home on Long Island, where I just returned from a recent vacation. Whitey lives in Lake Success, N.Y., not too far from where my sister lives in Syosset. He is employed for Saxon Industries in New York but still finds time to work with the young Yankee pitchers in the spring.

I asked him what he thought of the strike and he replied, "Terrible! I'm awful disappointed in both the owners and the players."

Neither Ford nor Mantle will admit to feeling cheated by missing out on today's lucrative salaries, but both expressed some dismay. For the record, Mantle's biggest salary was $100,000, while Ford's reached only $76,000. Mantle's assessment of present Yankee Dave Winfield's $20-million dollar contract was both funny and ironic.

"Last year Winfield bats .270, hits 20 home runs and gets $20 million. If I did that, I would have been cut," he said.

Mantle's off-years were better than that. He wound up with a .298 career mark with 536 home runs. His best season was 1961, when he whacked 54 home runs and batted .317. That same year, Ford won the Cy Young Award by posting a glittering 25-4 record. He won 70 percent of his games and at least 10 games every year. Only twice in his first 15 years with the Yanks did they fail to make the World Series.

"We were in the World Series so much my wife thought the pay was part of my salary," quipped Ford.

Together, Ford and Mantle accounted for eight World Series championships and 13 pennants. And there they were Monday night, sitting there at Shook's like any other John Doe who had just rolled in from the golf course.

That's exactly where they came from, the Elks Country Club. Watching them play with Bob and Mick Shook (who, incidentally, is named after Mantle), along with Gabby Davis was an experience in itself. The guys were constantly ribbing each other about their golf swings and occasional divots. Ford, Mick Shook and Davis ganged up on Mantle and Bob Shook in best-ball play, winning all bets.

Mantle jokingly complained about losing every time he comes here to a bunch of guys who tell him how lousy they are.

"All I know is that there are a bunch of lying' (bleeps) out here," he roared. "Every golfer in Indiana must by lying."

Mantle later got back at Ford when they were sitting with just a handful of locals at Shook's back bar.

"You can see how well Ford draws," he joked about the small gathering. "He really does pull them in. Last night (the main reception) was my crowd. This one is Whitey's."

Whitey just grinned and took it all in stride. You could tell he was used to Mickey's good-natured ribbing. Like regular guys, Hall of Famers drink beer, kid each other and enjoy being around people. They may not always make the best copy, but they make darn good drinking buddies.

Mantle's Battle with Alcohol No Surprise

It all caught up with Mantle in the end. How sad, so very sad.

Bloomington Herald-Times
April 1994

"I began some of my mornings the past 10 years with the "breakfast of champions" -- a big glass filled with a shot or more of brandy, some Kahlua and cream. Billy Martin and I used to drink them all the time, and I named the drink after us."

So begins baseball great Mickey Mantle in the April 18th issue of *Sports Illustrated*, an article he co-wrote with S.I.'s Jill Lieber.

It is a revealing look at Mantle's 40-year battle with alcoholism. It is a saga of memory lapses, embarrassing moments and foolish episodes. The revelation may come as a shock to some but not to me. I had some first-hand glimpses of Mantle's losing battle with the bottle.

In December, 1977, Mantle came to Kendallville for the grand opening of Shook's Lounge. Bob Shook, an enterprising Kendallville businessman, was a lifelong Yankee fan. He and his wife, Mary Lou, even named their first son Mickey Joe, after Mantle and Joe DiMaggio. As the grand opening of their family restaurant approached, the Shooks made arrangements for Mantle to be the guest of honor.

Mantle's pending visit to Kendallville caused quite a stir. The place was packed that night, a midweek night in mid-winter. I was there on assignment as sports editor for the *Kendallville News-Sun*. A winter storm delayed Mantle's arrival. When he finally burst through the door, he immediately accepted a beer, which he guzzled down with the excuse that he needed a drink after the turbulent flight. The watery look in his eyes suggested he already had some alcohol in him.

> "That was a part of the legend of Mickey Mantle. Everybody just expected me to start drinking. They'd buy me drinks. I think they expected me to get drunk. It was like this: Mickey Mantle couldn't hit it out of the ballpark anymore, but he could still drink 'em under the table."

"Everybody expected him to drink," Bob Shook said. "We knew. We read about it."

Mantle's charisma made it easy to overlook his overindulgence. People were drawn to him like ants at a picnic. That night he signed baseballs, posed for pictures and accepted more drinks from strangers.

I had made arrangements with the Shooks to interview Mantle later that evening, once the initial commotion subsided. It would be several hours before Mantle agreed to sit down with me. I admit I was nervous. I was only in my second year as a sportswriter and had never interviewed anyone of such notoriety.

I cautiously sidled over to Mantle seated at a table in the back. He barely even looked up at me as I introduced myself. He grunted and took a sip of his drink. I asked a few questions and he mumbled a few pat answers. Then I made the mistake of asking him a familiar question such as, "What was your greatest Yankee moment?"

Mantle snapped at me for asking such a routine question. I could tell he was drunk to the point of belligerence. The interview was terminated shortly thereafter. The last I saw of Mantle that night, he was dancing on top of the bar with Bob Shook.

I barely had enough Mantle material for a column. I was forced to focus on the spectacle rather than the person. The headline above the column read, "In Search of the Proverbial Exclusive."

> "When I was drinking, I thought I was funny -- the life of the party. But as it turned out, nobody could stand to be around me. I was loud, and I guess everything that came out of my mouth was rude and crude. After one or two drinks, I was real happy. People could ask me for autographs and I'd sign them. Then, after several drinks, I could be downright nasty."

It wouldn't be the last time I would speak with the Yankee great, however. Shook brought him back three more times for gala evenings at his restaurant. Those last three times he did not come alone. He brought his drinking buddies, Billy Martin and Whitey Ford. You could see that Mantle and Martin were two of a kind -- quick to drink, quick to laugh, quick to anger. I found Ford much more civil. He was more than willing to share some old Yankee war stories, while Mantle and Martin were rather guarded when it came to outsiders. I'm not sure Martin was a good influence on Mantle. He seemed to bring out the worst in him.

> "With Billy and me, drinking was a competitive thing. We'd see who could drink the other under the table. I'd get a kick out of seeing him get loaded before me. Alcohol made him so aggressive. He's the only person I knew who could HEAR a guy give him the finger from the back of the room."

Martin's influence on Mantle went back to the early 1950s, when they were Yankee teammates. Mantle used to boast of the times they stayed out past curfew, of their great tolerance for alcohol and their resistance to hangovers. He recalled one incident where Martin talked him into stepping out onto a ledge outside the window of their hotel room -- 22 floors above the pavement.

> "Billy and I were wild men. We drank up a storm and didn't get to bed until we were ready to fall into bed ... Billy and I were bad for each other."

"I remember one time when Billy dropped his pants here," Bob Shook said.

Mary Lou has a hunch why Martin could get Mantle to go along with almost any suggestion.

"Martin was a city boy; Mantle was a country boy," she said. "Mantle was like any young kid would have been. They were like sophisticated guys compared to him."

Mantle's drinking problem was no secret.

"You could tell," Bob Shook said. "He'd start drinking in the morning. He'd have a beer mixed with tomato juice."

In the *Sports Illustrated* article, Mantle pinpointed the origins of his drinking to the death of his father at age 39. Mantle had always wanted to please his father and never really got over the expected loss of his role model. He thought he would die at a young age, too.

"He truly believed he would never live to be this old (62)," Mary Lou Shook said.

On Christmas Day, 1989, Martin died in a pickup truck accident. Mantle served as a pall bearer at the funeral, but not even that sobering reminder stopped him from embarking on his frequent binges. It wasn't until his son Danny turned himself in for alcohol rehabilitation that Mantle realized he was probably the cause. He has since completed the Betty Ford rehabilitation program.

Perhaps Los Angeles manager Tom LaSorda was right when he said he could not bring himself to feel sorry for Dodger Darryl Strawberry, who is currently in rehabilitation for substance abuse.

"It is not a sickness," LaSorda said. "It is a weakness."

"There's a lot of people like that," said Mary Lou Shook of Mantle. "Maybe it will do some good. Like LaSorda said, it's time to stop overlooking this good ol' boy stuff."

> "It used to be that I was a role model for kids -- even older guys looked up to me. Maybe I can truly be a role model now -- because I ad-

mitted I had the problem, got treatment and am staying sober -- and maybe I can help more people than I ever helped when I was a famous ballplayer ... For all those years I lived the life of somebody I didn't know, a cartoon character. From now on, Mickey Mantle is going to be a real person."

A High School 'Love Story'

There are certain teams that even you can't help but get attached to. One of my all-time favorites was the East Noble High School baseball team of the early 1980s. I formed a bond with this team by joining them on a spring trip to Florida in 1980, back when most of them were sophomores. The "Knights" were championed by a lad with a fitting baseball name, Jay Grate, still the best high school player I have ever seen. He was later drafted by the Red Sox. In 1982, East Noble climbed to the top of the Indiana high school baseball poll and won the school's first regional title in any sport. The club was just one game away from a trip to the state finals when it fell to second-ranked LaPorte, 5-0. I was in the lockerroom following this crushing defeat. To this day, it is the only lockerroom scene that ever moved me to tears.

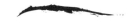

Kendallville News-Sun
June 21, 1982

There was a lot of love in the losers' lockerroom after East Noble bowed to LaPorte in the championship game of the Michigan City Semi-state Saturday night, 5-0. And just like in the movie, *Love Story*, "Love means never having to say you're sorry." Well, nobody was making any apologies or excuses for the Knights' disappointing defeat.

Jay Grate certainly didn't owe anybody any apologies, even though he absorbed a rare pounding by the LaPorte bats. And nobody dared to suggest that he let them down, because it was his arm that got them there. Standing motionless in the middle of the room with two wilted tulips in his hand, you could see that nobody felt worse about the loss than Grate himself did. He stared blankly into space, trying to come to grips with the fact that his remarkable high school career was over.

And nobody made any apologies for the six errors that led to Grate's demise, or the back injury that kept centerfielder Brian Fogg from playing a single inning. The painful silence, broken only by an occasional sniffle, was testimony to that bitter reality.

Many of the players sought solitude by seeking out a private corner of the dressing room to collect their thoughts. It wasn't until Coach Fred Inniger came in that a word was spoken.

"You people did too much good all year long to get down on yourselves tonight," he began. "You will look back and have some great memories. I'm so proud of you people. You seniors, come back around, baby. Don't leave us."

After those words, Inniger called senior Brad Holsinger up to lead the Knight in their final team prayer of the season. Holsinger had been of those who needed to be by himself for a few minutes, finding solace in the partially obscured stairwell near the exit. When it came time to lead the invocation, he did it with a poignancy that this writer will never forget. As the team drew close and joined hands around him, he thanked the Good Lord for rewarding them with an unforgettable year and wished the best of luck to Grate in his promising baseball future.

It was all Brad could do to keep from cracking up, and by the time he was done, there wasn't a dry eye in the room. The agony of defeat had found its way into the emotions of everyone in there, and it was an emotion called love.

After Holsinger finished, the players and coaches exchanged tearful, silent embraces. No more words were needed at this point, but Grate wanted to express his thanks for the support of his teammates.

"I couldn't have done it without you," he said.

Holsinger took the floor again and passed the responsibility of leadership over to the juniors, challenging them to keep the East Noble tradition going.

By then it was time to leave, and the players were anxious to get out of this heartbreaking scene. They voted against taking showers so they could get back home as soon as possible.

A small group of fans stood clapping as they boarded the bus, and they had tears in their eyes, too. Many of the parents came up and hugged their sons, and some of the non-parents hugged them as if they were their sons.

One fan made the statement, "They have become the sons of the community.

They are the sons we wished we had, never had before or maybe never will have."

On the ride back, silence prevailed again. Inniger went up to each player, assistant coach and bat girl and thanked them for their contributions.

At last he came over to me with his eyes red and swollen.

"Right now, these kids are showing the kind of class people they are," he said. "Back there in the lockerroom, there was no cussing, swearing or beating of lockers. So many positive things happened to us this year. I will really miss these kids."

Fred is not the only one who will miss them. The entire community will, too. As Athletic Director Tom Crist told them, "You people have brought this community together. You are the reason Coach Inniger and myself stay involved in high school sports."

Yes, it was a love affair between an entire community and a classy group of young men, and love means never having to say you're sorry.

This Kid Really Played Hardball

In addition to the excepts from the magazine article about Mantle, Sports Illustrated *also was kind enough to let me reprint this first-person piece I did for SI in 1987. Getting an article published in SI is still the highest honor a sports writer can ever receive, in my opinion.*

Sports Illustrated
October 12, 1987

Fathers must be the most frustrated species on the planet. From the time tots are old enough to insert the cat's tail into a wall socket, dads have big plans for them -- and are bound to be disappointed. For instance, my dad, a mechanical engineer, wanted me to be a rocket scientist. No sooner had I been toilet trained than he began surrounding me with technical toys. While other kids were getting baseball gloves and bicycles for Christmas, I was getting Erector Sets, chemistry sets and microscopes.

What Dad failed to realize was that I hadn't even the faintest interest in science or physics. The only thing I cared about was the Milwaukee Braves. From the time the Braves blew a three-games-to-one lead to the Yankees in the 1958 World Series -- and even after the Braves skipped to Atlanta -- I was hooked.

Radio station WTMJ in Milwaukee was my primary link with Hank Aaron, Eddie Mathews, Joe Adcock, Del Crandall, Warren Spahn and Lew Burdette. The radio became my constant companion after my parents sent my older sister away to boarding school.

My room became a sanctuary in which I would listen to distant baseball games and fantasize about future glory on the diamond. I would dream up games between the Braves and my other favorite National League team, the slugging Giants of Willie Mays, Willie McCovey, Orlando Cepeda, and Jim Davenport.

While listening to a game between the Braves and the Giants one day, I was toying with a marble on my desk. The marble got away and rolled to a stop against a pencil. My imagination took over. I wondered if striking a falling marble with a pencil was as difficult as getting a bat on one of Spahn's fastballs. To my satisfaction, I discovered the same hand-eye coordination was required. At first, I barely made contact.

Then I managed a few dribblers. With practice I was stroking soft liners. Soon I was smacking high drives off the bedroom window. The resulting "ping" brought Dad into the room.

"What was that?" he asked.

"Nothing."

"How can you write holding a pencil upside down?"

"I was just tapping to the music."

"What music? All you ever listen to is baseball and rock 'n' roll."

"I was tapping to the organ music in the background of the game."

Giving me a long suspicious look, Dad left the room. I locked the door. He was onto something. So was I.

Out came the Erector Set, the chemistry set, and the microscope. All the pieces remained inside, however. By placing the green Erector Set box on its side on the floor in front of my dresser, I fashioned my own version of the left field wall in Fenway Park.

The black chemistry set container made a nice hitter's background and centerfield wall, and the narrower microscope case made a convenient hitter's porch in right. Now I had a magical baseball park of my own. All I needed was a couple of teams.

I scrounged around for 18 pencils and saved the nine best ones for the Braves. They were mostly blue, my favorite color. The ugly orange and black ones were for the Giants.

I placed nine pencils around my homemade diamond according to the positions of the team in the field and allowed three swings per pencil (I batted Fungo-style while kneeling on the carpet; the plate was about seven feet from the outfield walls) for the team at bat.

The ground rules were simple. If the marble rolled against any one of the six "infielders," it was a ground out. All infield flies were pop-outs. Anything that went over the infielders and landed without hitting one of the "outfielders" was a single. Anything off the wall was a double. If the marble ricocheted off two or more walls, it was a triple. Anything over the barriers was a home run.

Oh what fun I had that summer! At first the home runs were few and far between, but the more I played, the more the marbles started flying out of my versions of County Stadium or Candlestick Park (I would face my electric fan against home plate to simulate the brisk winds of Candlestick). I later fashioned dugouts out of old shoe boxes and even supplied my own play by play, which came easily after listening to countless broadcasts.

About all I lacked was the roar of the crowd as I was accustomed to hearing it over the radio. That took some practice. I finally came up with a facsimile, which was half belch, half scream -- similar to the sound a person makes after eating something extremely hot. The first roar of the crowd brought Dad into my room.

"Are you teasing the dog again?"

"The dog's not in here."

"Then what was that awful noise? Are you listening to that rock 'n' roll trash again?"

Dad noticed the pencils scattered about the room.

"What are all those pencils doing on the floor?"

"Oh, those? I'm just trying a little experiment."

"Really, now. So what's the marble's role in this?"

"Uh, well, I'm trying to measure the trajectory of a spherical object when struck by a cylindrical object at various angles and speeds."

An eyebrow went up. But he left without further inquiry.

The games went on. And on. And on. I planned to complete a full 162-game schedule between the Braves and Giants before the summer was over, and each game took about an hour. I was careful to hold down the crowd noises when the folks were home, but I relished the times they were away. Then the room shook with noise -- and with flying marbles.

Holding down the cheering wasn't always easy, especially when Aaron launched one over the dresser or made a pencil-point catch in the outfield. At times like that, the noise was spontaneous. One time it was too loud. Dad charged into the room and caught me red-handed.

"Don't tell me you're experimenting with the theory of inertia," he bellowed.

I was forced to confess. I was a pencil baseball junkie. When I explained that the microscope, Erector Set, and chemistry sets were merely props, Dad shook his head and stalked out of my room muttering to himself.

My guilt didn't stop me from playing. I was addicted to this solitary game. It became a sore spot between us. When the fans roared in my make-believe stadium, I heard Dad moan, "Mother, that kid is making those ridiculous noises again. Two hundred dollars' worth of scientific equipment in there and the kid shuffles pencils like some moron."

Dad once stormed into the room and stepped right on Aaron, cracking him in half. It was a devastating blow to Milwaukee's pennant drive. I had no other pencils around with a barrel as big and as long as Hank's. I didn't even have a (Hurricane) Bob Hazel to call up as the '57 Braves did when Bill Bruton hurt his knee. All I had was a skinny one with no power -- Ty Cline I called him, after the outfielder who hit one home run in three years for the Braves in the early 1960s.

My worst fears came true. The Giants started closing in. An 11-game Milwaukee lead shrank to two in August. I always tried to swing with the same velocity for each team, and without Aaron's big bat the Braves could not match the power of Mays, McCovey, Cepeda, and Davenport.

Out of desperation, I decided to piece my heavy hitter together with model glue and friction tape. I held my breath as I swung the Aaron pencil the first time he came off the disabled list. To my utter delight, the marble put a dent in the Erector-Set-box-turned-Green-Monster.

No only had the tape made Aaron's barrel wider, it also had made it heavier. Like his real-life counterpart, my Aaron tore up the league, rocketing marbles all over the room-off the lampshade, off the upper bunkbed, and off my copy of *The Young Scientist*, which was collecting dust on the book shelf. Talk about poetic justice!

The most historic shot came in the pennant-clinching game. With the Braves trailing 6-5 in the bottom of the ninth, Aaron came to bat with the bases loaded and one out. On an 0-2 pitch, he zapped one all the way to the ceiling. It bounced off the glass light fixture, cracking it, and then dropped cleanly into the outfield, which made it a ground-rule double.

"Milwaukee wins the pennant! Milwaukee wins the pennant!" I screamed.

Within seconds, Dad came dashing into the room. The crack in the light fixture told him all he needed to know. The ensuing deduction from my allowance, however, was worth every single penny.

My Braves went on to avenge -- at least in my mind -- the 1958 World Series debacle by sweeping the wretched Yankees (now represented by the Giants' pencils) in four straight. Aaron finished with 50 home runs in the regular season -- despite his time on the disabled list -- and one in each of the Series games.

I was sorry to see the baseball season end, but it was late October and, to me, it just didn't seem right to play ball, even indoors, that late in the fall in the Midwest. As I dismantled the stadium for the last time, I stroked the marble into one of the cardboard dugouts. It made a loud pop. Before I knew it, I was making sweeping shots with my right hand and blocking maneuvers with my left. That day, pencil hockey was born, and you know what? Aaron had one heck of a wrist shot.

(Reprinted courtesy of Sports Illustrated *October 12, 1987. Copyright 1987, Time Inc. "Now This Kid Really Played Hardball -- With a Marble." All rights reserved)*

Where Have All the Sandlots Gone?

The movie, Field of Dreams, *had just about every baseball fan longing for the days you could just walk down the street and join in a ball game. As a kid I was lucky to have a jewel of a park in my own neighborhood.*

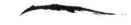

Bloomington Herald-Times
July 2, 1995

"If you build it, he will come," a whispering voice told Kevin Costner in the movie, *Field of Dreams*. So he created a magical baseball park in the middle of an Iowa corn field and, sure enough, along came the late, great Shoeless Joe Jackson and his cast of baseball legends.

That was fiction, of course, but not every field of dreams is mystical. There was a time when fields of dreams were commonplace around the nation's landscapes. My old stomping grounds, Fort Wayne's Ludwig Park, had a very real field of dreams during the early 1960s.

In the 1960s, Ludwig Park, a subdivision located on the northwest side of the Summit City, was not yet row upon row of houses. The streets were still dotted with empty lots, one of them owned by John Andrews Sr. Andrews and his son, John Jr., had a bond that went beyond blood -- baseball.

Young John and his friends, myself included, also shared in the Andrews passion for baseball and spent many a summer day playing on the spacious lot behind the Andrews home.

At first, the elder Andrews merely mowed the lot, which extended a couple of acres to a little-used tar road. As more boys from around the neighborhood began playing on a regular basis, Andrews began making improvements. The first thing he did was replace the cardboard bases with authentic ones. After that came a backstop, followed by a pitching mound.

The constant activity carved natural base paths. The outfield was uneven in spots, so Andrews rolled it and lined the foul lines with chalk. As the diamond took on a more finished appearance, the number of players and visitors mounted.

The improvements kept on coming. The gang showed up one day and discovered two rows of freshly built bleachers directly behind the backstop. The final touch was a dugout, with a roof and a screen to protect us from foul balls and foul weather. Mr. Andrews did all this on his own time and at his own expense.

The ground rules were simple. A ball hit in the road was a home run. A ball rolling into the road was a ground-rule double. On days we could not field full teams, the pitcher's mound doubled as first base. Any ball then hit to the opposite side was an automatic out.

Umpiring was left to the honor system, which didn't prevent our share of disputes. Somehow, we avoided bloodshed.

Word of our field of dreams spread to other subdivisions, luring visiting teams to challenge us on almost any given day. A team from Waterswolde, a housing complex further to the north, was a frequent challenger.

We even formed our own two-team league, comprised of Ludwig Park and its adjacent subdivision, Ludwig Circle. The two rivals played mostly on weekends and topped off the season with their own version of the World Series.

Loyalties were divided. Players with more friends on a rival team were liable to jump ship. One might say we were the original free agents, long before Curt Flood challenged the baseball establishment. Team-hopping became so frequent we finally devised crude "contracts" to declare our intentions in writing. There were no further transactions. A player was stuck with that team for the duration of the season -- win, lose or shunned by his peers.

One of the most infamous "defectors" was Mitch Bedree, who bolted for Ludwig Circle. Mitch went on to play college ball at Ball State. He caught the attention of scouts from the Tigers and White Sox, but never enjoyed a pro career.

Another one of the defectors was a loud-mouthed chap by the name of Roger Bir. Weighted down by baby fat, Roger had the annoying habit of broadcasting the game from his position, especially while he was pitching.

There was the time that Roger, a side-winding right-hander, threw away a sure game-ending grounder hit right back to him on the mound. With the tying run on first and two out, Roger cleanly fielded the one-hopper.

"Bir spears it and that should do it," he barked in his best Mel Allen before sidewinding the peg past first base and into the right field corner. Both runner and batter circled the bases to make him eat his words.

We would be still laughing today if Roger had not filled out to 250 pounds of muscle and played football for Indiana University. Now we live in fear of the times we made fun of him.

Roger was big enough to hit home runs down both lines, the farthest distance from home plate in our inverted pyramid of a park. The rest of us had to aim for center field, the most direct route.

When it became too easy to reach the road in succeeding years, a ball had to reach the other side of that road to qualify as a home run. That extra 20 feet made a big difference.

The summer we extended the home run boundaries, the leading sluggers turned out to be a couple of girls, Marianne Anderson and Mary Pequinot. Being ahead of the boys in terms of physical maturity, the girls could clear the road almost effortlessly. They were drafted early in those pickup games.

Usually chosen last was Steve "Casey" France. France wasn't much of a baseball player, but he had a mind for business. When he realized baseball wasn't in his future, France turned entrepreneur. He converted the dugout into a concession stand. The profits from "Casey's Concessions" probably went a long way toward paying for his college education.

There were days when we would play in the morning, break for lunch, return for more games in the afternoon, break for supper, and come back for a twilight doubleheader. Those who had Little League or Wildcat League obligations might play as many as five or six games in a single day.

The games went on until the summer we noticed that girls had qualities beyond hitting the long ball. Girls required cars; cars required jobs; jobs required time. Baseball no longer fit the equation.

Mr. Andrews understood and quietly surrendered the field back to Mother Nature. Not long after that, he sold the lot to the developers. Three houses now rest on what used to be our field of dreams. The road is paved and the neighboring lots also are housed.

Mr. Andrews passed away in 1972. He was a quiet man. About the only time we saw him was when he mowed the field or stopped by to watch us from the bleachers he built.

That was a different time. You rarely see kids playing pickup games anymore. You rarely see a sandlot anymore. Today, it seems all the games are played on a limited number of public diamonds in organized settings under adult supervision.

Today, in the name of development, our fields are drying up one by one. With them goes a part of our national pastime.

Is it a crime to leave one lot unfinished in each housing development? Is there still another Mr. Andrews out there, waiting to build a field of dreams and waiting for the kids to play the game the way it was meant to be played -- without uniforms, umpires, coaches or overzealous parents?

The kids are out there. The diamonds are not. Perhaps if we build them, they will come.

Ode to the Caps

In the summer of 1993, a bunch of over-the-hill softball players who called themselves "The Caps" were on the verge of a city league title, only to find themselves about to come up short in the final game. Their last hope came down to a spindly second baseman named Lee VanBuskirk, a lad not known for his power. In fact, he had never hit a home run in his life as he faced the ultimate challenge: two on, two outs, two strikes and down two runs. Well, the rest is the stuff of legend, inspiring me, a teammate, to write this limerick. I gave each player a framed copy accompanied by a team picture. Some of those copies still hang from office walls today, and we still greet each other with cries of "Flam Pang!"

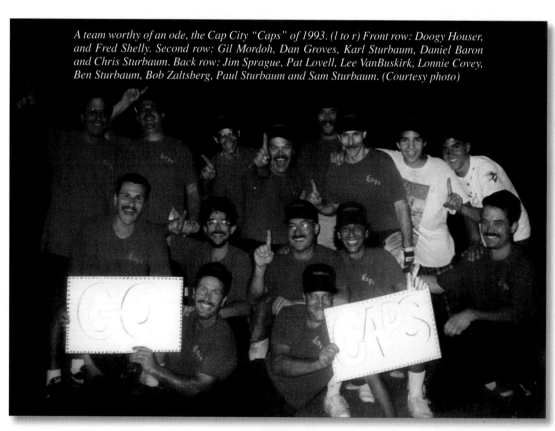

A team worthy of an ode, the Cap City "Caps" of 1993. (l to r) Front row: Doogy Houser, and Fred Shelly. Second row: Gil Mordoh, Dan Groves, Karl Sturbaum, Daniel Baron and Chris Sturbaum. Back row: Jim Sprague, Pat Lovell, Lee VanBuskirk, Lonnie Covey, Ben Sturbaum, Bob Zaltsberg, Paul Sturbaum and Sam Sturbaum. (Courtesy photo)

By Lynn "Doogy" Houser
August 1993

There once was a team they called the Caps,
Whose history had its share of collapse.
Then came the summer of '93,
When all the pieces did agree.

Fred Shelly would pitch and Karl Sturbaum would catch.
Bob Zaltsberg would field and Gil Mordoh would stretch.
Chris Sturbaum played left and Dan Groves played center,
A place where no missile dared to enter.

There was Lynn Houser in right and Dan Baron, too.
Jim Sprague and Pat Lovell supplied the glue.
Lonnie Covey would shout, 'cause he was their leader,
"Flam Pang!" he barked, and no one knew better …

Then Ben Sturbaum, the battle cry's inventor.
"Flam Pang!" they yelled, whenever they felt it.
"Flam Pang!" they cried, and VanBuskirk would belt it.
"Flam Pang!" they laughed, though no one could spell it.

One by one their foes would bow.
To this team they called, "those old loud mouths.'
"Flam Pangs" were heard from Cascades to Twin Lakes,
Rolling over the field like small earthquakes.

"Til only one team stood in their way
Of that long-awaited championship day.
But then it looked like all was for naught,
When the Caps were down to their final out.

Up stepped VanBuskirk, their very last hope.
With the tying run on first, Lee hit a rope.
The ball hit the grass and skipped on the dew
To the deepest part of the park it flew.

All the Caps gasped as Lee circled the bases,
Cheering each step as he took his paces.
As Lee hit third and headed for home,
The relay was looming from out of the gloam.

When for a moment it was bobbled,
VanBuskirk was homeward at full throttle.
He scored standing up, to his teammates' glee.
They hoisted him high in victory.

Arm-in-arm they marched away,
The finest hour of the Caps' finest day.
As they left the park t'was heard that twang,
"Caps win! Caps win! Flam Pang!"

A Duel for the Ages

From my imaginary games between the Braves and Giants to a real-life classic, played out in 1963. On the 40th anniversary of this gem in 2003, I was driven to write about it. Although I was able to reach only one of the players involved, it was a Hall of Famer Eddie Mathews. I reached him by phone back in 2001, shortly before he passed away. The rest of the quotes came from newspaper accounts of the game. The quality of the baseball played that night in 1963 warranted a look-back, no matter how late in coming. In 2011, Jim Kaplan wrote an entire book about it.

Bloomington Herald-Times
July 1, 2003

It was a baseball game that could not happen today, not in this age of pitch counts, pampered arms and steady parade of relief pitchers.

But 40 years ago tomorrow, July 2nd, 1963, a couple of future Hall of Famers engaged in one of the greatest pitching duels of all time. Juan Marichal of the San Francisco Giants outlasted Warren Spahn of the Milwaukee Braves, 1-0. In 16 innings.

With each hurler going the distance.

The 42-year-old Spahn, nearing the end of a brilliant 24-year career, matched the 26-year-old Marichal pitch for pitch until surrendering a walk-off home run to Willie Mays in with one out in the bottom of the 16th.

Unfortunately, most of America was unaware of this classic confrontation until the afternoon papers reached their doors the following day. Being a night game at San Francisco's Candlestick Park, the contest started after press deadlines for morning newspapers back East. And by the time Mays touched home plate at 12:28 a.m. Pacific Time, it also was well beyond the deadline of morning papers in Milwaukee and San Francisco. Had the game gone another half hour longer, it would have been called because of the 1 o'clock curfew San Francisco had at that time.

There was no ESPN or Baseball Tonight or Braves Baseball on TBS to take fans to the ballpark as the drama was unfolding. With no television commercials to drag it out, the game moved along at a good pace for a 16-inning affair -- four hours, 10 minutes. A crowd of 15,921 showed up on a night the Milwaukee *Journal* described as "much on the crisp side, even for notoriously chilly San Francisco."

For the month of July, it was a pitcher's kind of night. The gusts coming off San Francisco Bay held up a Henry Aaron drive in the fourth that had "home run" tattooed all over it. But not even the future home run king could beat the breeze at this point in the game. Mays was able to run it down by the fence in left-center.

"I don't think he could have hit the ball any harder," Marichal conceded later.

"You can't beat the elements," Aaron said. "I thought it was gone, too."

The Braves threatened again before the inning was over, but Mays ended it by throwing out Norm Larker trying to score from second on a single by Del Crandall. Milwaukee's only threat after that came in the seventh on another near home run - - this time by Spahn himself. As one of the best hitting pitchers of his era, Spahn nearly connected for the 34th home run of his career. The ball hit the right field fence and forced him to settle for a double, Milwaukee's only extra base hit of the game.

The Giants thought they had won the game in the bottom of the ninth when Willie McCovey lashed a Spahn pitch over the right field fence. Home plate umpire Ken Burkhart and first base umpire Chris Pelakoudas ruled the ball curved outside the foul pole. McCovey was so convinced the ball was fair that he had to be restrained by manager Alvin Dark.

"As hard as I hit the ball, it didn't have a chance to curve before leaving the ball park," McCovey told the San Francisco *Examiner*.

Had it been ruled a fair ball, baseball would have been deprived of this pitching gem. Today, both Spahn and Marichal surely would have been icing down their arms by the 10th inning and probably much earlier than that.

Reached by telephone a year before his death in 2001, Braves' Hall of Famer Eddie Mathews said that such a game is a thing of the past.

"First of all, 90 percent of them (pitchers) would not be good enough," he scoffed. "Secondly, there are only so many pitches the managers let them throw now. After seven innings, they start looking over their shoulders."

But there was Marichal and Spahn taking the mound in the 10th, the 11th, the 12th, the 13th, the 14th, the 15th and, finally, the 16th.

"I hate to see a pitcher go that long," Dark said to the *Examiner*. "I wanted to take Juan out, but he said he was strong enough to go on. Naturally, I left him in."

This box score from the July 3, 1963, Milwaukee Journal *tells it all.*

As the undisputed ace of the Giants' staff, Marichal was on his way to a 25-win season and a 2.41 Earned Run Average. Spahn was headed toward a 23-win season, the last of his 13 20-win campaigns. His 363 career wins is still the most by any left-hander in Major League history.

On his 201st pitch of the night, Spahn hung a screwball to Mays, who was 0-for-5 stepping to the plate. The greatest Giant of them all crushed the pitch for the game-winning home run.

"I knew it was gone the moment I creamed it," Mays told Curly Grieve of the *Examiner*.

The fans who were still in the ball park cheered for Mays as he circled the bases. They also applauded Spahn as he made the long walk toward the dugout.

"If ever a pitcher became a hero in defeat, it was Warren Spahn here Tuesday night," wrote Bob Wolf of the Milwaukee *Journal*. "Marichal richly deserved to win ... yet it was Spahn, the losing pitcher, whose name was on everyone's lips when the four-hour, 10-minute thriller ended at 2:25 a.m. Milwaukee time."

Historians were calling it the best pitching duel in over a quarter of a century. It fell on the 30th anniversary of another Giants' pitching jewel, Carl Hubbell's 1-0, 18- inning whitewash of the Cardinals in 1933, still the longest shutout in history.

"Greatest I've ever seen in all my experience," Dark said of the 1963 masterpiece.

In his 16 innings, Marichal allowed eight hits and four walks against a lineup that included the most prodigious home run tandem baseball has seen, Aaron and Mathews. He struck out 10 and threw 227 pitches. By today's standards, 100 pitches are cause for getting the bullpen ready.

How did Marichal feel the next day?

"Bad, tired -- sore everywhere" he told Grieve.

"I was a little tired, but my arm wasn't stiff or sore," Spahn told the Milwaukee *Journal*. "I wasn't throwing as hard at the end, but my arm was still strong."

While Marichal spent much of the next day in the whirlpool, Spahn was "running and exercising," the *Examiner* reported. As noted by Red Adams, the Candlestick clubhouse custodian, "He acts like a kid trying to earn his letter."

Spahn gave up nine hits and just one walk to a lineup that, besides Mays and McCovey, included Orlando Cepeda, Felipe Alou, Harvey Kuenn and other members of the defending National League champions -- Ed Bailey, Jim Davenport, Chuck Hiller and Jose Pagan.

"Spahn pitched a game that must rank with his best ever," Wolf concluded. "Facing a line-up loaded with power, he matched goose eggs for 15 innings with a man young enough to be his son."

"It's a shame we could not have won it for Spahn," Aaron told the *Examiner*. "I have been around a long time and that's the finest exhibition of throwing I've ever seen. It may be 10 years or 20 before you see another its equal."

It has been 40 years and baseball is still waiting. You might want to clip out the box score accompanying this piece. You probably won't see another one in your time.

Youth Baseball Makes Stars of Us All

On a slow news day during the 2009 Major League All-Star break, I decided to write about my first experience with baseball. Even though it was a total misadventure, it hooked me for life.

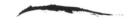

Bloomington Herald-Times
July 16, 2009

If you are a baseball fan, there is something about the Major League All-Star Game that turns you into a hopeless nostalgic. How can you watch the stars of today and not think of the times in your youth when stardom was beckoning?

For me it was the day I first encountered baseball. It wasn't even my own dad who introduced me to the sport. It was Fred Eakin, father of the Eakin brothers, Phil, Tim and John. They were a baseball family if there ever was one. They not only played it at every chance, they also invented a dice baseball game for rainy days.

I remember Mr. Eakin and the boys pulling up to my house on the south side of Fort Wayne on a summer night in 1958. They were piled into the family car, a purple Nash wagon. They told me they were going to play something called "baseball." It wasn't a totally foreign concept to me, but at age eight I had yet to experience it.

So I hopped in and away we went to Packard Park a few blocks away. They handed me this old, flat glove that looked like something out of a cartoon. However, it only took a couple of barehanded attempts at catching a hard ball to make me understand what the glove was for.

There was only one bat in the bag, a kid's-size Louisville Slugger held together by friction tape. It didn't hamper the Eakins. They hit awe-inspiring drives with it.

Then it was my turn. I tried to imitate the Eakins but could not even make contact. Lucky for me Mr. Eakin was patient. He kept tossing up soft, underhanded lobs from a few feet away, hoping I would eventually figure out how to put the lumber on the cowhide.

Finally, I managed a little foul tip. Then another. And another. I was getting close.

Then came the most magical moment of my baseball life. I hit a grounder right up the middle that startled Mr. Eakin. The ball had enough steam on it to make it past second base.

For a second or two, we all stood there in stunned silence. Then I heard the command, "Run!"

Running is something I knew how to do, but I was directionally challenged. I set sail for ... third base.

In my mind I was blazing along, but in reality I was plodding. Try running the bases in cowboy boots some time. How was I to know my Roy Rogers boots were made for the Wild West, not the ball field. Fortunately, they weren't on me very long.

Between third and second the first one came flying off. The other left me between second and first. It was a rather clever move on my part, though. By the time I lost boot No. 2, the Eakins were so paralyzed by laughter they were unable to field the ball.

But nobody told to me stop, so I kept running. I was in such a blissful trance I hardly noticed the Eakins.

By the time I rounded first and headed for home, I could feel my senses sharpen. I was so alive. I could see Mr. Eakins convulsing in laughter by the mound. I could sense the evening dew soaking through my socks. I could feel every muscle in my legs driving me to the finish line.

However, my feet could not keep up with my brain. The left foot got in the way of the right foot. Suddenly, I was airborne. It was such a strange sensation, being in the air long enough to think, "Help me, Mommy."

Good thing the grass was wet and soft. It helped me execute a perfect drop-and-roll long before I knew what the maneuver was. I barrel-rolled over home plate and laid there a few seconds, soaking it all in. My first baseball hit was an inside-the-park home run.

How kind of the Eakins to not ruin the moment by telling me I ran the wrong way. They were enjoying it as much as I was. The evidence helped me retrace my dash to glory: a boot between third and second, another between second and first, a divot between first and home. I was now a baseball player.

In the years to come, some other dubious firsts followed:

* First official baseball stat – HBP, "hit by pitch."

* First error: misjudged a pop fly and took it square on the cheek.

* First time threw glove: after failing to hold a three-run lead in the last inning.

* First time threw bat: after striking out to end the same game.

* First time chewed out by a coach: see above.

* First home run: a one-hopper that took a bad bounce over a fielder's head.

And to think none of this might have happened had it not been for that first night in the summer of '58. It doesn't matter now that I took a dyslexic journey around the bases.

I touched 'em all.

Chapter 3

Adventures and Misadventures

If a sportswriter fancies himself a true sportsman, he has to step between the lines once in a while. In my case, there were times when I should have stayed within the friendly confines of my office. Note how the movies of the day seemed to serve as suitable angles.

One City Slicker Who Horsed Around

Playing cowboy is about as easy as falling off a horse, you might say.

Bloomington Herald-Times
June 27, 1991

One of the hottest movies of the summer is *City Slickers*, which, as the title suggests, is about a couple of city dudes who discover the true meaning of life while working a cattle drive.

This dude had a *City Slickers* moment while vacationing last week in Michigan's Upper Peninsula. The "U.P.," as the natives call it, is truly one of our country's last frontiers. It is a wild, sparsely inhabited and often untamed land where the winters are long and harsh and the summers are short and sweet.

The first time I ventured into the U.P., the fall of 1986, I wound up on a bear hunt. It was an experience I will never forget, even though we never saw a bear. Just tracking one through the dense U.P. forests on a spectacular autumn day was enough.

My second trip to the U.P. brought me back to those forests, this time on horseback. For someone who had never ridden a horse before, it was every bit as exhilarating -- if that's the correct word.

Riding a horse was easy, I thought. All you do is hop on, grab the reins, give the horse a little nudge in the side and hold on. This much is true, but there is more to it than that -- much more. Stopping the horse is something else, especially on a dead gallop.

My brother-in-law, rancher Don Overmyer, thought it was safe to put me on his new Arabian, "Freckles." He bought the horse because it was renowned for its gentle disposition, perfectly suited for his 8-year-old daughter, Tricia. Watching Freckles willingly yield to Tricia's every command, I was convinced the horse was tame enough for this city boy.

Don gave me a 20-minute trial run on Freckles. "If he gets to going too fast, just pull back on the reins," he said.

Sounded simple enough. And it was -- for 20 minutes. The real test came a couple days later when Don's son, Tim, wanted to take his Uncle Lynn on a more challenging journey, a 2-hour jaunt up to their deer camp and back. The ease with which I handled Freckles the first time convinced me I was up to it. I borrowed a cowboy hat and hopped into the saddle feeling like one of the last great buckaroos.

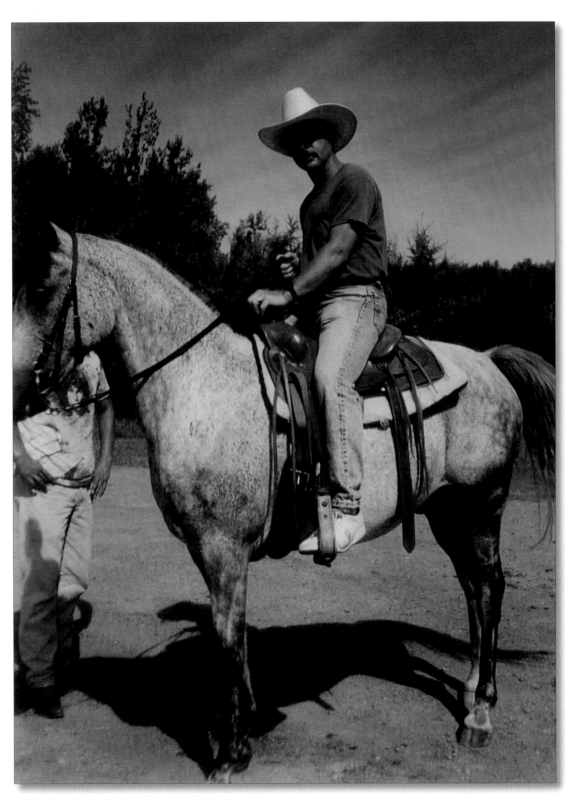

Lynn Houser saddles up on "Freckles," an Arabian who did not care for city slickers. (Courtesy photo)

"Just you and me, Freckles," I told my tireless steed, whose intelligence I underestimated. After about 45 minutes, Freckles discovered he knew more about horseback riding than his rider. The horse's first clue was that my rear end always seemed to be on the way down while his was on the way up. I was bouncing off the saddle like a golf ball on the cart path.

I think Freckles found some humor in this and proceeded to take liberties. I'm told that a horse will do as much as he can get away with if you don't take a firm hold of the reins. Freckles knew he had a rookie aboard and started to get downright sassy.

First he started wandering off the trail. I was starting to notice I had to do a lot more steering to do than the first time. Then he started to trot on his own volition, forcing me to keep pulling back on the reins. Then he got lazy and started to stumble, nearly launching me over his head.

As we entered a thick woods near the deer camp, I was beginning to lose my bravado. Complicating matters was the presence of horse flies, which acted as if they were on a mission to make Freckles' life miserable. I saw Tim take his ball cap and slowly brush a big black fly away from his horse's neck. I thought I would do the same with my cowboy hat.

Big mistake.

To my horse, this body language meant, "Hi ho, Freckles!"

The Lone Ranger never had a mask fit so tight as the hat which pinned itself to my face as Freckles exploded into high gear. The horse was going so fast the hat stayed right there, totally blinding me.

Talk about panic. With one hand I was trying to pry that hat away. With the other I was grabbing for anything that moved -- reins, saddle horn, Freckles' mane. I feared it was a matter of time before either Freckles bucked me off his back or a tree branch did the honor.

The bad news was that Freckles was going faster than I thought was possible for a creature made of flesh and blood. The good news was that, in so doing, the hat was swept away from my face. Quicker than any athletic move I ever made, I located the reins and gave them one massive tug, all the while screaming, "Whoa!" in a voice as shrill as that of the faithful Western sidekick, Gabby Hayes.

Freckles stopped almost as fast as he started. My heart was still going at warp speed, though. By this time Tim came galloping to the rescue and grabbed the reins to keep Freckles from having another surge of energy. I dismounted and almost kissed the ground in thanksgiving. We walked for about a quarter mile before I felt brave enough to get back on that wild Arabian.

There was one more scare when a school bus approached us on a rural road. This time Freckles reared up and stumbled into the roadway. Lucky for me the bus driver sized up the situation and wisely came to a stop.

I already was seeing the headlines: "No Children Injured As School Bus Flattens Horse, Rider." Or, "Sports Writer Has Fatal Dose of Freckles."

Once again I dismounted. I was perfectly willing to walk the last half mile if it meant I would live to talk about it. Then a sobering thought hit me. I was getting whipped by a horse, the same animal that was a piece of putty for my 8-year-old niece. I could almost hear my brother-in-law roll with laughter. To him I would be just another "Flat-lander," his term for any whimp from below the bridge at Mackinac. I really admire my brother-in-law, but I wasn't about to give him that satisfaction.

I boarded Freckles one last time and rode tall in the saddle for that final stretch. To my surprise, Don was quite understanding when I told him of my difficulties with a horse named Freckles, for pete's sake.

"Two more weeks here and you'd be handling him like you've been riding all your life," he said.

Thanks, but no thanks, Don. I now know it's possible to take the boy out of the city, but the jury is still out on whether you can take the city out of the boy.

The Snake and I

While cleaning out my storage shed one spring day in 1993, I was startled by an unexpected visitor.

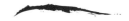

Bloomington Herald-Times
May 30, 1993

Moving to the country has been a lifelong dream of the Housers, who found the home of their dreams last fall. Nestled amidst tall oaks, maples, elms, pines and dogwoods, our rustic two-story has the feel of a state park shelter.

Making it even more park-like is the steady stream of wildlife parading by -- a beautiful doe escorting her fawn, a curious possum peering right through the glass door on the front porch, a bold raccoon rifling through your garbage.

Along with this slice of wilderness come some other less welcomed visitors -- rodents, bats and spiders big enough to carry away the cat.

In back is a storage shed -- one of those musty, aluminum shacks where spiders go to make cobwebs as thick as fishing nets. I always check for spiders before entering.

Entering the shed one day last week, I was relieved to see no eight-legged creatures. However, out of the corner of my eye I saw some movement on a ledge to my right. To my horror, it was a snake uncoiling from its resting place. I froze in my tracks. The brown, diamond-shaped bands on its back looked all too familiar. The Discovery Channel had taught me well.

Although common sense said, "no," my pounding heart said "yes." I dashed to into the house screaming, "Rattlesnake!"

I rushed to my stepson, Steve, a typically bold college student who would take a bungee jump on a dare. Ask him to help you hunt down a snake and he turns yellow. Snakes make cowards of us all, don't they?

Leaving Steve to wallow in his guilt, I rushed outside to see if there was a neighbor with the fortitude to help me expel the beast. There wasn't a soul in sight. I would have to go it alone.

Armed with long pants, hiking boots, gloves and a 3-iron, I took a deep breath and entered the shed. In the immortal words of Indiana Jones I moaned, "Snakes, I hate snakes."

As I moved in for the kill, a sobering thought struck me: "I haven't hit a decent 3-iron in years. If I can't hit a stationary object on a fairway, how can I hit an elusive target in the darkness of my shed?"

Proving that discretion is the better part of valor, I decided to call the sheriff.

"Are you sure it's a rattlesnake?" the dispatcher asked.

"I'm no expert, but this thing has all the markings of one," I replied.

"Well, if it's a rattlesnake, you can't just go in there and kill it."

"Why not?"

"They are an endangered species -- protected."

"What about my protection?" I cried. "I'm not out to kill it. I just want to get rid of it."

"I'll see if I can get somebody out from Animal Control."

"Animal Control," I mused, wondering if it wasn't the brigade of volunteer cops used to subdue the mobs at Varsity Villas during Little 500 weekend.

I went outside and maintained a vigil on the shack, waiting for the arrival of Animal Control, picturing one of those cold-hearted dog catchers with a butterfly net. Growing impatient, I ventured around the outside corner of the building and came face to face with my enemy. There, peeking out of a hole at the base, was the serpent. We made eye contact for several seconds before it mocked me with its forked tongue. I jabbed at it with my 3-iron. It retreated inside.

Round One was a draw.

About that time a van pulled up. Out stepped a burly fellow by the name of Rick Tracy.

"So this is Animal Control?" I observed. "This guy is big enough to control just about any animal, two-legged or four-legged."

In Tracy's hand was a long stick with pincers on the business end.

"Where is it?" he asked matter-of-factly.

I took him to the shed and pointed to the corner.

"You get outside in case it comes through there," he ordered.

"Oh sure, chase it right at me," I feared.

Tracy moved a couple of boxes out of the way and found his prey.

"I think it's coming your way," he warned.

Sure enough, the snake tried to escape from the hole at the base, but for once I made solid contact with a 3-iron. I pinned the reptile to the ground until Tracy came around with his snake-snatcher. He plucked it up as effortlessly as Edward Scissorhands.

"Is it a rattlesnake?" I asked.

"It looks a little like one, but I think it's just a Cow Snake," he said.

I'm not sure I was relieved or disappointed. He held the snake in the light and verified that it was indeed a Cow Snake, also known as a Bull Snake.

Suddenly, it dawned on me that I neither seen nor heard the dreaded rattle. We estimated length at about three feet. Some monster.

"Tell them it was six feet long with fangs yea big," laughed Tracy.

"Ol' Bull" wasn't laughing, though. The snake was snapping at anything that moved. It's a good thing he was toothless. He seemed genuinely disappointed at learning he wasn't a rattlesnake.

Tracy put the creature in a garbage bag and whisked it away in his van. Just like that, The Great Snake Adventure was over.

As I settled into my porch swing, I started to shake. My nerves were still telling me I had come face to face with one of nature's most feared creatures and, with the pressure on, safely hit a 3-iron.

In Pursuit of the Almighty Ticket

In November, 1993, No. 1 Florida State and No. 2 Notre Dame clashed in a battle of college titans, that decade's Game of the Century. Even though the game was a complete sell-out, that didn't stop some friends and me from going to South Bend and trying to work our way inside Notre Dame Stadium. Scalping is hard work, we found out.

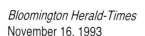

Bloomington Herald-Times
November 16, 1993

SOUTH BEND

One of the more moving scenes in the movie *Rudy* has the central character, walk-on Dan "Rudy" Ruettiger, wandering outside Notre Dame stadium, desperately looking for a way to get in. Rudy is so close he can hear the Notre Dame Victory March, the unceasing chant of the Notre Dame student body, and even the referee's whistle. The trouble is Rudy doesn't have a ticket.

He begs for admittance at each gate, only to be coldly turned away. The scene pans with a view from the top of the stadium, with all the splendor of college football on the inside, and a dejected Rudy walking with head down on the outside. So close, yet so far away.

Last Saturday, I was one of the thousands of Rudys experiencing the same frustration. All of us were looking for a way into perhaps the most hyped football game of all time, No. 1 Florida State vs. No. 2 Notre Dame.

Like all Notre Dame home games these days, it was a sellout. On lesser occasions, you can scalp a ticket for under $100. Not this time, however. The cheapest price quoted to me was $150, way beyond my budget.

I resorted to what I thought were all kinds of clever pleas. Playing upon the weather, balmy and wet, I reminded aging ticket-holders, "It's flu season. Why chance it?"

The only satisfaction I got from that was watching them bundle up. So the wise guy in me appealed to the conscience of every passing Catholic. I hollered, "Confessions for a ticket ... Papal blessings for a ticket."

Since it was obvious I was not a priest and certainly not the Pope, all that got me was some looks of disgust. The real problem was one of supply and demand. Notre Dame Stadium holds

Better late than never, a ticket into the 1993 Game of the Century.

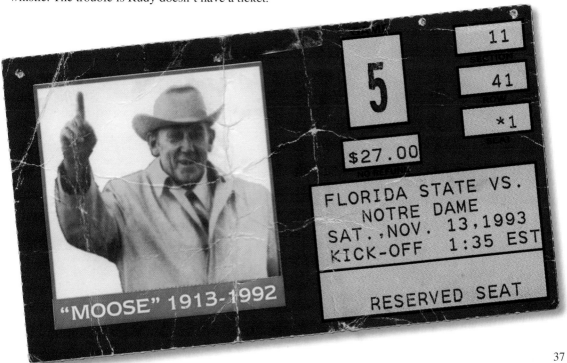

59,075. South Bend officials estimated that 80,000 fans had descended upon Notre Dame for the weekend. Let's see: 59,000 goes into 80,000 once with about 21,000 left over. That's how many extras were seeking tickets.

It was a scalper's paradise. The parking lot started filling up by Thursday night. By Friday night, people had to be turned away from the pep rally at the Athletic and Convocation Center, which holds 11,000. Earlier in the week, high-rollers were paying as much as $1,300 a ticket.

Our party of six arrived four hours before game time and scrambled to find a parking spot. Our plan was to fan-out in different directions, every man for himself. As kickoff approached, two of our comrades held up twin $100 bills. Money talks. They got in.

The rest of us filed into the ACC to watch the game on the big screen, along with about 7,000 others. It was almost like being in the stadium itself. People were leading cheers and stomping their feet as if the players could hear them. At halftime, we made one final sweep around the stadium. No one was selling. Our only hope was to sweet-talk our way in or use another proven tradition, the bribe.

Having never attempted a bribe, I was a bit awkward at it. I sidled up to one usher and mumbled, "I don't suppose 20 bucks would get me into the stadium, would it?"

Have you ever been scoffed at -- I mean really snarled at?

One member of our group tried to get in with a ticket stub he bought for $10, only to learn the ducat was counterfeit. We found out later that scalpers paid over $50,000 for counterfeit tickets. We also heard that scores of people were excused from the press box for having false credentials. The nerve!

My last hope was to prey upon the emotions of an usher. Using my best Rudy impersonation, I kept going from gate to gate with the heart-wrenching story of my 250-mile pilgrimage from Bloomington, longing to see the venerable stadium from the inside. My sob story had as much impact as the cheers inside the ACC. No gate was opened.

There I was, outside the stadium, a real-life Rudy, dragging my feet and hanging my head.

Finally, halfway through the fourth quarter, I spotted a couple of coeds leaving. I pleaded for a ticket stub. One wasn't about to part with her souvenir. The other had compassion. With some reluctance, she handed it over. I thanked her sincerely and sprinted to the proper gate.

By now, all the security guards knew me on sight. I had become a bit of a pest and they were more than happy to be rid of me. Like the parting of the Red Sea, the gate was opened. As I dashed into the daylight, I thought of how Rudy must have felt coming out of the Notre Dame tunnel.

I raced to my seat in time for the game's final eight minutes. It was worth the wait. It seemed everybody in the stadium had a story equal to or better than mine.

One fan from Florida State became ill. His wife, also a passionate FSU follower, saw him to the first aid station. She returned, minus her husband, to watch the thrilling finish.

Emotions flowed at the end of Notre Dame's 31-24 victory. One gentleman stood transfixed, tears welling up in his eyes. His ticket into the stadium was a 70th birthday present from his children.

"No one in this stadium is happier than I am," he said.

The feeling was mutual. Sometimes the end justifies the means.

He Dances with Squirrels

As an aging softball player in 2003, I traded my softball uniform for an umpire's uniform. It allowed me to stay involved with the game and could also be quite exhilarating, I discovered.

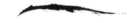

Bloomington Herald-Times
April 24, 2003

I don't know what drove me to sign up as a softball umpire this spring. I have never handled criticism well, nor have I demonstrated the kind of thick hide necessary to handle the ranting of an angry fan.

Maybe it had something to do with the fact that my softball skills have been steadily declining since the age of 30. Maybe it was the fact that umpiring offered a way to make a little money, contrary to the small fortune I spent trying to keep my aging body in shape. But I went ahead and signed up for the Bloomington Softball Association's mini-camp for rookie umpires. It wasn't long before I realized how little I knew about the game.

There was so much information thrown at us the first week. Fortunately, we had two excellent instructors in veteran umpires Randy Williamson and George Groff. The one thing they emphasized over and over was that, when you make a close call, be decisive -- "sell" it, they insisted.

Selling a call means taking two or three good strides toward the play, making a demonstrative "safe" or "out" signal, and backing it up with a booming voice. We all laughed at each other's wimpy first attempts. Groff and Williamson suggested we practice at home -- in front of a mirror, if possible. I had a better idea.

In my backyard is a family of squirrels that constantly raids the bird feeders. No matter how we try to discourage them with supposedly pest-proof cages and the like, the little rascals always seem to get the goods. My wife, Pat, tries to shoo them away in her best voice, but they almost laugh at her.

Being the loudmouth I am, I have had a little more success at running them off. It is only a temporary solution, however. Within minutes they are back in a feeding frenzy. If I was going to rid us of these nuisances, I was going to have to "sell" them on the idea I meant business.

So there I was in the backyard, taking three purposeful strides toward the bird feeder, winding up my right arm and bringing it down forcefully, accompanied with a hearty "yer out!"

One gray squirrel nearly had the big one right there. Another leaped about 20 feet to the nearest branch. Right then I knew I was on to something.

When I reported my experiment to Williamson, who happens to be the city's deputy chief of police, he looked at me as though I belonged with the squirrels themselves, or at least in a padded wagon.

Then came the day I had to sell a call on the ball field. Opening night found me more than a little nervous. There were so many rules and details and positioning mechanics going through my head that it was all I could do to make the obvious call.

Fortunately, the first night served up mostly routine plays. On my first and only real attempt to sell a call, a bang-bang play at first, my voice kind of cracked.

My really big chance came on my second night. I was behind home plate, calling balls and strikes for a men's D league game. In the third inning, one of the teams loaded the bases with nobody out. The batter hit a sharp grounder that the third baseman fielded cleanly and stepped on the bag, a no-brainer for out No. 1.

"Out there!" I snapped.

The third baseman then threw toward home. The catcher tagged the sliding runner for out No. 2.

"Out here!" I shouted with more emphasis.

Then I looked up and saw the runner from first base trying to leg it out to third. The catcher saw him, too, and gunned a throw.

I could sense the moment. In 30 years of playing softball, I had never seen a triple play. If there was ever a time to sell a call, this was it.

I practically danced toward third base, with arm cocked. As the third baseman applied the tag in a cloud of dust, I wound up like a tightly coiled spring, clenched my fist and unleashed the full fury of my voice as the hammer came down.

"Yer o-o-o-ut!" I roared, gleefully.

The players in the field shouted their approval. The players on the bases looked back in astonishment. To my utter surprise, nobody really challenged the call. Even those on the wrong side of a triple play appreciated its uniqueness. Groff, my partner that night, gave me an approving nod. My big moment came and I sold it, just like the manual said.

And somewhere in the trees behind the outfield fence, the squirrels scattered.

Fatigue Can Be Pleasantly Delirious

The mind can play some strange tricks on you at times, I realized one hot August night.

Bloomington Herald-Times
August 15, 1998

Have you ever been so exhausted you couldn't sleep? That was my condition when I roughed out this column at four o'clock in the morning, less than eight hours after a grueling city tennis match.

I was playing in the Men's 35 draw against Jeff Melton, a psychology professor whose lesson plan for the day was to put Lynn Houser through three hours of hell.

From the moment he took the court, Melton ran me from side to side, from front to back, from here to eternity. I had never played anybody who could hit with topspin so relentlessly from both forehand and backhand.

Melton had me down four games to love before I knew what hit me. I was so elated to finally win a game that I won another ... and another. The next thing I knew I was up 5-4 and serving for set point.

But I was already running on empty. It had taken so much energy to come all the way back that I had little left. A potential winning lob barely missed. Left off the hook, Melton bounced back to win the set, 7-5. And when he broke me to go up 3-2 in the second, I was starting to console myself on the idea of having given a noble effort. The thought revitalized me and I was able to play on.

Even though Melton was still jerking my around the court like a puppet on a racket string, I somehow won the second set, 6-3. The bad news was that there was still one more set to play.

Four games into that third set, my 48-year-old quadriceps muscles locked up in one massive cramp, hurtling me to the court like a bomb whistling from the sky. I had fallen and couldn't get up. In a state of exhaustion, my mind took me back to a time when I could have stayed on the court for another three hours …

It was the fall of 1970, my junior year at Indiana University. I was attempting to make the IU hockey team as a walk-on. I was 20 years old and, in my mind, chiseled by two summers of hard labor on an asphalt crew.

I reported to camp along with a couple dozen other wishful thinkers. Little did we know, we were about to begin hockey's version of Hell Week. We never saw the ice that first week. All we did for two hours each day after class was conditioning. The regimen consisted of this:

* 15 minutes of calisthenics - push-ups, sit-ups, chin-ups, jumping jacks;

* A 1-mile run;

* More calisthenics;

* Two trips up and down every step of old Memorial Stadium;

* Five sets of 100-yard dashes;

* Another mile run.

I kid you not. I remember every last push-up, every last lap, every single step of the stadium on Tenth Street. When I got back to the dorm after those excruciating afternoons, I was so exhausted I didn't even want to eat. All I wanted to do was collapse on my bunk. When the time finally came to hit the ice, we were more than ready.

But in came the returning veterans, mostly French Canadians. They actually resembled hockey players, unlike our ragged band of walk-ons. About all I remember of that week on ice was that I scored a couple of goals and played well enough to make the first cut.

But when the final list was posted, my name wasn't on it. I was crushed. All I had to hang my hat on was knowing I was in the best shape of my life. Nothing again would ever be as physically demanding, not even the seven weeks of boot camp in the Navy. That was a joke compared to hockey camp.

I did go on to play intramural hockey career at IU. In the final week of the season I skated into the corner too hard and too fast. The boards didn't give, but my ankle did – a fracture that kept me in a cast for seven long weeks.

A month into that difficult stretch, a pretty coed named Paula Holloway spotted a young man on crutches and volunteered to carry his books. She would go on to become my college sweetheart.

In my delirious mind the other night, I saw the kind face of Paula Holloway and even heard her voice. But it wasn't her. It was another thoughtful stranger, another pretty young lady, a spectator inquiring if I needed some assistance.

The moral of this story: If you want to get the pretty girl, you start with 15 minutes of calisthenics, followed by a mile run, then 15 more minutes of calisthenics ...

The Great Hoist

The last day of summer is not for sissies.

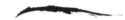

Bloomington Herald-Times
August 30, 2005

How many millions of kids are back at school -- or just returning this week -- and wondering where the summer went?

I know I had my share of forgettable summers, but there is one that stands out only because it was salvaged by the final day.

The summer of '61 was mostly uneventful in our neighborhood on Fort Wayne's south side. On the last day before school started, seven of us were just hanging around the garage.

It wasn't just any garage, though. This one had a loft full of sleazy detective magazines and books with dirty words in them. Because of this forbidden fruit, the loft was declared off limits to kids. Of course, we took that as a personal invitation.

The Caper

Also up there in that loft was a king-sized mattress, perfectly suited for wrestling. We got to rough-housing on the mattress that day and didn't notice it was sliding perilously close to the edge. But thanks to seven vigilant guardian angels, the only casualty was the mattress.

Over the side it went, crashing to the garage floor with such a force that a cloud of dust filled the stale air. At first we wanted to laugh, but then it occurred to us that the mattress was rock-solid evidence of our unauthorized presence in the loft. The only way to cover up our crime was to get the mattress back in the loft.

Lofty Goals

Mattresses back then were heavier than the fluffy, bouncy ones manufactured today. And this one was made heavier by the moisture it had absorbed in who knows how many years it lay there in the loft. It probably weighed more than 100 pounds -- way too heavy for a child to haul eight feet up a ladder. This was going to take some figuring.

We looked around the garage for a means. Hanging on nails right in front of us were some ropes and chains.

"We'll haul it up," we concluded.

Not so fast, kids.

As we tried to hoist the mattress, we made an unsettling discovery. Have you ever seen the biceps on a 10-year-old? They are about the size of robin eggs. Each time we attempted the great haul, we ran out of muscle about two feet from the top. And each time, the mattress, ropes and chains came plummeting back to earth.

Our plan needed rethinking.

Looking around for more answers, we noticed some cabinets and shelves. We figured if we could get the mattress on top of these supports, we could catch our breath and take it the remaining distance. Since the shelves and cabinets stood anywhere from four to six feet, we decided our best plan would be to raise the mattress in stages.

Stage One was to get the mattress off the floor. We dispatched two volunteers to use whatever objects were available -- buckets, gasoline cans, flower pots -- to slide under the mattress after the other five laborers raised it the first foot.

Stage Two would be much more difficult. We would have to raise the mattress five feet this time, then dispatch two volunteers to scramble down the ladder and hustle the shelves and cabinets in position while the others held on for dear life.

A Plan Comes Together

To our relief, Stage Two was a success. There was the mattress suspended in space, six feet above the floor.

Two feet to go.

By now we were already exhausted. Late-summer temperatures in a loft often approach triple digits, and this one was no exception. Our 95-pound bodies were glistening with sweat, and we were proud of it. This was manly labor, we said, while at the same time wondering if we had enough left in our little tanks to finish the job.

After guzzling some cokes -- the 1960s version of a power drink -- we geared up for the final pull. At least now we had our full complement of manpower, all seven playing a tug-o-war for keeps.

The Magnificent Seven

With one collective grunt, we began the final leg of our journey. Even though it was painfully difficult, we drew strength from each other. Seeing brows dripping with sweat and hands reddening from rope burns was enough to keep each young man persevering, unwilling to let his compatriots down.

We got the mattress to the top edge and knew the last few inches would be the hardest. But with one mighty last heave we lifted the mattress up and over.

For a few moments we sat there looking at our prize. The only sound was our heavy breathing. And then we met each others' eyes and cheered and laughed and clapped each other on the back as if each of us had belted a home run. For this bunch of puny kids, it was a grand slam.

Too bad we had to keep it to ourselves. It was tempting to tell our classmates about our final-day heroics, but we were sworn to secrecy.

But now it can be told that on the last day of summer in 1961, seven brothers-in-arms used blood, sweat, tears and brains to conquer matter. It just goes to show you what a group of kids can do when confronted with a common cause -- saving their hides.

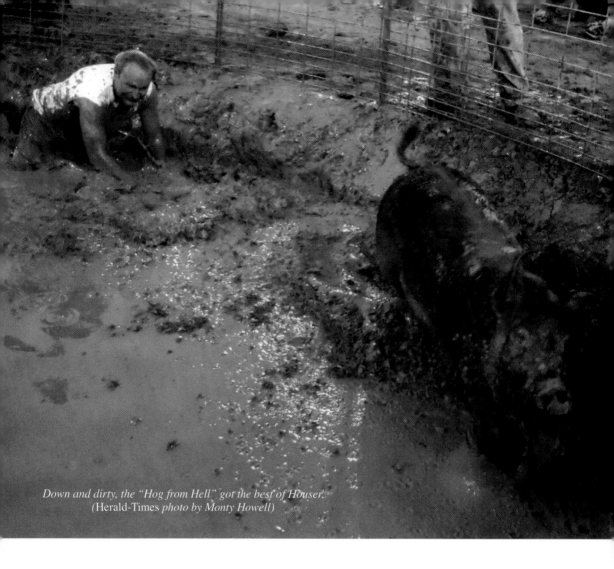
Down and dirty, the "Hog from Hell" got the best of Houser.
(Herald-Times *photo by Monty Howell*)

The Hog from Hell

This episode took mud-slinging to a new level.

Bloomington Herald-Times
July 17, 2007

Unwilling to stoop to the level of his critics, Lou Holtz once said, "Don't get in the mud with pigs. All you do is get muddy, and the pigs like it."

So what were two colleagues and me doing in a pig pen at the Greene County Fair Thursday night?

Blame it on staff writer Laura Lane. It was her article in the H-T that got us into our own little Bay of Pigs. Laura wrote a piece questioning whether hog wrestling and other county fair favorites constituted a form of animal abuse.

Boy, did that ever get the rural folks riled up. Ever since that article appeared in print, Laura has been besieged by angry fairgoers staunchly defending hog wrestling as a national pastime. It even prompted the editor of the Greene County Daily World, Nick Schneider, to write an editorial in which he summed up Laura's article as "hogwash."

Out of all the discussion, a gauntlet was thrown at Laura's feet: bring a team to the competition and see for yourself, the challenge went. Now, Laura is not one to back down from a fight, so she immediately started recruiting volunteers to fill out her squad, which by contest rules was limited to four.

Although one newsroom member after another wisely declined, Laura persevered until she found two suckers, Stewart Moon, a graphics designer, and myself, a sports writer in search of a column during the lean summer months.

Hey, we got uniforms out of it, plain white T-shirts with "H-T mud slingers" stenciled across the front — so people would know who to boo, I guess.

We had no idea what we were getting into. None of us was raised on a farm, so we wouldn't know a farm hog from a razorback. All we knew was that we would tangle with some form of the hog species weighing anywhere from 20 to 200 pounds. The object was to capture the hog, hoist it up and place it on top of a 55-gallon drum.

If our team drew the Fat Albert of hogs, we would be in big trouble. The heaviest thing I lift anymore is a 22-ounce beer. Stewart is no physical specimen himself, and Laura's orneriness can take her only so far. About the only thing we had going for us was life experience. Our average age was 49, easily the oldest team in the competition.

Fully aware of our limitations, we thought we might tame the beast with kindness. Why not just buy a corn dog at the fair and see if the pig will come to us, we reasoned.

Another strategy was to try and make eye contact with the pig in the hope of hypnotizing it the way Robert Redford tamed the unruly thoroughbred in the movie, *Horse Whisperer*. However, Redford's character patiently waited all day for the horse to come to him, and we had a mere 45 seconds to do our thing.

In these competitions, the hog is every bit as traumatized as the steed in *Horse Whisperer*. Did I mention the hog is often prompted by a kick in the hind end as it is ushered into the ring? If that doesn't scare the manure out of it, the sight of three or four crazed humans surely does.

There really isn't a sure-fire approach to catching a terrified pig who is all lathered up and knows where it is going. The piece of advice I received was, 'Hit him low."

That means you have to get down and dirty, down there where the pig feels right at home. Fortunately for the rest of our team, my stumpy legs are just as short as a pig's, so going low is no big deal for me. And one of my nicknames as a kid was Dirtball.

As we watched all the little kids catch frightened little piggy-wiggys for 90 minutes, we knew we were in for a much bigger challenge. Early in the evening, fair organizer John Beach went over to the chute operators and pointed us out. You could see them look our way and crack a wry smile.

When our time came, the pit was a vile soup of mud, sweat and whatever the hogs had left behind.

And by then the grandstand was packed. When the H-T team was announced, I couldn't really say if we were booed because my eyes were fixed on the biggest, baddest hog I had seen all night — a fresh one just for us. Fat Albert would have been a welcome substitute for Diablo, or whatever name this creature went by.

It didn't need any prompting to enter the ring. Snorting and snarling, it should have entered with bull-fighting music blaring over the loud speakers. Between its steamy breath, its sleek charcoal-grey coat and the sinister expression on its face, the beast could have passed for the devil himself. It had to be at least 200 pounds of hide, hooves, ham hocks and ill humor.

I looked at Laura and said, "Maybe we should rethink this." Then it was Laura's turn to snarl — something about my manhood — so it was game on.

Except when Laura entered the ring, she went left while "Satan" went right — right at me. This was one of those defining moments where you find out what you are made of, one of those Mano a Mano confrontations where you either back down or go for it. In front of some 2,000 people, I could neither run nor hide, so I did what any other man with an ego would do — foolishly go on the attack.

With a rush of adrenaline, I hit the hog broadside and pinned it against the fence for a couple of seconds, hoping that Laura and Stew would arrive in time for us to finish the task.

But this hombre was not going to have any of that. It exploded out of my grasp, giving me a swift kick in the chin as if to say, "Take that with ya."

Stunned, I belly-flopped into the muck, sending a wave of bilge directly into my nostrils. I can still taste it as I write.

I had no sooner pulled myself up and regained my senses when the brute came around again. By now I was just as possessed as it was. Whether it was classic "Little Man's Syndrome" or an excess of adrenaline, my soul descended to "a very dark place," Laura said later.

I hurled myself at the monster, drove it into the fence and was able to hold on long enough for my teammates to get there. Laura and I actually had its front half off the ground while Stew was working on the hind quarters when the clock mercifully expired.

Evidently, we made our point because the hog didn't need any coaxing to return to the chute, still snorting and snarling as it descended back into hell. It certainly wasn't hog heaven where he came from.

Although we didn't come close to completing our mission, we did receive the rousing approval of the fans.

As we made our way back to the horse barn to get hosed off, we were congratulated by fairgoers and other contestants.

Then we took inventory of our injuries. If there was any abuse going on, it was the two-legged animals on the receiving end of it. The kick on the chin drew blood, a noble red badge of courage for me. Both Stewart and I had abrasions from the hog's surprisingly coarse hide. Somehow, Laura didn't even break a fingernail. Go figure.

But we did ourselves proud, we think. Although the final score goes down as Hog 1, H-T 0, we can still sleep soundly, knowing we remain higher on the food chain.

Breaded tenderloin, anyone?

Chapter 4

Closer to Home

Every once in a while a guy has to get his mind off sports and consider matters closer to home. Over the years, I ventured away from the sports page to write some homespun columns, often featured in the Lifestyle section under the headings, "That's Life" and "Notes From Home." Up first, though, is a piece I authored in my first year at the Kendallville News-Sun, *a piece that has enjoyed more shelf life than any other I've written. Read on.*

Yes, Hannah, There Is a Santa Claus

Introducing Hannah Holstein, the legendary talking cow. Obviously, this will take some "splainin."

Hannah Holstein was the creation of the late Bill Fischbach, the man who preceded me as sports editor of the Kendallville News-Sun *in the 1970s. As the story went, Fischbach was passing by a pasture one day when heard a voice calling out to him. With no other human being in sight, Fischbach thought he was hearing voices of the wrong kind. But as he drew closer to the pasture, a cow of the Holstein variety sidled up and started talking – and never really stopped.*

Hannah Holstein ultimately became the alter ego of every sportswriter who ever worked for the Kendallville Publishing Company, and "she" still makes her high school sports picks to this day.

As Christmas approached in 1976, my first year on the job, I decided Hannah was the perfect author for this holiday message. To my utmost satisfaction, this spin-off of the "Yes, Virginia" Christmas story has been a tradition in Kendallville, published on Christmas Eve every year since '76, the gift that keeps on giving.

By Hannah Holstein
Kendallville News-Sun
December 24, 1976

It has come to my attention that certain readers out there doubt the actual existence of Hannah Holstein.

"Hannah is just a figment of some writer's imagination," they say.

Or, "Hannah is just a literary trick to write a sports column in the first person. No one has ever seen her, you know."

Well, let me ask you this, folks. If Hannah wasn't for real, why doesn't the United States Post Office strike me off the mailing list? I'll tell you why. Because I receive gobs of mail from faithful followers ever year.

Furthermore, I answer much of that mail personally, and many folks in this area have copies of my responses to prove it.

You know, I have a sneaky hunch that the same people who doubt the reality of Hannah Holstein also doubt the existence of another famous person who comes into the limelight this time of year. You know who I am talking about – Mr. Kris Kringle, otherwise known as Santa Claus.

Poor Santa. He has done so much for so many for so long, and yet he constantly has to defend his existence against scrooges, "realists," and beard-pulling children.

I sympathize with you, Santa, because I'm fighting the same kind of battle on a different plane.

To go a step farther, perhaps these same disbelievers also doubt the existence of another well-known person who comes to the fore at this time. His name is Jesus Christ, and He has been fighting an uphill battle since His birth 2,000 years ago.

That was a landmark occasion, and Hannah is proud to tell you that one of her ancestors was right there to warm that precious Babe in the stable. That was probably the most noble thing any Holstein ever did, and Hannah wishes she could have been the one.

But even though I wasn't there to see or meet the Baby Jesus, that doesn't stop me from believing in Him just the same. Why? Because Hannah possesses a gift much more valuable than the ability to predict the outcome of sporting events.

For you see, faith is not built on logic or factual proof. Faith is built on trust and personal conviction. For Hannah, her faith comes from looking at the world and seeing so much good. Only the Lord Himself could produce such a wonderful place, and that's good enough to get my vote.

And despite all of this, I believe in Him just because He told us that those who believe without seeing will enter that great pasture in the sky.

Now the point behind all of this is that no one has seen Hannah, either. I wish I could change that, but the nature of my work makes it impossible. It is essential for Hannah to remain out of the public eye because a talking cow would attract greedy profit-makers, and Hannah has no intentions of spending the rest of her days in a sideshow.

So let me conclude by drawing on the meaning of Christmas to defend the existence of Hannah Holstein. Christmas is a time to renew old friendships, the spirit of giving and the foundations of one's faith.

If one does not believe the Son of God was born at this time 2,000 years ago, Christmas has no meaning. But if one believes without seeing, one has everything to celebrate at Christmas.

By the same token, if one believes in lowly Hannah without seeing the Sacred Cow, one can enjoy her columns for what they are – entertainment.

Merry Christmas, friends.

Lost Your Pocket Knife? You Tool!

Losing my Swiss army knife in 1998 was like losing my entire tool box.

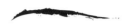

Bloomington Herald-Times
August 9, 1998

Ask any man and he probably has a favorite tool.

Get your mind out of the gutter, I'm talking work tool here. Look in any man's garage and there's probably an all-purpose tool within arm's length. It could be an adjustable wrench, an electric screwdriver, a heavy-duty scissors/wire cutter, a wood saw -- you name it.

I had a tool that could all but build the Space Shuttle, and it came in one tidy little package -- my Swiss army knife.

I say "had" because, after 23 years of faithful service, I misplaced it. I was so upset I went back the next day to look for it in the pouring rain. I think it must have slipped out of the hip pocket of my baseball pants the other night at Twin Lakes softball park.

What's a softball player doing with a pocket knife? Hey, I rarely left home without it. If it wasn't on my person, it was in my truck. On the occasions I didn't have it with me, I felt vulnerable. I called it Old Faithful.

I bought it in 1975 for $14 at the Navy PX store in Spain. It was one of the deluxe models that could service an entire aircraft carrier if need be. It had three screwdriver heads (two regular, one Phillips), two knife blades, a saw, a scissors, a magnifying glass, a can opener, a bottle opener, a nail file, a tooth pick and a tweezers. It came with its own instruction manual.

It seemed each little attachment had its own special story. I lost the toothpick and tweezers in the first six months. The tweezers disappeared at a Doobie Brothers concert. (Don't ask.) I dearly missed the tweezers for all those delicate jobs not intended for my clumsy hands.

In addition to opening many a heavy cardboard box, the saw came in handy one night when I blew a radiator hose. Not to worry. Old Faithful was in the glove box. With the saw I was able to cut away the bad section of hose and still had enough left to reattach it and get to a gas station before running out of water and engine coolant.

Besides the hundreds of fishing lines I cut with the knife blade, I also used it to whittle sticks for the grandchildren to roast marshmallows. And I don't know how many road maps I read with that magnifying glass. I even tried to start a fire with it on a camping trip but didn't quite succeed. In a pinch -- and with a little more patience -- I believe I could have done it, though.

I made sure Old Faithful was with me the first time I took a road trip to Penn State. Heeding the warnings of Indiana basketball coach Bob Knight -- that Penn State is a "camping trip" -- I was not about to venture into the wilderness without it.

I couldn't even begin to tell you how many bottles of beer I opened with Old Faithful. Too many brain cells are lost from the memory bank.

And even though a pocket knife could be construed as a weapon, Old Faithful was never raised in anger. It was instrument of peace, a conscientious objector among knives. After all, it had the white Swiss cross on its red handle, and we all know how much the Swiss value their neutrality in worldwide disputes.

I'm really going to miss Old Faithful. I'm sure there will be another Swiss army knife in my future (hint, hint, gift-buyers), but it will surely cost three or four times the amount of the original and I would be greatly surprised if it served me faithfully for almost a quarter of a century.

Old Faithful's final mission before its untimely demise was opening one last bottle of beer. When I get my replacement knife, I'm going back to that grassy knoll at Twin Lakes, pop open a Heineken, tip my hat and say, "Here's to Old Faithful, you old tool."

Air Conditioning Is Pretty Cool (or Not)

The 100th anniversary of air conditioning prompted this piece.

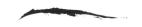

Bloomington Herald-Times
August 1, 2002

The summer heat of the last few days sure makes you appreciate air conditioning. How did we ever get along without it?

Well, with the help of some fresh air, the electric fan and the occasional summer breeze, we managed.

I just read where air conditioning celebrated its 100th birthday. It might have been invented a century ago, but it wasn't commonplace until the 1970s.

Thinking back to my childhood days in the 1950s, we cooled off by running through the sprinklers. At night the adults would sit on the porch, taking relief in the cool of the evening while the kids chased fireflies or each other.

In a neighborhood such as ours on the south side of Fort Wayne, nearly everyone spent their evenings on the porch. It was too hot to be in the house, so the great outdoors was your refuge.

Neighbors would often drop by for some conversation, a smoke or a cold beverage. People would stroll around the block, stopping every so often to chat with a familiar face. You really knew your neighbors then, whether you wanted to or not.

As you sat on your porch, the open window let you know your neighbors' business — what TV programs they watched, what radio stations they listened to, what instruments they played.

From my cousins' porch you could hear a young man who was aspiring to be an opera singer. The neighborhood was his audience. He was pretty good — up to a point. About the 10th time he sang "Figaro," the guy in the tank top who lived across the street would tell him to stick a sock in it.

In opening your windows you definitely opened yourself up to the world. On a quiet night you might doze off to the drone of the birds and locusts. On another you might have to endure a family quarrel. That was more than you ever wanted to hear.

If it got bad enough, you might hop in the family car and go for a drive. Cruising around with the radio on and the windows down was about as cool as it could get in more ways than one. If dad had some loose cash in his wallet, he might treat the family to an ice cream cone.

Our choice was the Humpty Dumpty, a popular ice cream stand on the corner of Fairfield and Packard. Across the street in Packard Park, you might catch a women's baseball game.

Fort Wayne boasted one of the finest women's fast-pitch leagues in the country. I still remember a game under the lights between the Daisies and Chicks. Although they suited up in blouses, short dresses, and knee socks, their skills rivaled the men's. Hundreds of fans would show up on a hot summer night to enjoy the evening air and marvel at their talents.

By bedtime the neighborhood had calmed down and the air had cooled. If you were lucky, you had a fan in your bedroom. If not, you slept in your underwear and didn't bother with the covers.

I don't remember many sleepless nights because of the heat. A more frequent nuisance was the mosquito. Entire squadrons would enter through holes in the screens and assemble in tactical formation around your head. As annoying as that was, part of me longs for that moment of time again.

Today, we practically have to drag ourselves out of our air-tight, air-conditioned houses, jump into our air-tight, air-conditioned automobiles, and dash into our air-tight, air-conditioned offices. Then we do it all over again in reverse, ending up in our air-tight, air-conditioned houses.

And many of today's houses don't even have a front porch. In their place is the garage, hardly a community gathering space.

We've lost a little with air conditioning. Now, when you step outside your house, about the only sound you hear is the hum of your neighbor's air conditioner.

That's not so cool, is it?

Daisy, He Only Had Eyes for You

Beach Boys, hot rods and a pretty girl. This column had it all.

Bloomington Herald-Times
August 18, 2002

> She's my little deuce coupe.
> You don't know what I've got.
> - The Beach Boys

Even though I knew the words to every Beach Boys' song about hot rods, I never fancied myself owning one.

Hot rods are for guys who can take a car apart and reassemble it in the time it takes for your average Indianapolis 500 pit stop. My mechanical expertise went no further than changing a spark plug.

But in 1976 I threw caution to the wind. I was 26 years old, single and carefree. That was before I saw "Daisy" – a sensuous, seductive, alluring lady in red, a real head-turner.

Daisy was a 1939 Oldsmobile sedan – but not just any sedan. She wore a brilliant shade of lipstick red, and strutted around in chrome wheels. She was powered by a 327 cubic-inch Corvette engine. And even though she belonged to another man, I had to have her.

I was in the Navy at the time, a lonely young sailor stationed in Brunswick, Maine. She was the pride of a dashing lieutenant. For me it was love at first sight. For weeks I longed for her, a distant dream.

Then it happened. The lieutenant put her up for sale. He was asking $2,500, a lot of money in 1976, especially for a car almost 40 years old, but I didn't even bother to negotiate a lower price. Money was no object. I burned rubber all the way to the bank in my old "beater," a banged up, battleship-gray Mustang.

I plopped 25 $100 bills in the lieutenant's hand and ran off with Daisy. Can't tell you how I came up with the name. It just seemed to fit.

You should have seen the lust in the eyes of my fellow enlisted men. Whenever an occasion called for a "road trip," Daisy was first choice.

She offered plenty of room. With bench seats in front and back, she could easily accommodate six passengers. On one occasion, we crammed eight in the compartment. We liked to rumble down Main Street in Brunswick honking Daisy's powerful horn as if we were on parade. We used to refer to her as "The Buglemobile."

Even with all that Corvette horsepower under the hood, I never engaged in any drag races. Daisy was above that. She was a showgirl.

You would have thought I was a man dating an exotic dancer, the way I showed her off. And like a woman in show business, she was "high maintenance."

I discovered it took a lot of money to keep a lady looking her best. Spare parts for vehicles of her vintage were not easily located.

And Daisy was so temperamental. On her maiden voyage to Indiana, she broke down somewhere in upstate New York. But since she was such an eye-grabber, it wasn't long before help was on the way. A state trooper stopped, marveled at her, then quickly radioed for assistance.

About 20 minutes later, two teenage boys pulled up in a pick-up truck. Daisy wowed 'em.

A half hour later, they came back with a used fuel pump, slapped it on and sent us one our way. I practically had to force a couple of twenties into their hands. The privilege of working on such a treasure was payment enough, they said.

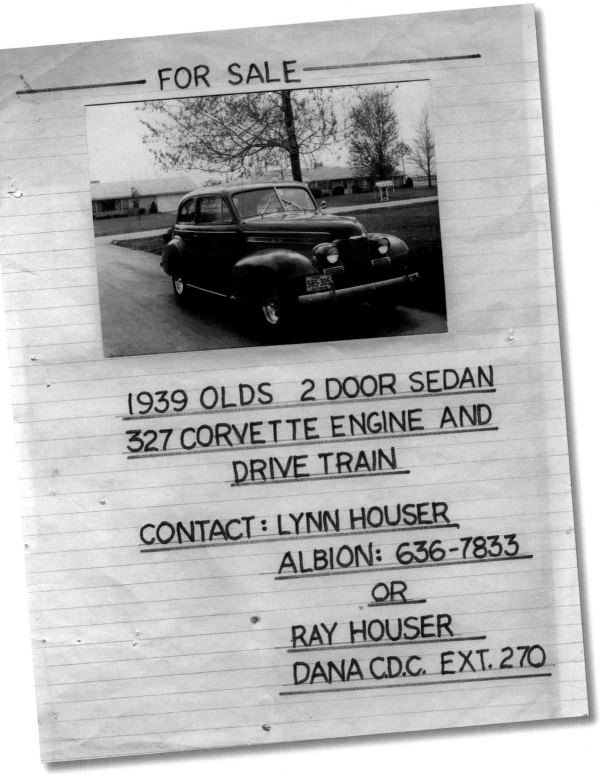

FOR SALE

1939 OLDS 2 DOOR SEDAN
327 CORVETTE ENGINE AND
DRIVE TRAIN

CONTACT: LYNN HOUSER
ALBION: 636-7833
OR
RAY HOUSER
DANA C.D.C. EXT. 270

It broke my heart to break up with the girl of my dreams

My love affair with Daisy burned on for an-other year, until the upkeep became too much. The Corvette engine drank gasoline the way a sailor on liberty drinks beer. And those repairs just kept mounting.

Finally, like the man who trades in a society dame for a woman of more substance, I opted for a more practical car – a Ford Pinto, for pete's sake.

I can't tell you how it pained me to turn Daisy over to another man. Average guys like me don't often get the pretty girl, the girl of their dreams.

Hard Labor Is Hard on the Nerves

If it wasn't for two summers on a road crew, I would not have been able to pay for the college education that made me the fine writer I am today. OK, so maybe my writing isn't so hot, but those summers on the asphalt were.

Bloomington Herald-Times
July 1, 2003

Is it just me, or is all of Monroe County under road construction? There is no escaping it.

If you live on the west side, your day starts with trying to weave through Ellettsville, where old Ind. 46 remains under construction. If you live on the east side, College Mall Road remains under construction. And smack in the middle of Bloom-ington is the project known as Miller-Showers Park. It too remains under construction.

As you proceed through downtown, you en-counter more lane restrictions from, guess what? Construction -- this time, of new hotels and apart-ment complexes.

No need to build another parking garage. Dur-ing rush hour you can jump out of your car, dash into the courthouse, register to vote, grab a cup of coffee on the way out and catch up to your car in the next block.

If you think Bloomington is bad, have you been to Indianapolis lately? The streets of Bagh-dad have to be less restricted.

It doesn't do any good to honk your horn, pound your steering wheel or swear at the con-struction crews. The latter work at only once pace -- their own. I speak from experience, having spent two summers on a road crew while working my way through college.

We shoveled asphalt with the speed of volca-nic lava. Of course, asphalt is a form of molten lava, reaching a temperature of almost 400 degrees when it is fresh out of the mixer. That's why you see road crews wearing thick-soled boots. Try standing on hot asphalt for any length of time. You might as well walk barefoot on hot charcoals.

In my first summer on the job, I had a fore-man of Kentucky roots who I will identify only as "Lonnie." That's in case he has a score to settle. Lonnie used to delight in putting me and the other "college kids" through torturous trials.

One 90-degree day, after we'd already been out in the sun for some nine hours, Lonnie decided there was still enough daylight to put down some curb. The laborer's job was to jump into a dump truck full of steaming asphalt and feed the curb machine with continuous shoveling. Although the asphalt was not 400 degrees in the truck bed, it was still a good 140. After about five minutes your boots would be smoking. The laborers would "tag-team" to keep from passing out.

On this particular day, I was the only laborer available. I gave it my best shot, but after a half hour the sky started swirling. I guzzled a can of pop, but that did not stay down. It was all I could do to climb out of the truck and find some shade. When Lonnie made some comment as to my man-hood, I secretly vowed to get even.

On my last day of the first summer, we were putting the finishing touches on a freshly paved parking lot. By then I was pretty good with a shov-el, accurate up to about 20 feet with a level scoop. From about 15 feet away, Lonnie called for a shov-el-full near the curb where he was standing. I lev-eled off the proper amount, took aim and nailed a bull's-eye -- his crotch.

So sorry, Lonnie.

You could hear him screaming all the way to Kentucky. Talk about going out in a blaze of glory!

Although my days on his crew were over, I was allowed to return the following summer. I wound up on a stone crew. The stone crews did the preliminary work before the asphalt crews came through. Instead of shoveling asphalt, we shov-eled rocks -- big, gnarly rocks -- lots of 'em. It was like hard prison labor, breaking big rocks into little ones. This was the cost of a college education, I kept telling myself.

The foreman, who I will identify only as "Big Jim," was another good ol' boy who did not have much use for "#%&+ college kids," as he called us.

And for good reason. We were always screwing up. Well, at least I was. Fortunately, I saved the worst for last.

On the Friday before I was to return to college, my crew was prepping the turn lanes for a stretch of road near St. Charles Elementary in Fort Wayne. Big Jim assigned me the simple task of stringing a path for the paver to follow. I was handed a wad of string the size of a beach ball. After about stringing about 30 feet, I encountered a knot. In trying to free it I only succeeded in making a larger knot -- one about the size of Big Jim's pickup truck.

He saw my futility and came up swearing. When he pulled out his pocket knife, I feared my last day on the job would also be my last day on Earth. Big Jim ripped the tangled mess out of my hands and sliced it off, muttering the usual "#%&+ college kids."

I was relieved from my post, but I was only warming up.

As we were about to wrap up the project, a trucker needed somebody to move a back-hoe that was blocking his path. Even though I was not properly licensed to operate such a piece of equipment, I felt confident I could move it a short distance.

I fired it up and got it in gear with no problem, but as I pulled away I felt a tug. I looked behind me and saw that the upright section of the back hoe had snagged a support wire of a schoolyard basketball goal. The backboard tilted at a 45-degree angle. I could hear the trucker snickering. Hoping nobody else was watching, I put the machine in reverse and retreated until the wire snapped back, then maneuvered the machine out of the way of both the goal and the truck.

I was quite proud of myself until I saw Big Jim frantically waving at me. I heard shouts from fellow workers. Why such a commotion over one little basketball rim, I wondered. I climbed off the back hoe and saw a much greater disaster. In front of me was a 20-foot patch of chewed-up asphalt. In my haste I had failed to raise the machine's heavy front bucket.

I figured that was as good a time as any to call it a day -- and a career. The last thing I heard as I sprinted toward my car was "#%&+ college kids."

So the next time you feel yourself boiling over because of road work, show a little patience. It might be some #%&+ college kid's last day on the job.

Life Is Good on the Lake

Owners of lake cottages can probably rattle off names of moochers like me. For those who I imposed on, and there were many, consider this an long overdue thank-you note.

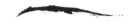

Bloomington Herald-Times
August 19, 2004

Coming from the flatlands of northern Indiana, I have found much to like about southern Indiana. The hills, the trees, the rock formations and sweeping landscapes have been enough for me to call southern Indiana home for 20 years now.

But come this time of year, there is one thing I really miss about northern Indiana, the abundance of natural lakes. In the northeast part of the state, you can drive in any direction and encounter a healthy body of water in 15 minutes or less. We do have some nice lakes down here in southern Indiana, but they do not match the ones up north in scope and number.

Up north, the lakes are so plentiful and available that even Hoosiers who aren't fortunate to have a lake cottage will know somebody who does. Dropping in on these poor souls is an art I once mastered.

My fondness for lakes started with my favorite childhood vacation, spending an entire week with my cousins at Big Long Lake in LaGrange County. When we weren't swimming, fishing or skipping stones across the lake, we were playing Kick the Can. The cottage didn't even have a television, but we didn't miss it.

When I got old enough to drive, my high school buddies and I would routinely crash somebody's cottage almost every weekend. All those generous people ever asked of us in return was to bring some food. Being the poor teenagers we were, that sometimes amounted to stopping on a country road and raiding a corn field.

I was most proud of one particular "harvest" until the gracious host pointed out that it was field corn, not the kind meant for human consumption. Of course that didn't stop a bunch of growing boys from eating it because, as you might already know, being around water all day makes you hungry enough to eat ... well, field corn.

A typical day might find us water skiing and "tubing" until we could no longer hang onto the rope. We used to play a water tubing game called Rodeo, where the objective called for the boat driver to criss-cross the waves like a wild bull until he bucked the helpless tuber.

I remember being on the business end of one of those wild rides and seeing this enormous wave hurtling at the tube. I hit the wave with such force I was airborne long enough to look down onto the water and wonder what the impact was going to feel like on splashdown. Is that fun or what?

In the shallow water we would play football or volleyball, contests that deteriorated into all-out wars. You could elbow, poke, gouge, clutch, bite, scratch and the go for the ultimate defensive tactic -- grab the other guy's swimsuit. The only rule was, if you grabbed a swimsuit, you better not get too grabby, if you know what I mean.

Not all of the day was devoted to mayhem. Sometimes you would just sun yourself on one of those wooden, anchored rafts floating about a hundred yards off the shore. Or you might take a boat ride out to a sand bar where the other lake-goers were hanging out.

Better yet was a moonlight boat ride. The lake would usually be perfectly still then, except for the frogs croaking. Hunting frogs also was a favorite past time. Catch enough of them and you had a frog leg feast, a true delicacy on the lake.

So are bluegill. Ever had a meal of fried bluegill, sweet corn and ripe Indiana tomatoes? That's about as good as it gets, folks.

After a day on the lake, you would not have any trouble sleeping. Your muscles would be so water-logged they would just conform to the shape of any bed, couch or hammock.

And when the time came for you to leave the lake, you really didn't want to go. When we were kids we would go kicking and screaming, not at all ready to leave our aquatic playpens. Come to think of it, I had to be shown the door a time or two as an adult.

You think they owned the place or something.

Nothing Routine about This Procedure

Those of you who have had their colon scoped out will relate to this.

Bloomington Herald-Times
October 18, 2004

Whatever happened to the good ol' "routine" physical examination?

You know what I'm talking about. The doctor listens to your heart, makes you say "ah," thumps you on the back and taps you on the knee. And as a bonus for men who have reached middle age, the good doctor straps on a rubber glove and thrusts an index finger all the way up to the prostate which, I've painfully concluded, must be located somewhere near the tonsils.

I was prepared for all that when I recently signed up for a physical, but then the doctor had the nerve to ask me when was the last time I had my colon checked. The writer in me wanted to make a joke about knowing my colons from my semicolons, but I knew the doctor would not be amused.

Unable to give the physician a satisfactory answer, he suggested a colonoscopy. I wasn't totally sure what he was talking about, but I knew any procedure involving the words "colon" and "scope" could not be pleasant.

I learned a colonoscopy is true to its verbal roots. A tiny camera is threaded up your colon for a little look-see, checking for abnormal growths called polyps. Webster's Dictionary defines a polyp as a "smooth, projecting growth of hypertrophied mucous membrane in the nose, bladder, rectum, etc."

Correct me if I'm wrong, but isn't that just a polite way of saying "booger?"

Checking my intestines for such disgusting objects would be a waste of time because I stopped picking my nose in the second grade. The only thing in my intestines other than food products might be the dirty note I had to swallow to avoid detection in high school.

The doctor, of course, went ahead and scheduled the colonoscopy. I was told the procedure itself would be brief but that the necessary preparations would take some time. The "prep work," I found out, entailed a thorough purging of the entire digestive system. This would be accomplished along two fronts. Make that one front and one rear, actually.

The first part called for a 24-hour fast -- no solid foods of any kind leading up to the procedure. The other half of the equation called for ridding the system of existing food products through powerful laxatives.

Got the picture yet? In other words, your body's exports were going to exceed its imports. And those exports turned out to be quite urgent. When told to not make any plans after taking one of those laxatives, I found out the doctor wasn't kidding. You wouldn't dare wander too far away from your friendly commode.

That wasn't even the worst of it, though. The hardest part for me was not eating. Not only do I love to eat; I live to eat. The day I go without eating a single bite, well, you better start up the hearse. (I was permitted to eat clear liquids, hard candy and popsicles, but try making a meal out of that.)

I did my best to keep my mind off food during The Longest Day but didn't get much help. We have a popcorn machine in the cantina and about once a month somebody fires it up. And wouldn't you know it, somebody got a yen for popcorn that day. Is there a more tantalizing smell than hot, buttery popcorn? The aroma had my nose on speed dial.

"Why don't you guys just fry up some bacon while you're at it!" I snapped.

That afternoon I went to the cantina for one of my piddly little popsicles, only to happen upon some fellow employees enjoying some birthday cake. I stared at it with lust.

Temptation was everywhere. While running errands I saw a billboard advertising Hardee's "Six Dollar Burger." I hope my truck's tinted windows hid the drool oozing from lip.

I tried to lose myself in some mindless television that night, only to see one commercial after another taunting me with a beckoning food item. As if that wasn't enough, I had to set my alarm clock for 3:30 a.m. to take another laxative. By the time I arrived at the medical facility, my intestines had to be cleaner than a new garden hose.

I don't even remember the procedure. They injected me with an anesthetic that almost instantly put me in Little Lynn Land. Before I knew it, I was coming to in the recovery room. A familiar voice was speaking to me. As I tried to focus, my eyes saw "wife," but my brain saw "meat."

Patricia Ann Houser will never know how close she was to becoming a blue plate special. Good thing she treated me to a milk shake on the drive home.

For the rest of the day I ate everything I could get my hands on, giving the kitchen cupboards a spring cleaning in the fall. Even the canned beets were calling me. There's nothing like an empty colon to make the taste buds grow fonder.

Pass the beets, please.

Raking It All In

Living on a wooded lot since 1992, I grew accustomed to tackling the leaves every fall. As you will see, it wasn't so bad.

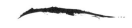

Bloomington Herald-Times
November 4, 2004

Is there a more beautiful season than autumn? Look at all those colorful leaves floating gracefully to the ground — over and over and over and over. Hey, they don't call it "fall" for nothing. I'm convinced the Houser yard in Ellettsville is the final resting place for leaves from four counties.

Not only does the yard get smothered with the leaves from its own trees, but by being at the north end of a cul-de-sac, it is the final resting place for the rest of the leaves in the neighborhood, thanks to the southwesterly winds that blow almost daily in the fall. That's right neighborly of everybody.

I can handle it, though, thanks to my trusty rake. The yard tool was a housewarming gift to the family when we moved into our current home in the fall of 1992. This wasn't one of those cheap, wooden rakes that leave splinters in your hands and snap in half when you try to move a pile weighing more than a feather. This rake was made out of heavy-duty wood with a wide, plastic head and, best of all, a padded handle. Not only have I yet to suffer a splinter, I haven't even had a single blister.

Don't ask me for a brand name. The only marking on the rake reads, "Made in the USA." Bless you, Uncle Sam, for not out-sourcing this product. The efforts of a few American laborers have been channeled into years of good clean work by this American laborer.

How many man-hours in 12 years I can only guess. From mid-September to Thanksgiving, I rake my yard at least once a week, averaging about four hours. Over 10 weeks that is a minimum of 40 hours, a solid work week. Multiply that by 12 (years) and you have 480 hours, or 60 eight-hour days. And that's a conservative estimate.

Think of the thousands upon thousands of strokes and the millions upon millions of leaves. And the old rake is still going strong, aging better than its owner. The only sign of wear and tear is some duct tape on the throat for support and one bent "finger." We are talking the rake now, not me.

We make quite a team, the rake and me. With one flick of the wrist I can shoot a one-foot pile of leaves about 10 feet to its final destination. I don't play hockey any more, but thanks to countless repetitions with the rake, I bet I still have a pretty good wrist shot.

Raking your yard is plenty of exercise. A lot of people don't know that because of the rake's biggest competitor, the leaf blower.

I personally detest this machine. The noise — the unceasing, high-pitched drone — is enough to make both the ears and head ring well into the night.

I much prefer nature's leaf blower, a good, stiff October gust. The blustery day we had on Halloween Eve was just what the yard doctor ordered to move a mountain of leaves from my yard.

A wind howling at its loudest is never as annoying as a leaf blower a block away. I don't even turn on the radio much anymore because I enjoy the peace and quiet. It gives me a chance to lose myself in my thoughts. A lot of the stories I have written over the years have been conceived while I was alone with my rake.

The rake is not only a very good listener, but also a good tour guide. Each time I rake I get to revisit my yard.

The rake guides me on a tour of the flower beds, where my wife and I spent one entire Fourth of July putting them in.

The rake takes me over by the porch swing, which hangs under the elm tree that has supplied us with plenty of shade for those mellow afternoons with a book and a cold beverage.

The rake also takes me to a place under some pine trees we call "Our Lady of the Pines." Buried there are two precious cats, Odie and Molly. Watching over them is a little statue of the Mother Mary. I usually find myself saying a Hail Mary for the kitties as my rake gently touches their graves. (If I have been a bad boy I might say an entire Rosary.)

As the rake moves across the yard, it has been known to uncover a thing or two — maybe a toad, a quarter or one of my wife's earrings that she spent days looking for.

Then there was the time the rake uncovered a nest of yellow jackets. I got stung three times before I could run out of harm's way. I couldn't hold it against my partner, however. It was only doing its job like it has for a dozen years now.

When I am done writing this piece, I will head out to the garage to the spot where my rake hangs, waiting for me to put it to good use once again. The leaves just keep falling and falling, but I don't mind.

I just look at it as an excuse to spend some quality time with an old friend.

Price Was Right for This Bonding Experience

In attempt to bond with my grandson, I took him to a brawl and watched a hockey game break out.

Bloomington Herald-Times
November 16, 2005

You've probably seen the MasterCard commercials claiming that no price is too high (nor credit too steep) when a sport memory is made.

The making of a sports memory was what I had in mind for the 11th birthday of my grandson, Alex, a young man who knows his sports. Alex plays them the year-around and watches Sports Center the way other kids watch cartoons.

Trying to find something unique for his birthday present, I came up with what I thought was a novel idea – a professional hockey game. Alex lives close to Fort Wayne, home of the minor-league Komets, who have thrived for more than a half century.

Talk about memories. I have a good 45 years of Komet gems stored away.

There was my first Komet game in 1960, a game halted by an all-out, bench-clearing brawl. Although this bloodbath left my overly sensitive sister seemingly scarred for life, I was hooked. That was not to like about a sport that offered speed, skill and mayhem?

With Alex's age now numbering in double figures, I figured it was safe to expose him to sometimes violent sport of ice hockey. The chosen date featured a game against the Rockford

IceHogs at Fort Wayne's Memorial Coliseum. To keep it civilized, I also invited Alex's grandma, my wife Pat, who has had to humor my Komet cravings over the years.

For $50 I landed three seats directly behind the visitor's bench. Before the game even started, Alex had two souvenirs, a Komets' ball cap he purchased with $19 of his own money and a practice puck one of the team managers was kind enough to toss our way.

Before the game I cautioned Alex that, in the heat of the action, tempers and fists could fly. I don't condone violence in hockey or any other venue, but a man has to defend himself, I told Alex while privately hoping for a "friendly" fracas to prove my point.

Be careful what you wish for.

A mere three seconds after the opening face-off, a Komet player dropped his gloves and started pummeling a hapless IceHog. I looked over to Alex for a reaction and saw him engulfed in a full belly laugh.

"How cool is that!" he squealed.

That's my boy.

Even grandma was enjoying this sudden dispensation of civilities, but it was only a sampling of what was to come.

The second period saw an eight-man brawl that had the fans shaking the Plexiglas barriers and shouting such unpleasantries as "Sit down, you puke!"

It took 20 minutes for the referees to restore order. Three players were excused from the game. Before the curtain came down on a 3-1 Komet victory, there were four fights, 123 minutes in penalties, three game misconducts and three 10-minute misconducts.

How's that for some wholesome family entertainment?

On the drive home, Alex challenged us to come up with one word to describe the game. Grandma submitted "chaotic." I was still searching for my answer when Alex blurted out "bashing."

It was a bash all right, and the damage was minimal.

Three rink-side seats ... $50.

One souvenir cap ... $19.

Making a hockey fan for life ... priceless.

My Home Away from Home

I wish everybody had the fortune of having a second family and a second home like the one Charles and Dora LeGras provided. This story was published in both the Bloomington Herald-Times *and the* Kendallville News-Sun.

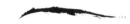

Bloomington Herald-Times
November 23, 2006

Thirty years ago this fall, I was fresh out of the Navy and beginning my career in journalism as a rookie sportswriter for the *Kendallville News-Sun*. On short notice, the best I could do for living arrangements was a trailer by the railroad tracks in Albion.

It wasn't long before I discovered that trailer life wasn't for me. The daily train whistles at 5:15 a.m. quickly convinced me of that.

So I started checking the classified ads for apartments in the area and came across one that claimed to be a "homey cottage" on the Angling Road north of Kendallville.

Sounding almost too good to be true, I had to check it out. To my utter surprise, the "cottage" turned out to be a converted chicken coop.

I kid you not.

It was a flat, one-story dwelling barely six feet from roof to floor. But being a height-challenged person of 5-foot-6, I did not consider that a deal-breaker.

On the inside you would never suspect a chicken ever had called it home. It was immaculately clean with natural wood floors and paneled walls. It was furnished with simple but functional furniture.

The owners of this property were Charles and Dora LeGras, a couple in their 50s whose children already were out of the nest. We seemed to hit it off from the start, even before I asked them how much they wanted to rent the place. The words "$125 a month" had barely left their lips before I said, "I'll take it." Even by 1976 standards, that was an offer I couldn't refuse.

It also was the start of a beautiful friendship. Living in a two-story farm house just a few paces away, the LeGrases always had the welcome mat out for me. I wore that path out, too, especially when the aroma of Dora's homemade pies made its way to my kitchen window.

I could not have asked for better landlords. Not once did they ever complain about the times I cranked up my stereo or the times when my noisy friends stayed too late. They didn't even complain when I, against their wishes, allowed a big ol' farm cat named Herman to come in from the cold. They had every right to complain about that after Herman marked his territory with a foul-smelling spray in the corner.

The LeGrases even felt as if they were imposing on me by asking for the rent when I was a little tardy. There would be a timid knock on the door and a reminder that went something like this: "Uh, Lynn, the rent was due last Monday, but if you need another couple of days it's OK."

They really felt bad when they had to raise the rent a mere $10 during the recession of 1978. Speaking of '78, that was the year of the Great Blizzard. Without them, I might have been marooned by myself for days. As it turned out, we had a pretty good time riding out the storm together.

It was during some of those cold, desolate winter nights that we became family. A hot meal is one thing; a warm house is much more.

By "warm" I mean "warmth" — as in the genuine, caring, warmth that family members have for each other. As the years passed I claimed the LeGrases as my surrogate parents, and I think they looked at me as an adopted son.

Charles and Dora welcomed just about any friend of mine with open arms. They were the kind of people who did not have it in them to harbor malice, not even against the drunk driver who left them with health issues for years.

Even after moving to Bloomington in 1984, I continued to drop in on them during return visits to Kendallville. It was around Christmas last year when I stopped in to see them along with my wife Pat, who they also "adopted" from the time I first introduced her to them in 1981.

We had heard that Dora's health wasn't good, but we wouldn't have known it by the way her eyes lit up when she saw us. It was a truly wonderful visit — lots of laughs about blizzards and cats and good times around the kitchen table.

Before leaving, Charles took us aside and privately thanked us for stopping by. I told him it was the other way around, that it was us who should be thanking them for being there all those years.

In September, we received one of those dreaded phone calls. Dora had succumbed to her long battle with cancer. The family wanted us to be among the first to know.

If circumstance would have allowed, my wife and I would have immediately hopped into the car and motored all the way to Kendallville. We would have made that turn onto the Angling Road and driven the three-mile distance to that familiar house with the chicken coop in back. We would have loved to have shared some stories about Dora over apple pie, coffee and tears.

It would have been a joyful gathering because Dora wouldn't have had it any other way. Although she would have moved on to an even better home, her family will see to it that the warmth lives on as long as the house remains standing.

Give Me Some Skin, Man

When this hit the front page of the Lifestyle section, some of my buddies demanded I turn in my "Man Card." But I showed them I'm thick-skinned in more ways than one.

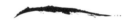

Bloomington Herald-Times
September 23, 2007

When learning that my stepdaughter, Robin, had taken a job with Arbonne International, a company that specializes in cosmetics, I didn't realize her career move would affect me as well. It was Robin who convinced me to try a line of men's skin care products distributed by Arbonne.

I know what you're thinking, that only girlie-men use creams and toners and what-not, and I have to admit the testosterone in me was screaming, "just say no." But Robin needed the business, so I decided to help her out on the condition it remain our little family secret. The stuff might even work, I reasoned. Lord knows my skin could use a little help after more than 50 years of neglect.

We men have never paid much attention to our skin, other than the occasional splash of aftershave and a little sunscreen. Our dads never said anything about skin lotions and exfoliating washes. At the risk of violating those unwritten "man rules," I now admit to using all the above.

My kit from Arbonne included no less than four items with instructions for each. The package didn't come cheap, either. The four units averaged a little over $16 an ounce. But, hey, it went for a good cause — one of Robin's first sales.

So there I was, staring at three tubes and one bottle of spray, wondering where in the heck to start. I might still be staring at them if it hadn't been for my wife, Pat, who, as a woman, knows something about every skin-care product under the sun. She had me begin with the exfoliating wash, a cream containing some grainy particles to help remove the dirt and dead skin cells. Think of it as liquid sandpaper.

If you still have some skin left after the stripping process, you are ready to shave. You squeeze out a small dab of the shaving gel and work it in. You have to trust the gel because it is so thin you can read a road map through it. But it's there, all right, and a little bit goes a long way, too. Razor burn is rare.

Now you are ready for the toner, a clear spray that you "spritz" onto your face. If the word "toner" doesn't smack of "sissie," then "spritz" certainly does. I'm still not sure what that toner does, but the label says, "This cool, revitalizing tonic leaves skin feeling squeaky-clean and helps to restore firmness, balance and vital nourishment."

Now that is getting your money's worth (out of a 4-ounce container, no less). You let that soak into the skin for a minute or so, then remove with a wash cloth.

Still with me? The final step is applying on the moisturizing lotion/sun screen, which is supposed to slow the aging process by limiting the damage of the sun's rays.

Each day for a month I repeated this four-step process in the secrecy of my private bath. I wouldn't dare do it after basketball at the Boys Club. I couldn't bear the snickering as I spritzed up. The guys would really get a laugh if I suggested they visit the Arbonne Web site, which — I do not lie — is "PictureMeBeautiful.com."

I must say I had my doubts. After 30 days, the face looking back in the mirror did not look all that much different. I was just about to write it off as a waste of time, money and manly pride when, in the span of a single week, two lady friends complimented me on my skin.

Snicker now, fellas!

Since then, it has been one big coming-out party for me. I mentioned my skin-care ritual at a recent after-hours party and drew looks of astonishment from some female co-workers who were surprised to learn that I, a sports writer, would pay that much attention to my skin. Hence, the suggestion to do a story for our Lifestyle Section.

At first I was reluctant, knowing the abuse I would take from my male colleagues, but maybe it's time to get the information out there so other men can start taking better care of themselves.

Guys, you may not know this, but your skin is your body's largest organ and the first line of defense against infection. And with our ever-decreasing ozone layer making our skin more vulnerable to the elements, it is high time we took care of it.

Laugh if you may. Call me a wuss. Call me a nerd. Call me a "metrosexual," if you will, but that's my story.

And I'm sticking to it.

Houser in the Hall? Yeah, Right

In 2008 I was inducted into the Herald-Times City Golf Tournament Hall of Fame. *It had nothing to do with my achievements on the golf course, unless you consider covering the city tournament a ticket to the Hall of Fame. As you will read, it was my ONLY ticket. I've been told this was the funniest column I ever wrote. Hope you get as big a chuckle reading it as I did writing it.*

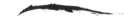

Bloomington Herald-Times
July 22, 2008

Ah, the H-T City Golf Hall of Fame, home of such household names as Talbot, Mullins, Martin, Burris, Foddrill, Houser, Lawson, Karcher, Gillespie, Gates.

Hold on. Back up a few names. Houser? As in Lynn Houser, the guy who merely covers the tournament for the H-T?

That would be me.

I know what you're thinking, "What in the name of Otis Foddrill is Houser doing there?"

Now just a minute. I'll have you know I have performed some legendary feats on the golf course.

For instance, I'd like to see you make a fairway shot hang a 90-degree turn around a tree 30 yards away and find its target.

I pulled off that improbable shot at Limberlost Country Club in Rome City in 1979. My playing partner, Tom Markle, should have thought twice about walking ahead to locate his ball. I cautioned him to stand behind a tree. Young Thomas wisely agreed, but the tree couldn't save him. I hit the most wicked snap-hook in the history of Limberlost.

Like a heat-seeking missile it zeroed in on the hapless lad's knee, ending his day. After thanking him and his kneecap for keeping my ball in bounds, I played on.

But that ain't nothin.'

I may be the only man in the history of golf to lose a ball while putting. Swear to God.

It came on No. 4 at Hidden Hills, Rodney Ritter's course near Owensburg. I was attempting a 15-foot putt for par when I must have passed a kidney stone in mid-swing. How else can I account for what happened? Oh, the horror!

I watched in disbelief as the ball did a wheelie as it raced past the cup, ran through a stop sign at the edge of the green, put the pedal to the metal as it descended down the slope, burned rubber as it sped down the cart path and finally skidded into a ravine, never to be seen again.

From putting for par to triple-bogey. I wish I could say alcohol was involved, but I was as sober as a nun.

The triple-bogey and its dreaded cousin, the "snowman," are familiar visitors to my score card. Birdies are rare, and eagles have yet to be spotted.

Needless to say, a hole-in-one hasn't appeared either, although I almost got lucky on the par-3 No. 8 hole at Pine Woods when a misguided tee shot deflected off a bank and grazed the stick, stopping six feet away. I wound up three-putting for a bogey.

There is one area of golf where I may have no peers, the art of club tossing. I have mastered the Helicopter (whirly bird), the Tomahawk (end-over-end) and, my personal favorite, the Moon Shot (Houston, we have a problem).

My most infamous Moon Shot came at Riverbend in Fort Wayne. After chunking an approach with an 8-iron, I launched the club straight up the air, only to discover that what goes up does not always come down. The 8-iron — a brand new one, I might add — lodged in a tall oak.

A member of my group suggested I shake it free. I'm not sure what was more absurd, getting that spanking new 8-iron caught in an unforgiving tree or having the delusion I could dislodge it with my own two hands. Picture this: a troll trying to shake a 100-foot oak. Last I heard, that club is still dangling from the tree, a course landmark.

I did play in one city tournament. Qualified in the illustrious 11th flight and got beat 4 and 3.

OK, so I'm not match-play material. Big deal. I've had my moments in scrambles.

Teeing off first for one luckless foursome, I failed to drive past the ladies' tee. Amidst all the guffawing and needling that I would have to walk past said tees with my britches down, each of my three playing partners proceeded to hit out-of-bounds. So, in the end, we had to play that little girlie drive.

If this isn't the stuff of Hall of Famers, I don't know what is.

Truthfully, I've witnessed a lot of Hall of Famers in my 24 years covering the city tournament and have had the privilege of writing the induction story for 37 of them. And now that I have to write my own, it is a bit awkward, especially when you have a handicap as high as the price of gas.

However, there is precedent for a non-golfer to be entered in the Hall of Fame. Bob Hammel, my mentor, was inducted in 1988 for his many years of coverage and devotion to the tournament. It was Hammel who, upon his retirement in 1996, handed me the keys and said in so many words, "Houser, I give you the City Golf Tournament. Try not to screw it up."

Well, the tournament just turned 80. And at least on my watch it hasn't gone the way of that ill-fated putt at Hidden Hills.

Never Too Late to Get Back in the Game

Having turned 60 in 2010, I was starting to hear the clock ticking, prompting some serious reflection on the golf course one day. It now amazes me how many men my age responded to this column – some even clipping it to their bulletin boards.

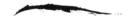

Bloomington Herald-Times
July 20, 2010

While covering the H-T City Golf Tournament this weekend, a member of the gallery approached me and asked if I was playing much golf.

"Not much," I said, knowing I could count the number of rounds on one hand the last two years.

"What about tennis — you used to play a lot of tennis," the man asked.

"Yeah, used to," I answered, knowing I have played only three times this year.

Later that same day, a former bridge partner approached me.

"Still playing bridge?" he asked.

"Not lately," I said, knowing I haven't played in almost two years.

And then it dawned on me: "used to" play golf; "used to" play tennis; "used to" play bridge. I started making a list. Under the heading, "Things I used to do," I scribbled:

Golf.

Tennis.

Softball.

Bridge.

Fish.

Tailgate.

Take exotic vacations.

Go to rock concerts.

Go hiking.

Go dancing.

Have a life.

The more items I listed, the more depressed I got. It was starting to look more like a Bucket List — you know, the kind you make before you "kick the bucket."

Mine was sort of a Bucket List in reverse. For me the question was, "How have I managed to subtract so many enjoyable things from my life?"

Not all of it has been of my own choosing. The trickle-down effect of the struggling economy has dipped into my "fun money" fund, forcing me to eliminate some of the more expensive pursuits. Scratch golf, exotic vacations

and rock concerts. It also has prompted me to take a part-time job. I now umpire softball instead of playing it.

But perhaps the biggest reason for the decline of the fun things is the departure of some close friends. My two best golfing partners moved away, and my most steady tennis partner passed away.

That was Bob Millican. He suffered a fatal heart attack on the tennis court — while playing with me. I lost interest in tennis that day and never really got it back.

Bob also was my fishing buddy. Haven't fished since.

Death even took a member of my bridge foursome, and we never found a reliable fourth after that.

So I used to have a circle of friends, too, a circle that continues to shrink. In the last year and a half, the couple my wife and I hung around the most with moved to Florida. We haven't been able to replace them, either.

You just can't go out and replace long-time friends, people you have so much history with, people who are as comfortable as a pair of old flip flops. Someone suggested we find younger couples to hang with, someone whose youth would energize us, but we are finding that younger couples are usually consumed with their children and don't have much time to cultivate friendships.

I was bouncing these theories off a colleague Sunday, H-T photographer Monty Howell, who was riding in my golf cart as we headed to the next photo opportunity. If I was looking for someone to invite to my pity party, Monty was the wrong guy. At the age of 56, he is in the process of reinventing himself — as a nurse. Going from professional photographer to male nurse is a bold step at any age.

But Monty listened patiently to my rant, nodded his head, and then admitted he had his own mid-life crisis a while back. How did he deal with it?

"I decided that every day I was going to do something a 9-year-old would do," he said.

"Say what?"

"Really. A 9-year-old can make fun anywhere, and he is old enough to know to not do the wrong thing.

"Think about it," Monty continued. "If a 9-year-old is hiking and comes across a stream with a log bridging it, what does he do? He takes the log. Just the other night, the '9-year-old' in me drug my wife outside to watch the lightning in the sky."

I looked at Monty in total wonderment. Here I am, wallowing in a very dark place, looking for some fun in my life, without realizing the opportunities are still there.

What is keeping me from taking a hike or taking my wife dancing? What is to keep me from grabbing that fishing pole out of my garage and dropping a line off the pier at Lake Monroe? What is to keep me from calling some of the guys I used to play softball with and inviting them to join me for a tailgate party?

Only me is keeping me from those things.

And maybe my wife and I can't afford an exotic vacation, but there are some friends in Florida who I know would love to have us visit any time.

So, the answer to my problem is as simple as fording a stream or looking up into the sky.

Thanks, Monty. Today I am going to take that Used-To-Do List and make it into a To-Do List.

Before it becomes a Bucket List.

Chapter 5
On the Beaten Path

There is more to covering a beat than just showing up on game night. The games themselves are often garden variety, although I have included two here that were a cut above the normal regular season contests. While serving as the H-T's point man on the IU basketball beat from 1998-2000, I had a lot more than basketball to write about. A couple of features dealt with matters of life and death.

One of those is the story of William Gladness, who came to IU from junior college with some excess baggage – a bullet in his side. In April of 1999, there was the sudden departure of Luke Recker, a homegrown golden boy. Recker bolted a month after IU's season ended in the second round of the NCAA Tournament. I discovered then that there is no such thing as a quiet offseason at Indiana, not under Bob Knight.

A month later, I found myself in a little Tennessee town. Shortly before Mother's Day, a tornado took the life of the mother of sophomore Kirk Haston. The H-T sent a team to Tennessee to cover the tragedy. It turned out to be one of the more solemn assignments I ever had.

The two games that defined Knight's final season were overtime battles with eventual national champion Michigan State. The columns that ran with each cover package best captured the drama and emotions of those two thrilling contests.

Aloha from Paradise

As the 1998-99 college basketball season dawned, I was named the lead man on the IU beat. Just one week into the season, I got to travel with the Hoosiers to Hawaii. Right then I knew I was going to like covering the Hoosiers on a full-time basis.

Bloomington Herald-Times
November 29, 1998

"The weather is here,
wish you were beautiful."
- Jimmy Buffett

MAUI, HAWAII --
Aloha, Bloomington

The Good Book says God rested on the seventh day. I now know where he spent his R & R -- Hawaii.

It is 6:45 a.m. here, almost noon in Indiana. I come to you from a balcony looking out on the Pacific Ocean, which at the moment is calm and beckoning. Hawaii is very much that way.

The isles seduce you with their calm, even though the wind never ceases. A breeze perpetually swirls through the palm trees, making a rustling sound that seems to say, "Shhhh ... quiet, please ... God at rest."

I am sitting here in my gym shorts, tank top and sandals. I would guess the temperature is around 70 degrees. If I were sitting on my deck at home, I would be clothed in a heavy sweat shirt, sweat pants and thermal socks.

From here I can hear the waves breaking on the beach, rocking you with nature's most perfect lullaby. You could easily lapse into dream land, but here you already are in dream land in your waking state.

Let's talk about the sounds, or lack thereof. There are no semi-tractor trailers grinding through the gears, no cars honking, no construction equipment pounding, no stereos blasting. In their place are the voices of birds singing. When is the last time, Bloomington, that you really noticed birds singing?

And then there are the smells -- salt water, wild flowers and fresh air. Have you forgotten, like me, what fresh air really smells like? Fresh air is the absence of smell, which allows you to smell the salt water and wild flowers.

As I look to the east I see mountains. In southern Indiana we enjoy our rolling hills, but you could stack them all on top of each other and they would not rise to the wonder of these mountains, formed out of volcanic thrusts millions of years ago.

Are those clouds cruising over the mountain tops or volcanic wisps? Whatever the veil is, it is delaying the sun's grand entrance. I spent 12 hours on a plane Monday heading westward, trying to outrace the sun trailing in the east. Now I am eager for the sun to catch me.

Ah, there it is, the Creator's most brilliant ember, Hawaii's unofficial alarm clock. You don't need clocks here. The sun will tell you what time it is. It is time to stop and smell the flowers, man, time to forget some of those daily routines and enjoy life. We are so wrapped up in living to work that we forget to work at living.

Speaking of work, I've got to cover an Indiana basketball game later in the day. Before I left Bloomington, I was watching the Hoosiers practice when coach Bob Knight sidled over and said, "Houser, you ought to put me in your will for showing you the world."

The U.S. Navy showed me Paris, Madrid, Rome, Amsterdam, the Azores and Bermuda. Now I can say Bob Knight has showed me paradise. A half day here and I would put gladly put him in my will on the condition I can make Hawaii my Western bureau. I will file an IU basketball story every day for as long as my lap top holds up.

Out in the harbor is a cruise ship and some fishing vessels. Four years in the Navy as an airman left me longing to feel the sea under my feet. There must be some sort of odd job I could do to earn my keep on one those crafts. I believe I could tend bar on a cruise ship, or, with a little practice, learn to tie a double-hitch knot.

What's that? A raindrop? No big deal. These clouds will soon pass, unlike the ones in the Midwest that hang around for a solid week.

It's going on 8 a.m. now. The sun is blazing away in the rich, royal blue sky. Lovers are holding hands on the beach. Joggers are going through their paces. Surfers are trying to catch a wave.

Let's see, the Hoosiers play at 4 o'clock, Hawaii time -- 9 o'clock, Indiana time. I can file this column and be on the beach in 10 minutes. If you see an *Associated Press* story in place of my game story, forgive me. I lost track of time while smelling the flowers.

Flying the Not-So-Friendly Skies

Maui represented the good side of travel along on the IU beat. There were other occasions when I wished I had never left Bloomington.

Bloomington Herald-Times
December 14, 1999

In the year and a half I've been on the IU basketball beat, I wish I had a dollar for every time I was asked, "What is the hardest part about your job -- dealing with Bob Knight?"

The answer is "no," although you never want to run afoul of the Big Guy. Trust me on that one.

No, the real difficulty is just getting to the doggone games themselves, especially when it involves air travel. Sometimes we fly commercial and other times we charter a flight.

The charters are owned and piloted by 66-year-old Ralph Rogers, a veteran of Vietnam missions. You won't find a better pilot. He could fly a kite here to Kitty Hawk if need be.

We call this method of travel, Air Ralph. Usually, Ralph picks us up at the Monroe County Airport in a sleek, twin-engine Cessna 310. That craft has plenty of storage space and ample leg room.

And then there are times when the 310 is in the shop for repairs and Ralph shows up in a borrowed contraption we call The Flying Coffin, a single-engine job that, from outward appearances, is held together solely with duct tape and bailing wire.

We have had some anxious moments flying Air Ralph. As we were cruising along one time we asked Ralph about the coat of greasy film on the windshield.

"Oh, that's just a little engine oil," he said.

Unflappable guy, that Ralph.

Another time the engine sputtered to a complete stop in mid-flight. Ralph was whistling along as if it were business as usual, while the rest of us were thinking, "Houston, we have a problem."

Ralph calmly switched over to the auxiliary fuel tank. The plane started right up -- along with our hearts.

Ask fellow scribe Andy Graham about a certain flight to Iowa City. Not known for having a strong stomach to begin with, Andy made a very bad choice for breakfast that day, a burrito. The flight wasn't 15 minutes old before the burrito wanted out. Again, and again and again.

We finally let Andy off in Muscatine, Iowa, and picked him up on the way back, whereas he commenced to enjoy that breakfast all over again. Andy's episode gave new meaning to the term, Air Ralph.

For our trip to Missouri last week, Rogers showed up in a borrowed plane that he proudly revealed was 49 years old, an even older version of The Flying Coffin. It just happened to be the 58th anniversary of Pearl Harbor. For all we knew, this plane could have been flying reconnaissance on that Day of Infamy.

We quickly knew we were in for it when Ralph pulled out a roll of duct tape during pre-flight. Gaps around the door were allowing cold air to pour into the plane, he said.

Speaking of the door, we had a little problem with that. After takeoff we noticed the door was ajar -- on my side of the plane, no less. Back to the airport we went. It took us several tries to get it completely shut. The only thing holding it in place was a thin slide bolt. It almost goes without saying that I tightened my seat belt to the point I couldn't exhale.

It was smooth flying for the next 90 minutes. Ralph was as professional as ever, constantly checking instruments, making calculations and charting his course. However, as we made our descent into the airport at Columbia, Mo., an alarm went off.

Apparently, the landing gear hadn't engaged. Ralph immediately pulled up and circled the airport, repeatedly flipping the electric landing gear switch -- to no avail. He could sense the wheels had not deployed.

By now he had radioed the airport about his difficulty. Ground control recommended a pass by the tower so they could have a look. Ralph's hunch was right. The wheels were still up.

Plan B was to use the manual landing gear release, but it was stiff and unbending. Ralph managed to get it halfway forward and felt some movement in the wheels. But were they completely down?

For the first time we could see a real look of concern on Ralph's face. Feverishly, he kept applying pressure to the manual control.

Houston, we really have a problem.

Finally, with one mighty push, he shoved it all the way forward. We all exhaled at the sound of the wheels unlocking. Another pass by the tower confirmed it.

Come to find out this has happened before to Ralph.

"I once had to hang out the plane and move the gear forward with a tow bar," he claimed.

This is information you don't need at 2,500 feet.

Awaiting us on the air strip must have been every fire truck and emergency vehicle in the Show Me State, a scene right out of one of those airport disaster movies. The emergency wasn't over until the wheels touched the ground ever so smoothly, one of Ralph's typical landings.

However, as we were taxiing down the runway, the electrical power went out. It came back on, but there was a very good chance the landing gear problem was more electrical than mechanical. It was enough to keep us from flying out of Columbia until repairs were made the next day.

As we disembarked, a rescue worker in a fireproof suit rushed over. I half expected to see the face of Bruce Willis or some other Hollywood hero.

"Everyone all right?" the stranger asked.

Never a doubt. Just another adventure in the friendly skies of Air Ralph.

Gladness Means 'Happy to Be Alive'

Writing player features becomes almost routine on the beat, but this one was special.

Bloomington Herald-Times
February 8, 1999

He is in and out of lineups. His game runs hot and cold. He is all over the court one minute and nowhere to be found the next.

As an Indiana basketball player, William Gladness has been exasperating and exhilarating. What could be more exasperating than air-mailing a potential game-tying five-footer against Kentucky in 1997?

Exhilarating? How about 16 points, 14 rebounds, five assists and two steals in the season opener against Seton Hall.

If you researched Gladness' numbers, you would find the good minutes far outnumber the bad, yet his contributions often go unnoticed.

Gladness can handle it, however. The streets of West Memphis, Ark., have prepared him for any adversity life can throw at him. Growing up on the "wrong" side of the Mississippi River in Memphis is not like growing up in Bloomington.

"You see people jogging in the street here," Gladness said before a recent practice. "You don't see anybody on the streets (of West Memphis); they would get mugged."

Or shot.

Know what it's like to get shot? Been there, done that, Gladness can say. Gladness did not take the normal channels to Indiana University. He never played high school basketball -- never finished high school, for that matter.

"I was considered a troublemaker," he said.

So Gladness took his game to the streets and became a sort of playground legend at an area called Balfour, a place where you better have game. A 6-foot-8 player with good hands, good moves and good hops, Gladness did indeed have game.

At Balfour, the big game wasn't Gus Macker 3-on-3 basketball. The game was against a rival 'hood from Memphis. The stakes were a little higher than the average high school game. You might say it was a matter of life and death.

One night a couple years ago, Memphis crossed the Mississippi to West Memphis and lost. Sore losers, those Memphis dudes, who followed the West Memphis guys home. Gladness and a friend were walking back when they found themselves in a hail of bullets.

The friend took one in the leg. Gladness took one in his left side. Badly wounded but operating on adrenaline, Gladness mustered up the reserve to drag himself and his friend to the Gladness home two blocks away.

"I was numb, just trying to get home," Gladness said.

Gladness had seen the look on the face of his mother, Luevernal, as her heart broke the night one of his older brothers came home with a bullet wound. "I didn't want her to worry about me," he said.

There was no hiding the seriousness of the wound. He spent the next 10 days in the hospital. Fearing damage to the spine, doctors did not surgically remove the bullet. So there it resides in his side to this day, not the usual hardware for winning the big game.

As Gladness lay on that hospital bed, all sorts of thoughts entered his mind, but the most frightening thought was, "Will I ever play at Balfour again?"

Basketball means that much to Gladness -- everything.

He recovered and went back to Balfour and to the Boys Club, the only organized basketball he had ever played until Ron Murphy discovered him in one of the local tournaments, the Bluff City Classic. Murphy, the coach of Carl Albert Junior College in Oklahoma, took one look at Gladness and practically signed him on the spot.

By his second year in the junior college ranks, Gladness was the MVP of his region, averaging 20 points and 11 rebounds. But while soul-searching on that hospital bed two years before, Gladness had set higher goals.

"I wanted to go somewhere where I would have my name on the back of my shirt," he said.

Along comes Bob Knight, who doesn't believe in any name on the jersey other than "Indiana." On the surface, Knight and Gladness do not appear to be a good fit. There is no room for playground basketball in the Indiana system, and Gladness occasionally forgets that. When he does, he finds himself on the bench, which he fears even more than a drive-by shooting.

"In junior college I averaged 38 minutes," he pointed out. "For me to get in a flow, I have to play a chunk of minutes at a time."

Some chunks are bigger than others at Indiana. Recent games serve as an example. At Purdue, Gladness played all 40 minutes and contributed 13 points and 10 rebounds. At Penn State, Gladness played 11 less-productive minutes before giving way to freshman Jarrad Odle.

"There are only five spots out there," Knight said after the game. "We brought Odle in for Gladness, and (Odle) was the most effective player we had on the floor at that time. If a kid comes in and plays well, that's the guy who is going to stay out there."

A starter 20 times this season, Gladness wasn't in the starting lineup Wednesday night for Wisconsin, yet he was Knight's first choice off the bench when freshman Kirk Haston took a defensive siesta in the opening minute. Gladness never came out.

As the lone forward in a four-guard lineup, he had nine rebounds by halftime and finished with 14.

Gladness is averaging 26.3 minutes, third-highest on the team behind A.J. Guyton (33.6) and Luke Recker (30.7). He is contributing 8.8 points and 6.0 rebounds. He is second in steals with 39 and fourth in assists with 42. Projected over 40 minutes, Gladness would be averaging 13.4 points, 9.1 rebounds, 2.6 assists and 2.4 steals.

No wonder minutes on the floor are precious to Gladness. Playing an average of 12 minutes less a game than he did in junior college has been a tough adjustment.

"I can't get used to it, but I have to keep the mindset of playing," he said.

Basketball has helped Gladness keep his sanity in a year in which he has buried both his father and his 26-year-old brother, Nathan. Nathan also had the misfortune of catching a bullet, but, unlike his younger brother, did not survive. He was killed on the same October night Gladness was taking the court for Midnight Madness at Indiana. Nathan was gone before William finished his season-opening paces at Assembly Hall.

"He got into it with somebody," said William. "The guy came back and shot him in the yard. They were calling me all night, but I didn't get the message until 1:30."

In July, the head of the household, Rufus "Jack" Gladness, died of a heart attack, denying him the chance to watch his son play another year at Indiana.

"One reason I came here was so my folks could see me play," William said. "My father was getting to watch me on TV. He was jacked up about it. All of West Memphis was jacked up, people who used to see me around town playing at Balfour."

Luevernal also has had heart trouble, requiring multiple heart bypasses. In addition, she has lost a leg to diabetes. For William, who just turned 25, the best way to deal with succession of tragedies is to plunge further into basketball.

"I just try to stay busy. Playing basketball has helped me out," he said.

So you can understand how important basketball is to Gladness and how it pains him to come out of any game. He accepts his role, however, and doesn't pout. Replay the Penn State game and watch Gladness celebrate Guyton's winning shot.

"I guess I've got to do whatever the team needs," he says. "When I'm in there playing, I can do a lot of stuff."

With the completion of nine more academic hours, Gladness will be the first in his family to graduate from college. The learning process began the moment the bullet entered his side. There it remains, a permanent reminder that life is only a matter of minutes.

Editor's Note: That bullet in his side got Gladness in the end. In May, 2008, Gladness passed away unexpectedly from flu-like symptoms. It was believed the removal of his spleen following the shooting in 1996 left him vulnerable to infection and ultimately shortened his life.

This Cool Hand, Luke, a Slap in the Face

If ever there was a Hoosier Golden Boy, Luke Recker was it. A highly prized recruit out of Auburn, Ind., Recker committed to IU after his sophomore year of high school and then dazzled Hoosier fans for two years, inspiring chants of "Luke, Luke" around Assembly Hall. Then, one month after the conclusion of his sophomore season, Recker abruptly announced he was leaving school. The sudden departure broke the hearts of the Hoosier Nation, leaving me to write this column.

Bloomington Herald-Times
April 15, 1999

Luke.
     Lu-u-u-u-ke.
The way your name used to echo around Assembly Hall is now one long moan around Hoosierland.

That is some bombshell you dropped on us, Luke, saying you are leaving IU. We never saw it coming. Yeah, sure, the rumors of your departure never went away, but didn't you just look me in the eye and deny the rumors three times within the last month? What was that? A cock crowing?

This hurts, Luke, really hurts. Do you have any idea what you mean to IU basketball fans?

For two years, you have been the best thing that to happen to IU basketball since Damon Bailey. Like Bailey, you were a Hoosier high school legend, a Mr. Basketball, a matinee idol, a G.I. Joe and Leonardo DiCaprio all rolled up in a 6-foot-6, fair-haired package.

We enjoyed the way you strutted around the court, pumping your fists and winking at the crowd. You made basketball fun again.

What happened to you? What happened to the eager teenager who committed to Indiana his sophomore year, making him the youngest recruit ever? What happened to the player who said Indiana was the only place for him, and Bob Knight the only coach?

Don't tell me Knight was too hard on you. You knew he was going to demand a lot out of you before you ever suited up at Indiana. I attended enough practices to see that he treated you fairly. Couldn't you have at least told him of your decision face to face? You owed him more than an overnight fax when he was out of the country. That's about as gutless as the Colts stealing out of Baltimore in the dead of night.

You say your decision to leave was because you were not pleased with your "development as a player." Just what sort of development did you expect? You went from averaging 12.8 points your freshman year to 16.2 points your sophomore year. The offense was structured to get you and A.J. Guyton more shots. In fact, you got 132 more shots this year.

"I blame no one but myself for this," you said, while adding that you think you can prosper elsewhere. What greener pastures do you have in mind? Where else will you be featured as much as Indiana? Where else will you be as popular and admired?

And why now? You already are halfway through a four-year career, certainly the toughest part behind you. Look at what is on the horizon -- a veteran team coming back, including Guyton, plus some athletic recruits. Your last two years at Indiana could have been very special, Luke.

And where is the loyalty, not just to the fans of Indiana basketball, but to your teammates? Have you been able to look all of them in the eye and say, "I don't want to be your teammate anymore?"

It's one thing to leave school early for the NBA. That is often just good business. But to drop one school for another, well, that's personal.

If you only knew the hearts you have broken. I overheard one father saying, "My daughter cried all the way to school."

Forgive me for being a little harsh here, Luke. You sure had me convinced you were staying when you went on the record saying so in no uncertain terms. I went to the bank on those comments, wrote them up as the gospel truth. I realize you were put on the spot, but at least you could have taken the road Guyton did by admitting the possibility of leaving.

To wake up with the news of your departure Wednesday morning was like being served divorce papers. It will take a while to get over the feeling of rejection and deception.

But Indiana basketball will go on without you, Luke, much as we rather it didn't. It reminds me of the famous scene from the movie, *Hoosiers*.

Being a Hoosier, I'm sure you will remember the part where coach Norman Dale benches star guard Rade Butcher, who defied the coach by refusing to run the offense. After another Hickory player fouls out, leaving the Huskers with four on the floor and Butcher the likely substitute, Dale refuses to put in Butcher -- or anybody else. When the referee comes over to remind Dale he has just four players in the game, the coach makes a profound point with this reply: "My team's on the floor."

With or without you next year, Luke, our team is on the floor.

A Mournful Mother's Day

What a terrible way to lose one's mother, and what a courageous way for a son to handle it. The day after the tragedy happened, the Herald-Times *flew a photographer and me to this tiny Tennessee town for a first-hand account of how the community responded.*

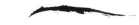

Bloomington Herald-Times
May 9, 1999 (Mother's Day)

LINDEN, TENNESSEE

This town of 1,300 could pass for the average small town in Indiana.

It is a place where people greet each other by their first names, a place where they don't feel the need to lock their doors, a place where they give a lift to a stranger without hesitation, a place where they still go to church on Wednesday evenings and, like most small towns in Indiana, a place where the high school basketball team brings them all together.

On this day, Mother's Day, a far more serious cause brings them together. This Mother's

a real world. Things happen. Life is a journey. We are subject to diseases, accidents and freaks of nature.

"I not only lost my daughter, and a kid his mother, we lost our best friend. She went the extra mile to be a good teacher. She devoted extra time to her son. She is the apple of my eye and the apple of her son's eye."

Mother, Daughter, Friend

For a young man of 20, Kirk Haston has his grandfather's wisdom, as well as his inner strength. He seemed to be holding up well in the aftermath of the tragedy.

"Having a lot of people around helps," he said.

Among those at his side were his IU teammates and coaches, including Knight. It didn't surprise Haston that Knight would be there.

"He is always geared up the same," he said of the coach. "He doesn't just turn it on and off. I really appreciated him being here.

"I'd like to thank the school and the people for all the flowers and support," Haston added. "The university has really been good. Bloomington is my second home. They have embraced me as much as anybody could."

Hoyt was just as appreciative.

"Indiana and Bloomington have been kind to my boy," he said.

But the sense of loss remains.

"She was my teacher in school and my teacher in life," Haston said. "I couldn't imagine a closer mother-son relationship. You never know when something like this is going to happen. We live in the real world where the forces of nature can't be controlled. There are no reasons to look for. God needed her now more than we needed her here. That's the only way you can have any peace."

Hoosiers to Find Out
What They Are Made Of

On another "Air Ralph" flight up to East Lansing this January night, I came across these words of encouragement from former IU president William Lowe Bryan. After the Hoosiers lost a heartbreaker in overtime, Bryan's words made for an appropriate column lead.

Bloomington Herald-Times
January 12, 2000

EAST LANSING, MICHIGAN

William Lowe Bryan, one of Indiana University's earliest college presidents and a baseball lettermen in 1884, took Hoosier losses as hard as any Big Red fan.

After a particularly crushing defeat, he wrote, "One of the compensations for defeat, and every man must sometimes lose, is to find out for yourself whether you are made of steel or pewter. If you are one kind of man, defeat will crumple you up; you will whine or sulk or swear at somebody else; and you will quit. If you are another sort, you will discover in yourself, under the chagrin of defeat, one of the deepest joys of man, a joy of finding that you possess an unbeaten heart."

Tuesday night at Michigan State, the Hoosiers fought like warriors. The Spartans fought like ... well, Spartans. In the end there were no losers, although the scoreboard said Indiana fell six points short of winning, 77-71.

The Hoosiers were so close to a victory not many believed they could achieve. They went into the "Izzone" and nearly denied coach Tom Izzo his 100th victory and, more important, undisputed possession of first place in the Big Ten. Only a desperation 3-pointer by Morris Peterson stood between Indiana that precious victory. Izzo himself said the Hoosiers deserved better.

"A lot of credit goes to Indiana. They played harder than us the second half. That doesn't happen to us very often."

Not at home, not at the Breslin Center, not in front of the Izzone, the crazed student section. But Indiana had victory in its grasp and just couldn't squeeze the fist tight enough.

There were no goats in a game like this. Not center Kirk Haston, who struggled so mightily after scoring 28 points at Penn State Saturday. Not Michael Lewis because he missed a free throw in the last minute that could have given Indiana the extra cushion it needed. Not A.J. Guyton because his shots started coming up short after laboring through a game-high 42 minutes. Not Dane Fife after throwing his body all over the floor before fouling out.

Fife, a Michigan native, was the primary target of abuse from the Izzone. His brother, Dugan

Fife, played at Michigan, and Dane spurned recruiting efforts by Izzo to play for Bob Knight.

Fife hasn't become quite the scorer the fans anticipated, but he does so many other things to keep the Hoosiers in games. Scoring 10 points Tuesday night was almost out of character for him and his six-point average. But true to form was his defense, his hustle, his diving for loose balls and his infectious intensity.

Izzo took note.

"Dane is not the same," he said of the Fife he recruited. "He's going through a deal like Charlie Bell went through. He was a great scorer in high school, a great, great player. I love Dane Fife, love his toughness.

"Now he's doing a little more defending, setting up people. I give him a lot of credit for accepting his role on the team. If you want to look at one guy, other than A.J. Guyton, who had a lot to do with their 'almost' win, it's Dane Fife. He got steals. He got loose balls. He got this, he got that. He did a great job. He's not the player I recruited, but neither is Charlie."

Bell had his hands full with Guyton, making the Hoosiers' leading scorer toil for all of his game-high 28 points. Bell himself had a season-high 22.

"A guy (Guyton) scores 28 points and you're proud of your guy," said Izzo. "When you have to go through 8,913 screens -- and I counted them -- you've got to give Charlie credit. At the end he was running on fumes and so was Guyton, who I have a lot of respect for. It was like two prizefighters -- whoever had something left at the end."

It was that kind of game, one that Indiana could have and probably should have won.

So now the Hoosiers must look themselves into the mirror, realize they gave their all, and learn from this defeat.

President Bryan would liken it to the kind of defeats that haunted George Washington, who lost a lot of battles before winning the war.

"The great thing about Washington is not his victories," Bryan wrote. "He won few victories. The thing which lifts him into place with the few great world leaders is that through years of defeat upon defeat, he kept together a little army of men who were always ready for a fight. It was the unbeaten heart of Washington, more than anything else, which won American independence."

So what is it, Hoosiers, steel or pewter?

Spartans Came a Knockin' and the Hall Was a Rockin'

Six weeks later, the Hoosiers found out they were made of steel, avenging that first meeting with Michigan State.

Bloomington Herald-Times
February 27, 2000

It was like old times at Assembly Hall Saturday.

The Hoosiers were playing like men possessed.

There were unsung heroes coming off the bench. There were Hoosiers throwing their bodies all over the floor. There were Hoosiers standing firm to take a charge. There was that look in their eye, an absolute refusal to lose. And then it all came together at the buzzer, causing the delirious crowd to spill out onto the floor.

It was a beautiful thing.

There haven't been many scenes like that at The Hall in recent years. In fact, the entire decade of the '90s passed by without a celebration like the one that followed this 81-79 win over fifth-ranked Michigan State.

Assembly Hall used to be where highly ranked teams went to see their rankings topple, but the last top five team to fall at Assembly Hall was Kansas in December, 1994. However, that was a 20-point Hoosier victory, a victory that, while thoroughly enjoyed by the fans, didn't inspire them to storm the court.

To find a spontaneous eruption like that, you would have to go back to 1989, when Jay Edwards turned defeat into victory with a buzzer-beater over Michigan. The way the students poured onto Branch McCracken Court Saturday, you would have thought Indiana had won the Big Ten.

The fact that the Hoosiers only succeeded in the spoiler's role Saturday indicates the hunger that burns in their fans. Coming off three losses in their last four games, the Hoosiers were reeling, knowing their chances of a Big Ten title had vanished. But the Indiana crowd was there for them in a big, big way Saturday. No one was more appreciative than Bob Knight himself.

"Nowhere else in the world would fans have supported a team the way our fans supported us today, with the way we had struggled in the previous three or four games," he said. "I really do believe that. I thought it was incredible."

With the help of the crowd and some breaks that finally went Indiana's way, victory was achieved. Long before Lynn Washington grabbed A.J. Guyton's air-ball and converted it into a winning putback, bounces were going Indiana's way.

There were the two Michael Lewis 3-pointers from long distance, a good city block from the basket, taken and made out of necessity to beat the shot clock.

There were the two free throws by Larry Richardson clanging around the rim and backboard for what seemed like an hour before disappearing into the basket like a snake seeking the refuge of a hole.

There were the many bounces that found Hoosier hands, especially the hands of reserve guard Kyle Hornsby. If there was any one player who swung the game in Indiana's favor, with the obvious exception of A.J. Guyton and his 34 points, it was Hornsby, the red-shirt freshman.

Until Saturday, Hornsby's meaningful minutes could be counted on your hands and toes, but every single one of the 26 minutes he played Saturday was meaningful. How is this for play off the bench: 10 points, five rebounds, two steals, two assists, no turnovers.

"Hornsby had a heart as big as a warrior today," Spartan coach Tom Izzo said. "That was an individual effort of mammoth proportion."

In the face of a defeat which probably cost his team a title all to itself, Izzo showed his customary class.

"In a lot of ways, it was one of the better college basketball games I've been involved with. Unfortunately for me, the wrong team won. I don't fault our kids. They played extremely hard. It thought Indiana played extremely hard. They took it at us pretty good, caused us to get out of sync, offensively."

Indiana got back to playing the kind of defense that made it a Big Ten contender. The Hoosiers denied the passing lanes, pushed the Spartan offense away from the basket and hustled back to keep the Spartans from cranking up their high-octane running game.

"We wanted to establish ourselves defensively, as we had all year, which was something that we had gotten away from the last three or four games," Guyton said. "That was a big emphasis in practice and I thought we executed it pretty well, except for the start of the second half."

Guyton had the defensive assignment on Mateen Cleaves, the league's two-time player of the year, an honor he shared with Ohio State's Scoonie Penn last year. Penn was Guyton's assignment last week, not one of his better defensive efforts. But Guyton's defense on Cleaves was a factor in the latter's nine turnovers, an unusually high number for a player on pace to become the league's all-time assist king.

"They did a good job on Mateen, jumping out on our screens and rolls," Izzo said. "They took some things away. Every time we forged ahead, we had a problem that has plagued us all year, turnovers. When we were up nine, they had two steals in a row and 3-point plays. That was critical."

Another surprising statistic was Indiana's 13-11 edge on the offensive boards – against the national leader in rebounding margin. The Spartans average 14 more rebounds a game than their opposition.

"That's the leading rebounding team in the nation," Guyton pointed out. "We knew they can just beat you on the boards alone. We had a lot of blocking-out drills in practice, and I thought that helped us."

No offensive rebound was more important than Washington's.

"They always tell you, it's not the shot taken at the end; it's the rebound," Izzo said. "We talked to our five guys about rebounding. I don't know whose mistake it was on the far side. It's kind of a shame the game ended that way, but it did."

With the exception of the finish, the game had a lot of similarities to the one played at East Lansing in January. In that game, Indiana saw a six-point lead get away in the final 90 seconds, with the tying shot coming on a 3-pointer by State's leading scorer, Morris Peterson. And that game also was won by the home team in overtime, a 77-71 decision for the Spartans.

"The truth is, (Indiana) could have -- maybe should have -- beaten us at our place," Izzo said.

Coming out of timeout inside the three-minute mark, Knight was reminded of the game at East Lansing.

"The score was 70-65, and as we were going out onto the floor I said, 'The last time we were up five, we got beat. Now let's turn it around.' "

That they did, possibly saving a season that was starting to nosedive.

"It's just the flip side," Guyton said. "We were real down after that loss in East Lansing, because we made a lot of mistakes to lose the game. They didn't take it from us. We gave it to them. Today, we finally took a game from somebody in the last five minutes."

The Hoosiers were due for some breaks. They saw 3-pointers bounding off the glass and into the basket in losses to Purdue and Minnesota. They saw Peterson's 3-pointer off the dribble tie the game with 10 seconds left at Michigan State. They saw almost every offensive rebound fall into the hands of Purdue at West Lafayette. They didn't get last-minute calls at East Lansing and Minneapolis.

But this was more than luck. It was about finding a way to win rather than lose.

"These kids hung in there and fought back, which is unusual for this group of kids," Knight said. "To do that, to get down and come back after playing as poorly as we did in three of our last four games was really a good thing for these guys."

"Indiana deserved to win the game," said Izzo. "They outplayed us a little bit down that one stretch, but other than that, both teams played their ass off. Nobody is going to walk away thinking this anything but a great basketball game."

Chapter 6

The General's Last Stand

For Bob Knight, a.k.a The General, it started to unravel when, just before the 2000 NCAA Tournament, Sports Illustrated broke a shocking story. It focused on accusations made by former Hoosier Neil Reed, claiming Knight choked him during a practice in the 1996-97 season.

From that point on, the Bob Knight ship sprung more leaks than an old Spanish wreck. Over the next month, there were more reports of physical or verbal abuse. Given the newspaper's strong, 29-year relationship with Knight, the reporters were inclined to rally to his defense, leading to a steady diet of damage control.

Although the mounting claims were refuted by other teammates and assistant coaches, the accusations created a whirlpool that eventually sucked Knight into the abyss. And once IU president Myles Brand imposed a restraint as unrealistic as "Zero Tolerance," it was just a matter of time.

Knight Cool under Fire

Knight's press conference on eve of the 2000 NCAA Tournament showed what a cool customer he could be. Shooting straight from the hip for a solid 30 minutes, he quieted the critics for the time being.

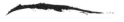

Bloomington Herald-Times
March 17, 2000

BUFFALO, NEW YORK

It was Show Time in Buffalo Thursday night, and Bob Knight was the main event. A throng of newspapers, magazines and television stations was buzzing in anticipation of what Knight had to say in the aftermath of this week's CNN/SI report charging him with choking former Hoosier Neil Reed, waving soiled toilet paper at his team and booting the university president out of practice.

Even though many other Hoosier players, past and present, stepped forward to refute the charges, the masses wanted to hear it from the man himself. When it came time for Knight to speak at the press conference scheduled for each of the eight head coaches here in Buffalo for the first round of the NCAA, he was asked for opening remarks.

You can bet your boxer shorts that many of those in attendance were expecting -- hoping, surely -- for Knight to throw toilet paper into the audience and launch into an angry tirade.

But Knight's opening statement was nothing of the sort. Speaking candidly but calmly, he answered the charges. And he did it all without benefit of notes. Here, with the exception of a few inconsequential tangents, is Knight's statement in its entirety.

"Apparently, there's been a lot of time given to Indiana basketball in the last couple of days, and so I'll talk about Indiana basketball," he began.

"Let me give you a little rundown on our team. Our team is responsible for almost the total support of the Boys and Girls Club in Bloomington and Monroe County, by virtue of a dinner that raises funds for those programs. Our kids go to hospitals, our kids go to schools and talk about drug and alcohol problems. A lot of teams across the country do that, which I think is one of the things that is so good about college athletics. We are certainly not the only team to do that, but we do a lot of it.

"Basketball, according to the latest estimate from our president, has raised about $5 million for the university library -- $5 million that benefits all students and all faculty. All of our scholarships through the golf tournament we have and some contributions that have been made, have endowed all of our scholarships. So about $250,000 a year goes back in the athletic budget for other sports.

"We operate on the lowest recruiting budget of any school in the Big Ten. Our graduation rate... From what I see and read from time to time, I think, 'Man, you must not graduate anybody. What the hell are we in this for? Everybody quits Indiana.'

"So we made a study. We've given 117 scholarships since I've been there, and out of those 117 scholarships, 80 have played four years. We've lost 37 kids. Now I'm not real good at math, so I had a friend of mine figure it out. That's 31 percent. The national average in Division I in loss of kids is 38 percent. So not only are we not near the bottom, we are at the upper half in terms of retention.

"Then it really changes a lot. Of the 80 that played, 77 have a degree. You're going to have a hard time matching that anywhere. Among those are teachers and lawyers -- I'm not all that proud

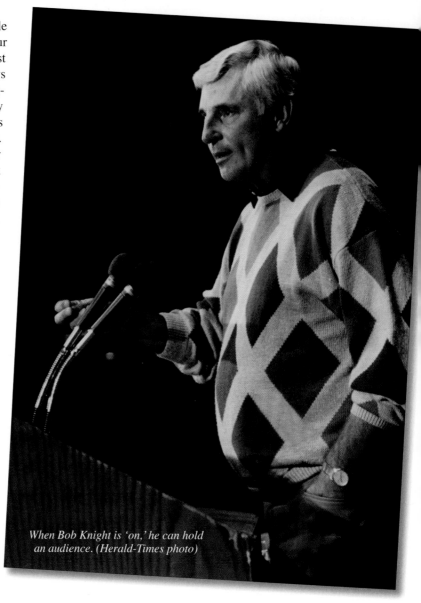

When Bob Knight is 'on,' he can hold an audience. (Herald-Times photo)

of the lawyers (pausing for laughs) -- but teachers, doctors and businessmen are pretty good in representing the university.

"Our graduation rate in basketball in the '90s, published by the NCAA, of those kids entering on basketball scholarships and those graduating, was just about 79 percent. The graduation rate for our university, the same period of time, was 68 percent. We've always tried to maintain a level above university standards.

"In the time that I've been there, we've never had NCAA violations for recruiting or academics or anything else. And yet, during the same period of time, our teams have been able to win more games in the '70s, '80s and '90s than any team in the conference.

"I don't expect everybody to agree with everything I do. Hell, my mom didn't. I bet I've done a thousand things to motivate kids as individuals and teams, and I guarantee you that a lot of them I wouldn't want to talk about at a church social, a PTA meeting or a garden party. But we're not teaching kids how to play Canasta. This is a game where kids get bloody noses, and they get broken legs, they get hurt, they compete, they dive on the floor. They're playing like hell to win.

"I don't know that I can say I'm proud of everything I've done to motivate kids, but if I think I did wrong or somebody has told me I did wrong, then I try to find something else to do. I guarantee you I'm pretty damned inventive at doing this over the years. And yet, my basic thought is to make this kid the best player he possibly can be, so that leads us to be the best team we can possibly be.

"If my kids left, weren't successful and didn't have degrees, and they're in the bread line or out selling drugs, or in jail for one thing or another, then I would have a lot of questions about just what the hell my methods were all leading to.

"But I've had kids come back and talk about their experience here. I'm not sure what I'm supposed to apologize for. It always amazes me when something like this comes up, people don't talk to Calbert Cheaney or Quinn Buckner or Mike Woodson or Randy Wittman or Scott May or Kent Benson. I could go on and on -- (Ted) Kitchell, (Tom) Abernethy, Damon Bailey, Greg and Pat Graham. It seems it's always some malcontent that has something to say.

"I don't know why Indiana was picked for this. You could go to any school in America and find kids who were bitter, unhappy, malcontents. I just asked a very good player, from a very good school today, 'How quickly can you come up with three kids who played while you were in school that would be bitter about their experience basically because they didn't play very much, or weren't as good as people thought they would be?' He just laughed and said, 'It would take me about three seconds, Coach.'

"So, I don't know why there isn't a series on this. Why not a series on kids who have really represented their schools well? I don't know if you people understand this -- a kid (Neil Reed) that was voted off the team by returning players by an 8-0 vote.

"There was another kid (Richard Mandeville) who the players kind of laughed at, because

of his work ethic. I suggested after his junior year of competition that he go to a Division II school, because I didn't think he had developed well. Whether it was his fault or my fault, he hadn't. But he needed to go someplace and he begged to stay.

"Now I'm not going to go through these things, other than to make a couple of comments. I think there is a real positive aspect to this. Brian Evans (the former Hoosier) heard about it in Italy. Indiana basketball must be pretty big if he heard about it in Italy. He was so upset about it he called our newspaper.

"So the positive thing was the feedback I got from players and coaches that had been with us. The players, coaches, trainers that were involved in this, when anything would have happened, have all come forward to refute it. So I'm not going to get into that.

"One thing that just makes the thing so ridiculous was that I demanded our president to leave practice. Now, you're not ever going to look at me as the smartest guy you ever dealt with, but I'm damn sure smart enough not to throw the president out of practice. I've had a few people leave, but I've had three good presidents -- John Ryan, Tom Ehrlich and now Myles Brand. They have been very interested in basketball. They speak to the basketball team at least twice a year. They each have come to practice a half a dozen times. Ryan and Ehrlich have both retired and each time they're back on campus they come to practice, as do a lot of professors, men and women.

"It amazed me in this TV thing, what is an 'unnamed source?' Is an unnamed source me standing up here and saying, 'I was just told outside by somebody not wishing to be named, that 65 percent of the men in this room are having extramarital affairs with sheep.' (More laughs.) Is that an unnamed source? As far as you ladies are concerned, I look over you and I can't see one of you in here that an unnamed source would accuse of an extramarital affair. My wife told me to say that.

"The last time I saw Isiah Thomas was in November. He was working out with our team. He talked to our players after practice. As we were talking out on the floor, he started away and he walked up to me, grabbed a hold of my shirt. I probably taught him that. He grabbed a hold of my shirt, looked me in the eye and said, 'Coach, don't you ever change. Kids need you. Don't change.' So, I don't think I will."

Knight, Brand Backed into a Corner

A week after IU was knocked out in the first round of the NCAA Tournament, the storm around Knight had yet to subside, even overshadowing the passing of the great Herman B Wells, the revered university chancellor. This column tried to capture the absurdness of it all.

Bloomington Herald-Times
March 24, 2000

One of the great injustices of the last decade was when Mother Teresa had a most untimely death, leaving this earth on the same weekend that Lady Diana perished in a car crash.

Here was a modern day saint put on the backburner by a woman who, though a charming member of British royalty and a loving mother, did not belong in the same breath.

And now we have Herman B Wells, the man who made Indiana University the great institution that it is today, almost lost in the storm swirling around the university's basketball coach.

And here is the university's president, Myles Brand, forced to call an investigation in a matter involving Bob Knight, a day after burying Wells.

"The last two days, the university has been in mourning for our beloved chancellor, Herman Wells," Brand said at a Thursday press conference. "We are addressing this as expeditiously as possible, given the present circumstances."

Some of those swept up by the CNN/*Sports Illustrated* piece on Knight, which just happened to air on the eve of the NCAA, would have had Knight suspended on the spot. He did strangle Neil Reed, right? The former Hoosier said so on CNN, so it must be true.

Forget the fact that the university looked into the allegations in 1997, back when Neil Reed was first dismissed from the team -- by an 8-0 vote of the returning players, mind you.

Forget the fact that everyone from assistant coaches to trainers to past and present players could not recall a choking incident. The fact that an accusation was made before a national television audience is enough to force the university's hand. It is a proven formula. Take one disgruntled player, ask him to come up with a Bob Knight tale, sprinkle in a few half-truths and presto! You have a full-fledged scandal.

It doesn't take much for the public to assume the worst when it comes to Knight. Whether right or wrong, just or unjust, he has given his adversaries enough ammunition to keep the potshots coming.

O.J. Simpson could point the finger at Knight as the killer of Nicole Simpson and Ronald Goldman and the public would buy it. The Serbs could accuse Knight of war crimes in Yugoslavia, and the Croatians would issue the wanted posters. The economics committee could blame Knight for the rise in gas prices and the consumers would cry for his scalp.

So here is Reed claiming he was choked, forcing a reopening of a case that had been closed for three years. For what purpose and at what cost? Just think of the dollars wasted on this investigation if it goes the full 90 days Brand has set aside for it, dollars better spent for education.

Some dare to see it as a power struggle between Brand and Knight. Brand bristled at the absurdity of the suggestion in Thursday's press conference in which he announced the follow-up investigation.

"I am calling for the review," he said with a cold stare. "This is Indiana University. There are no sacred cows at Indiana University, including the basketball program. We will run this institution with integrity at all times."

Not only was Brand's character impugned, but also that of the appointed investigators -- attorneys John Walda and Frederick Eichorn. Being members of the Indiana Board of Trustees makes them incapable of conducting an impartial investigation, some implied.

"The object of the review is one simple thing and that is to get to the truth," Walda said. "We want to be fair to all parties involved and want to determine if any additional measures are required. I'm very mindful of the seriousness of the allegations that were aired. The integrity of Indiana University is at stake and that's why this will be a full and fair review.

"Our dedication is to the institution, and to determining the truth," Walda added. "I can promise you that is the guiding principle Mr. Eichorn and I will live by."

Knight told Brand he is willing to suffer the consequences.

"I told him (Knight) how we were proceeding," Brand said. "He listened carefully and said, 'I will do whatever is in the best interests of the university.' And he was comfortable with our proceeding."

It is a no-win situation for Brand. If the allegations are supported by fact, he will have to take severe measures against the most visible coach this university has ever known. If Knight is cleared, the anti-Knight faction will claim the investigation was a sham.

If Brand has read Wells's book, *Being Lucky*, he might recall this passage: "The presidential role, to be successful, is demanding. It demands all of one's life, energy, thought, enthusiasm and vision, and still one cannot fully realize its potentials. I think it is the most difficult top leadership post in America other than the presidency of the United States, more difficult than that of being a governor or head of a large corporation or the presiding bishop of a religious congregation."

Our late chancellor said it best. It is lonely at the top.

Feinstein: Knight Once Again 'On The Brink'

At the 2000 Final Four in Indianapolis I caught up with John Feinstein, author of Season on the Brink, *his first-hand account of IU's 1985-86 season. This column covered Feinstein's take on the Knight situation.*

Bloomington Herald-Times
April 4, 2000

INDIANAPOLIS, INDIANA

Fourteen years ago, a 29-year-old sports writer for the *Washington Post* approached editor Ben Bradlee with a book proposal that didn't exactly captivate Bradlee the way Watergate had 15 years before.

The proposal was this: a six-month sabbatical to spend the entire 1985-86 season with Bob Knight and his Indiana Hoosiers. Knight already had given his consent to the writer, John Feinstein.

"Nobody really gives a damn about Bob Knight," Bradlee grumbled to Feinstein. It was with some reservation that Bradlee ultimately gave his approval. Bradlee wasn't alone in his reluctance. Five publishers rejected Feinstein's proposal. Finally, McMillan advanced him $17,500. Feinstein went to Bloomington and delivered the book that became a national best-seller, *Season on the Brink*.

Ten books later, Feinstein is sport's most recognized author. Monday, the U.S. Basketball Writers Association recognized his achievements by making the 43-year-old Feinstein the youngest inductee into the USBWA Hall of Fame. And Feinstein owes it all to *Season on the Brink*.

"It never occurred to me I had a best-seller," he said after the induction ceremonies. "All I wanted was that the book be good enough, reviewed good enough, that I would have a chance to write another book. To every one's surprise, it took off like a rocket. They couldn't keep it in stores. They had to go back for three more printings before the official publication date."

Since then, a million copies have been sold, making it the all-time No. 1 seller among sports books until 1995, when Feinstein published his inside look at the PGA Tour, *A Good Walk Spoiled*.

What made *Season on the Brink* so unique was that it took the reader into the inner sanctum of a college program that previously had been closed to outsiders. Knight granted him unlimited access with only one ground rule: Feinstein couldn't write about Knight's personal life. Everything else was fair game, including the language, Feinstein said.

"Knight knew I would leave in the profanity. I don't think he knew what it would look like in print. Writing a book without it, that would have been like writing a book about Bob Knight without the word 'basketball.' It's a part of who he is."

Knight let it be known he did not care to have all the salty words of the lockerroom put down on paper. For eight years, there was no further contact with Feinstein. It wasn't until a chance meeting in the 1994 Maui Classic that the coach extended an olive branch. Knight was there with his Indiana team and spotted Feinstein walking along with Maryland coach Gary Williams.

"Knight just came up and started talking," said Feinstein, who was glad for the opportunity to break the ice. Later, Williams asked him, "After all the things he (Knight) has said about you, why did you talk to him?"

"Because he built my house," said Feinstein, who now describes his relationship with the Hoosier coach as "cordial." Having seen Knight and the program on a daily basis through an entire season, Feinstein has had a hard time believing the allegations put forth by the CNN/*Sports Illustrated* piece in which former Hoosier Neil Reed claimed Knight once choked him.

"The CNN/SI thing is overblown," Feinstein said. "The crux of the study is three years old. Neil

Reed made those charges when he left the program (in 1997). CNN/SI said they investigated the story for 11 months and came back with three-year-old charges. I don't think that is enough to merit a piece like that. "I'm guessing Knight put his hands on Reed and said, 'Get over here.' That's the way Knight is. He's a very physical person. He shows affection physically, always putting his arms around people. The closest I ever saw Bob Knight being physically abusive was when he slapped Sam Alford (the Iowa assistant coach) on the back this year. He almost put him in the next county."

Feinstein also saw nothing in the way of the charges made by Ricky Calloway, a freshman on the '85-86 team, who claimed Knight punched Steve Alford and slapped Daryl Thomas at some point during Calloway's three years at IU. Alford, Thomas and two other teammates, Keith Smart and Joe Hillman, have denied the accusations.

As Feinstein recalled, "There were times I cringed, but there was never a moment I thought a kid was in physical danger. If Knight had a penchant for that sort of thing, it would have come out at some point during that year."

The one thing *Season on the Brink* proved beyond a doubt is that Bob Knight sells. Feinstein has a theory about that.

"I think it is the fact that Knight can be so good and so bad. You see all these extraordinary qualities -- he's brilliant, caring, a great coach. He plays by the rules, he's charitable, he's generous. And then he is also a bully, with a temper out of control. People look at him and say, 'Why?' I'm not sure any of us have an answer. I'm not sure Bob Knight has an answer. That's why I named the book, *Season on the Brink*. You never know which direction he's going."

Knight Ready to Tackle 'Zero Tolerance'

When Brand handed down the "Zero Tolerance" ultimatum, Knight was OK with it at first. In his first public discussion of it, Knight invited only a handful of media to hear his say. I was among the chosen few, later labeled The Sympathetic Seven. The others were my Herald-Times *colleague, Mike Leonard, along with Dave Kindred (The* Sporting News*), Billy Reed (Sports Illustrated), Ursula Reel (New York Post), Hubert Mizell (St. Petersburg Times) and William Guildea (Washington Post).*

Bloomington Herald-Times
May 31, 2000

Bob Knight has had to face many a challenge in his 34 years of coaching. Now he will try to confront another -- himself.

In his first meeting with the press since sanctions were imposed on him by Indiana University May 15, Knight was confident he could still effectively coach within the framework established by President Myles Brand and the university trustees. That means operating under a "zero tolerance" policy prohibiting physical abuse or angry outbursts beyond the scope of accepted behavior.

"I don't have any problems with guidelines," Knight said to a small group of reporters who were at IU's Assembly Hall by invitation only Tuesday. He later went on ESPN in a live television interview with Roy Firestone and Digger Phelps. Knight did not go into any detail concerning the physical abuse allegations made by former players Neil Reed, Ricky Calloway and Chris Lawson that surfaced in the past 60 days.

"I really don't want to dwell on what's happened," he said.

Knight did comment on the CNN/*Sports Illustrated* tape of the alleged choking of Reed.

"You take the accusations that are made and compare those accusations to the practice tape ... and you draw your own conclusions," said Knight, who has not looked at the tape himself since that 1997 practice.

"I don't need to look at the tape to know I didn't choke anybody," he said.

Knight said he was more upset by the accusations of another former player, Butch Carter, that he used racial slurs.

"I really take a lot of pride in what I've done over the years ... as far as minority kids are concerned, whether they are playing basketball or sometimes kids not even involved in athletics," Knight said.

Knight did recognize his combative side, though.

"There are times when ... I feel I'm so right that nobody can prove me wrong. There are times I seem to be a lot more confrontational on things. That bothers me because that should be something I should be able to control. I can't control what somebody else says, but I can control what I do. That's a part of what's in the future, my trying to do that," he said.

"Anybody who knows me has said many times, 'Hey, I get the point.' I've got the nail in the board but I try to drive the nail through the board sometimes," he said. "I have always been competitive and part of that is getting in the last word."

Although skeptics doubt if the 59-year-old coach can curb his temper at this stage in his life, Knight is convinced he can, because "I think I know me better than they do."

Knight said his temper outbursts are not as numerous as the public is led to believe.

"There are a lot of times I have done things the right way and times when I haven't. It is the times I haven't that are always being discussed. I think I have to do basically all the time what I think I do most of the time."

Knight thinks his wife, Karen, is all he needs in the way of anger management. He said he is not seeking any professional counseling at this time.

"My wife is as good an anger management instructor as anybody could have," he said. "She is really good at looking at things. She is a great observer. There are probably five magnets around the house saying, 'The horse is dead; get off.' A lot of people have problems with anger. I have obviously made a mistake here and a mistake there, but I don't think (anger) defines me as a person."

What about the first time a fan or sportswriter deliberately tries to provoke him, Knight was asked.

"Is that new? ... A key word for me is 'approach.' I can approach things one way, or approach them another, or still approach them a third way. Going at things, or taking on things, has always been my style. Well, there are pitchers, guys who last in the major leagues long after they can't throw 90 miles per hour because they develop a split-finger (fastball) or something else. Sometimes there are changes in style, changes in approaches. I will be surprised that there's anybody who can bait me into any kind of difficult situation.

"How many times have you seen me walking off the floor with my head down, no matter what was said? This whole thing becomes a challenge. Through the whole thing, I just wanted to coach basketball. I have been dealt a hand of cards. How I feel makes no difference. What I have to do is play these cards.

"I think I can live with any set of parameters as long as I don't have my mouth taped shut. I don't have any problem with the guidelines. If a kid keeps making mistakes, I bench him. If I continue to make mistakes, it's nobody's fault but my own."

Knight feels a special obligation to Brand and to his players for the chance to continue coaching.

"There are basically two reasons why I'm the Indiana coach today. One is our players. They have been very supportive throughout this whole thing," he said. "The second thing is our president. I mean the president has made a decision here that not everybody agrees with. I want to do the absolute utmost that I can to show everybody that the president was right in his decision."

In order to limit the chances of violating the sanctions, Knight said he might cut back on his public appearances.

"Some of these sanctions will inhibit me from doing some worthwhile things -- fund-raisers and speaking to groups. If I talk to a group, some people might be offended. If you want to be careful, you want to eliminate those situations that can cause a problem."

In closing the ESPN interview, Knight promised to do his best.

"To all of the people who have supported us, keep rooting for us. Because of your support, the extent of that support, I'm not going to let you down."

Knight's Dismissal Rekindles Student Unrest

As mentioned earlier, it was just a matter of time before Knight exceeded the boundaries of Zero Tolerance. A brush with a student led to a final clash with president Myles Brand. I was on my way to cover an Indianapolis Colts' game when the news came over the radio that Bob Knight had been dismissed. I quickly called my editor for instructions and was redirected to the press conference in Indianapolis. I did a player reaction piece from there and then returned to Assembly Hall for more reactions. The scene there was riotous. Fortunately, this was Bloomington in the Year 2000, not Chicago, 1968. Cooler heads prevailed.

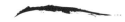

Bloomington Herald-Times
September 12, 2000

The enormity of Bob Knight's dismissal from Indiana University really didn't hit home until a visit was made to Assembly Hall Sunday night.

Gathered there were several thousand students on the verge of rioting. Braced to discourage them were police in full riot gear. Played out under a full September moon, it was an eerie reminder of the mid-1960s and early 1970s at Indiana University. The university back then was perceived as a Midwest version of Berkeley, the tumultuous campus at the University of California, a hotbed of student unrest.

Only this time the cause wasn't Vietnam, or civil rights or women's lib. And the figures burned in effigy weren't Lyndon Johnson or Richard Nixon. Instead of an American president being the target of student anger, it was a university president, IU's Myles Brand.

There were times when the crowd seemed to be on the verge of turning violent. When one protester became dangerously belligerent and had to be restrained with handcuffs, there was a breathtaking moment when the mob turned toward the police line in a confrontational stance.

The police, some of them not older than students themselves, had looks of resolve and fear. The students had looks of anger and distrust. But instead of venting their frustration on law enforcers, the students turned and marched away en masse, presumably toward Showalter Fountain, site of many an IU basketball celebration.

That was a much safer rallying point because fountains are fireproof. In one of those stormy IU protests of the '60s, the old library and its priceless books went up in flames at the hand of an arsonist.

Staying behind at Assembly Hall Sunday night was a handful of students awaiting the appearance of Knight and his players, who were huddled inside for a farewell meeting. One by one the players trickled out, eyes clouded by tears, genuine heartfelt tears, exposing these rugged young men as yet vulnerable boys.

As each one passed, fans would beg "Stay here, guys. Don't leave IU. Stick with us."

Some of the players paused to give interviews. Others waved them off. Junior guard Dane Fife described the emotional meeting with their coach.

"It was sad, very sad," said Fife with a broken voice. "Coach expressed to us how much he cared for us and how much he wanted us to succeed. He said he was sorry for what happened and that he would help us on the court as well as off the court."

"This is a very trying time for us, very emotional," said junior forward Jarrad Odle. "Coach showed a lot of love for us and we showed a lot of love for him. It's a tough situation, something that will never leave our minds. You could see it on the guys' faces as we were walking out. We all cried in the lockerroom, cried with Coach Knight and hugged Coach Knight."

"I have been to funerals before and not witness the emotions that were in there last night," said assistant coach Mike Davis. "Man, it was tough."

"You could feel it when Coach walked in," Fife said. "He saw the looks on our faces. We are a family."

"Coach was as emotional as I've ever seen him," said junior forward Kirk Haston. "He said he was sorry he couldn't coach this team because he felt it was a special team. He said he hoped that by coming here we would be better players and also a success in life. I can say that is a definite fact."

This truly was a side of Knight that only the most intimate IU family members see.

"We claim him as our coach," sophomore guard Kyle Hornsby said earlier in the day. "He does so many good things for us. You see the bad things he has done, but we see the good things."

"What person isn't going to have minor discrepancies throughout life?" said freshman guard A.J. Moye, who had yet to attend his first practice under Knight. "Coach is not a prophet. He's not Moses or Jesus. He's a man like you and me. A man should have margins for error. We (players) are the only ones that he interacts with daily. We are the only students that really count in this decision."

"He was Indiana basketball," said junior forward Tom Geyer. "We wanted him to finish his legacy here. He said he would coach again. I hope he does."

"He's the best coach in the country and he's not just going to sit around on his hind end," Odle said. "He's going to find a place in America that wants him."

IU Program in Limbo

Knight's sudden departure left a lot of unanswered questions and uncertainties. This column tried to address some of those.

Bloomington Herald-Times
September 12, 2000

Will he or won't he?
That was the prevailing question coming out of Day 1 in the year A.K. -- "After Knight."

* Will either assistant coach Mike Davis or John Treloar be named as interim head coach to replace their mentor, Bob Knight?

* Will junior guard Dane Fife pick up his gear and head back to Michigan?

* Will freshman guard A.J. Moye head South, back to Atlanta?

* Will there be other Hoosiers to follow?

* Will Indiana lose recruits because of the dismissal of Knight?

Answers to these and other questions were few and far between on a wild day at Assembly Hall, a day when stories and subplots unfolded hourly. Hoosier players met with the coaching staff in the morning and then took their cause before athletic director Clarence Doninger and vice president Terry Clapacs in the afternoon. The players made their pitch for the assistant coaches, hoping to keep the "family" intact as much as possible.

Fife and Moye already had made it known they were leaning toward leaving the university, although they later left their options open. Not even Fife's father, Dan, knew whether his son was staying or leaving.

Judging by this personal letter from Bob Knight, written five months after he was fired, Lynn Houser earned his trust.

INDIANA UNIVERSITY

DEPARTMENT OF
INTERCOLLEGIATE
ATHLETICS

January 29, 2001

Lynn Houser
The Herald Times
1900 South Walnut Street
Bloomington, IN 47401

Dear Lynn:

I wanted to take this opportunity to tell you how much I enjoyed having you as a part of Indiana Basketball. I really enjoyed you covering our basketball program and I thought you did an excellent job. I was disappointed that you weren't going to do it this year but would have done everything I could to include you with things along the way. You have an honesty and understanding that I find a real rarity in your profession.

If I can ever be of help to you, just give me a call.

Sincerely,

Bob

Bob Knight

BK:md

Assembly Hall
1001 East 17th Street
Bloomington, Indiana
47408-1590

812-855-2794
Fax: 812-856-5155

"I just got off the phone with him and I honestly can't tell you now," Dan said by phone from his Clarkston, Mich. Home Monday evening. "Dane did say earlier he was leaving, but when I got home from work, he called and said, 'Dad, If I did all this, does that mean I've got to leave?' Dane is torn, acting on emotion."

"Dane's decision is not official," Haston said. "He told me, 'It's not official until I sign.' It's all words right now. Emotions are high right now. I know I said some things and my teammates said some things we wish we could take back."

"Dane has it in his mind that he's out of here," said junior forward Jarrad Odle. "It's going to take a drastic change. Dane's parents will have to change their viewpoints."

"Dane is so upset by it all," Dan Fife said. "The problem for juniors like Dane and (Kirk) Haston, (Jarrad) Odle and (Tom) Geyer is that they are going to be faced with an interim coach for one year, then another coach next year. That's not a good situation for the kids. Most coaches want their own players, want to bring in the players and win with their own kids."

With tensions running high, Moye thought better of attending the team meeting with Doninger and Clapacs.

"I want to keep this thing civil," Moye said. "I'm so emotionally frustrated I might say some things that would jeopardize my career here at Indiana. I'm staying out of the process."

Asked if leaving was a real possibility, Moye said, "Very much so."

The one thing that would keep him at Indiana would be naming of Davis the interim coach. Davis recruited Moye.

"That's the only way. He's got to be head coach," Moye said. "You can't bring someone else in and leave him (Davis) as an assistant."

Davis already has stated that his only interest is being a head coach, not another coach's assistant. In a Sunday night meeting with Doninger and Clapacs, Davis and Treloar were told they could stay on as assistants.

"They said John and I could stay during the search and that we were candidates," Davis said. "From my point of view, it's not fair to ask me to stay on as an assistant coach."

Treloar was not available for comment, but Davis said his fellow assistant "feels the same way about the players. He loves these guys."

The players are reciprocating.

"We all know there's no chance Coach Knight can come back, but you have to maintain a part of the family," said sophomore center George Leach, also lobbying for the assistants.

The players are in a quandary. With the first semester well under way, they would have to await roughly three semesters before they would be eligible following a transfer. In the case of Leach, who missed all of last year as a partial academic qualifier, it would leave him with barely two years worth of eligibility.

"That would mean two years to achieve my goal, my dream of going pro," Leach said. "Two years, that would take a hell of a lot of miracles to develop that fast. That is screwing up my life."

Also in limbo are some possible future Hoosiers, recruits Sean Kline and Kei Madison, as well as other players in the recruiting process.

"The sad part about it is that we were headed in the right direction," Davis said. "I had guys lined up waiting to come that would have been outstanding for the program, players they haven't had here since the Isiah Thomas days. Put all these guys together and, boy, you've got a hell of a team."

Davis, a former player at Alabama and an assistant to Treloar in the CBA, is convinced he could take over the program.

"No question," he said. "I can coach. I can teach. Will I be another Coach Knight? There are a lot of coaches who won't be a Coach Knight. Coach gave me the opportunity to coach in college. Without having any experience in recruiting at a major, major program, Coach brought me in. He didn't know me from Adam. A lot coaches wouldn't hire you unless they knew you."

The longer the administration waits to make a decision, the greater the chances of losing players, Davis said. "If it goes a couple more days... you have other schools calling these kids. You may say that's against the rules, but I'm telling you. For a kid to transfer somewhere, somebody has to call him. "They said they would know something in the next week or two," Davis added. "In my opinion, an interim coach has to be in place immediately."

Will common sense prevail over emotion?

"The majority of us are saying we want to stay," said freshman Jared Jeffries, also recruited by Davis. "We hope everything works out. We just have to sit back, take a look at what we want to do and not let our emotions run as high as they are now."

Chapter 7
Old Generals Never Die

When it became evident that Knight was going to resurrect his career at Texas Tech, the Herald-Times *sent me to Lubbock to cover the story. After enduring some rocky moments with Knight in his final days at IU, I found him extremely generous with his time when I showed up in Lubbock. Over lunch he granted me a 1-on-1 interview, a rarity for Knight under any circumstances. We parted on such good terms that it paved the way for a return trip in November, the weekend he coached his first game at Tech.*

Texas Gives a Big 'Howdy' to Knight

The size of the welcome mat Tech threw down for Knight was the kind normally reserved for football coaches in this state.

Bloomington Herald-Times
March 24, 2001

LUBBOCK, TEXAS

The state of Texas prides itself on doing things in a big way. Friday night, Texas Tech threw a Texas-size welcoming party for its new men's head basketball coach, Bob Knight.

An estimated 7,500 fans showed up to greet Knight at an open news conference set in United Spirit Arena. That was 3,500 more than the average home attendance for Red Raider men's games this year. The women drew an average of 12,500 fans.

As Knight made his entrance into the arena, it was as if he were heading to his customary seat on the bench at Assembly Hall. Only the noise level was louder. Fans were chanting, "Bobby, Bobby."

The pep band, cheerleaders and pom squad were on hand, as well as 12 local television stations and two national networks. It was March Madness in Texas and it had nothing to do with the NCAA Tournament, although it had a lot to do with college basketball.

"This is without a doubt the day we get to break the worst-kept secret in Texas," said Tech President David Schmidly as he introduced Knight, who delighted the Red Raider fans by giving the traditional "Guns Up" salute with his thumb and index finger.

Athletics Director Gerald Myers then presented Knight with a Texas Tech sweater vest. Knight slipped it on and said, "This is the most comfortable red sweater I've had in six years."

Knight has signed a five-year, $1.25 million deal with Tech. With other incentives, the salary comes to about $400,000 annually.

Friday wasn't Knight's first appearance in United Spirit Arena. In November, 1999, he brought his Indiana team in for the grand opening of the 15,500-seat facility. That night he took some abuse from the Tech fans, many of whom showed up in camouflage attire to poke fun at the coach's recent hunting accident. On this night the coach asked for a show of hands from those who had donned the camouflage.

"I'll feel a lot better walking out on this floor knowing you're going to be for me than against me," he said.

There was no question as to the support on this occasion. Knight further endeared himself by announcing he was going to start a library fund similar to the one he established at Indiana and volunteered to contribute the first $10,000. He then asked his wife, Karen, to say a few words. She also was warmly received.

"I feel like I'm home already," she said, followed by a personal plea. "Some people say he has a temper. What I see every day is a passion for living. I ask just one thing: Please don't judge him until you get a chance to know him. He's very loyal. If he's your friend, he's your friend for life."

As Knight fielded questions from the media, it was obvious the deck was stacked in his favor. Any question the fans deemed too harsh was drowned out by boos until the interviewer retreated.

The harshest jeers went to the CNN/SI reporter Tom Rinaldi, who asked Knight about the Neil Reed incident, the story CNN/SI broke a year ago this month, the story that started Knight's downfall.

Another reporter was booed for asking if Knight had undergone any counseling in his year away from basketball. Most of the questions were softball lobs. One pertained to his issues with the media.

"I sometimes entertain a sense of humor with the media that hasn't always gone over well," Knight said. "Let's just start from scratch and see where we go. If you have a problem with me, tell me about it before writing it. Or come see me. You might be surprised by the results. My objective is to have a team here you can be proud to watch play."

Before exiting the stage, Knight told his new players to get a good night's sleep because he was ready to get down to business. A team meeting was called for Saturday morning at 7. Junior center Andy Ellis could hardly wait.

"The only time I've seen this place this full was when he was here the first time," he said. "When you just think about the game getting ready to start and he walks in and the crowd goes crazy, I can't imagine what it's going to be like having them going crazy for us."

Travel Guide to Loveable Lubbock

Going from Bloomington to Lubbock had to be a shock for Knight. It sure was for me. I had fun describing the experience tongue-in-cheek.

Bloomington Herald-Times
March 23, 2001

LUBBOCK, TEXAS

Before you pack up all of your belongings and follow Bob Knight out to Texas Tech, you might want to know a few things about your new home.

Lubbock is located in a part of west Texas known as the Texas Pan Handle. If you hang a frying pan on the wall and use your imagination, you can see an outline of Texas. If that doesn't work for you, try thinking of the love handles looking back at you in the mirror from eating too much pan-fried food.

In order to get to this Texas outback, you have to board the same plane that Lubbock native Buddy Holly allegedly went down in, the Spirit of St. Louis from the looks of it. We say "alleged" because rumor has it that the great rock legend isn't dead at all. Buddy is simply circling endlessly on Loop 289, the belt around the city that has no marked exits.

A Hoosier with no pride will finally stop and ask for directions to Texas Tech, an agricultural school located in the heart of a city. This is proof that you don't need farmland to study farming.

Texas Tech students like to believe their institution is more than just an "ag" school, as is rival Texas A&M, whose nickname actually is Aggies. The rivalry goes very deep.

How deep you ask? On the Texas Tech campus is a statue of Will Rogers (yes, the great American humorist) riding eastward on a horse. Upon further review, the statue was turned around so that the horse's backside was pointing to the southeast, in the direction of College Station, home of the hapless Aggies, who also happen to be down-wind.

Speaking of wind, Lubbock is home to the American Wind Power Center, the world's largest collection of windmills. These huge, futuristic-looking structures are powered by a single man, a very large Texan eating bean burritos. It is believed he is the lead singer for the country band, the Mavericks.

Speaking of musicians, Holly isn't the only one to come out of Lubbock. Others include Tanya Tucker, Waylon Jennings, Mac Davis, Joe Ely, Natalie Maines (Dixie Chicks) and Richie McDonald (Lone Star).

Lone Star is not only the name of a country band, it also is the brand name for the most popular beer in Texas. It is popular because it is rare. You can't buy it. The hard reality is that Lubbock is a dry city -- no liquor stores, by local ordinance.

You can't keep a Texan from his beer, though. Just outside the city limits, a matter of inches outside the city limits, is an area called The Strip. This is nothing more than one continuous liquor store. You don't even have to get out of your car. On The Strip you can buy your liquor at drive-through windows. Is the country going to heck or what?

Thanks to The Strip, there is no shortage of fire water at tailgate parties. The male students, who greatly outnumber the female students at an "ag" school (ask Purdue), like to down a few Lone Stars, march into the stadium and form a traditional cheer block known as Saddle Tramps. When the Red Raiders do something good, the Saddle Tramps form the "Guns Up" salute, a gesture made by making a "pistol" out of the index finger and thumb.

The problem with the Guns Up salute is that too many Lone Stars often lead to confusion over the index and middle finger. Many an A&M fan has seen the middle finger from a Red Raider, we are told.

Before and after each game, the Saddle Tramps get sappy and sing the "Matador Song" for old Alma Mater.

> Fight, Matadors, for Tech!
> Songs of love we'll sing for thee...

There is another problem here. While matador is a noble term in bullfighting, it is a slam in basketball. If a guy is playing "matador" defense, it means he is allowing his man go past him like a raging bull. Knight, always a firm believer in defense, might not care to hear the Matador Song before he sends his team out to defend Texas A&M.

Knight will find plenty to like about Lubbock, though. A typical day in the off-season might see him rising early and heading for the nearest fishing hole, Buffalo Lake, perhaps. Along the way he might stop at Sugar Baker's, known for its fresh cinnamon rolls, a Knight favorite.

If fishing isn't in the cards, Knight might want to play a round of golf at Meadowlands or at the Lubbock Country Club.

If it's hunting season, he can head in any direction and rustle up some quail, pheasant or dove.

For dinner he might want to grab a big ol' Texas steak at Cagle's, which is worth a stop just to meet the owner, John Cagle himself.

"He is everything you want to know about Texas," said Blayne Beal of the Texas Tech athletic department. "He's got the Gunsmoke hat, the Wrangler blue jeans, the handle bar moustache, the cattle boots, you name it."

To wrap up the perfect day, Knight might want to take his wife, Karen, out for an evening with the Lubbock Symphony or the Lubbock Ballet. Lubbock is not without its fine arts.

The working day will find Knight at United Spirit Arena, the glittering new home of the Red Raiders. As long as he stays away from the Loop, he shouldn't have any trouble finding the facility. It's located on a street named "Indiana."

Home at last.

Knight Begins a New Day

Here is that 1-on-1 chat with Knight. After a few softball lobs, he fielded some harder questions.

Bloomington Herald-Times
March 25, 2001

LUBBOCK, TEXAS

The day after Bob Knight was hailed as the new head coach at Texas Tech, he sat down to talk about his latest challenge.

Q: Bob, the reception you had (Friday) night was unbelievable. What did that mean to you in light of what has happened to you in the last year?

Knight: "Well, it didn't have any real correlation with last year. There were a lot of good things that happened to me prior to the last five years. But this was kind of a confirmation of how I felt about this community, this institution and the people here. When I was here last week they were really, really good people, very enthusiastic of what we might do with the basketball team here, so that just confirmed my thinking about the people."

Q: You could feel the goose bumps, even around the members of the media. Could you feel the electricity?

Knight: "I wouldn't go as far as to include the media, but I think there was a great atmosphere there, a great feeling of anticipation. I just hope we will be able to put something out there that they can enjoy."

Q: You are taking over a team with not many players coming back. You always feel you can win right away. What will it take to get things turned around at Texas Tech?

Knight: "We are going to have to have some good kids come in here as recruits. There is a lot of opportunity to play here right now, probably more opportunity by far than on any team I've ever coached. When I came to Indiana, there were some really good players there. We added some players like Steve Green, Steve Ahlfeld, John Kamstra, and then those kids the next year, Quinn Buckner and Jimmy Crews, then (Bob) Wilkerson and (Scott) May the next year. We started out with really good players, added good players, and added more good players.

"So the first three years I was there we had a really good foundation. We don't have that here. We've got to add players to what we have."

Q: What do you see as your recruiting base and will the state of Indiana be included?

Knight: "I think we will recruit across Texas, beginning with West Texas. There were four really good kids here in the last year that went elsewhere. We've just got to expand from there. I would think we would recruit Kansas, Oklahoma and recruit more in the junior colleges than we did before. I think we will do a lot of recruiting in California. And we will obviously touch on some kids in Indiana. There will be some kids there that will want to go where we are. We've already had an indication from some kids. We'll see."

Q: What would you say to the person who says, "Knight should retire. Why would he want to coach again?"

Knight: "Because I like it and it's something I do about as well as anybody does. I've got to have something to do that's interesting, something to do that is challenging. I can play golf a little bit, fish and hunt. But coaching provides me with the kind of thing to be interested in, the kind of thing that challenges me. It makes up and takes up a big part of my life. I think it will be tough getting things started here, but once we do, I think it will be something I will enjoy."

Q: Have you found any places to hunt and fish yet?

Knight: "There are a lot. This is a great area. In fact, when I first talked to the athletic director and president, they spent about a half-hour talking about the opportunities to hunt and fish."

Q: How do you like the people of West Texas?

Knight: "These are great people. They are hard-working people, so they appreciate hard-working people. They are honest. They don't have hidden agendas. They are not trying to do something at your expense."

Q: People across the country today are going, "Why Texas Tech?"

Knight: "Why not?"

Q: Texas Tech doesn't jump off the page to the average basketball fan ...

Knight: "I don't think Indiana did when I went there, either. Check Indiana over the previous 10 years (the 1960s). Did that jump off the page at you? This is a great place to play. We have one of the two best arenas in America. Here and North Carolina State are probably the two state-of-the-art arenas in America. "And Texas Tech at one time enjoyed the same reputation in the Southwest Conference for basketball that any good team in the country did. Texas Tech and SMU were the dominant teams in the Southwest Conference. People here like basketball."

Q: Do you feel energized by this new opportunity?

Knight: "I think this is great. I wish I felt a little bit more strongly about how we can get started in terms of the kind of team we can have right away, but we will just see what breaks in that direction. But, yes, this is really a nice town, an extremely nice place to live. If I just had another player that looks like he's going to be another Steve Green or another Mike Woodson, that always got my juices going with a player. You've got a Calbert Cheaney and you look at him and say, 'Man, this kid is going to be as good as Woodson.' That really increases your enthusiasm right there."

Q: Were you hurt when things fell apart at Indiana?

Knight: "Hurt would not be the correct word for that because I knew what I was dealing with. I will continue to follow the kids I recruited. My interest will hold. I think perhaps the biggest sense of disappointment I had was not being able to coach this team we had put together. "I felt going into this season that we would win between 28 and 30 games. We were going to play a lot of games. We were going to play in the preseason NIT, the Big Ten Tournament and on top of that the NCAA. I felt the minimum number of games we would win the next two seasons would be 60-some. I didn't think this year's team would be a national contender, but I thought next year's team would be a prime contender. That's something I wanted to have a part in bringing back to the people of Indiana."

Q: How closely did you follow the team this year?

Knight: "Just that I knew what they were doing, where they were and whether they won or not.

Q: Did you ever watch them on TV?
Knight: "No."

Q: Have you got an idea of who's going on to be on your coaching staff?

Knight: "No, not really -- Pat (Knight) and work from there."

Q: Do you feel under your new administration, that you have to walk the straight and narrow?

Knight: "No, I just have to be myself. I was pretty well accepted at Indiana for a long time and I think I will be here."

Q: In a (televised) interview with Charlie Rose you talked about being maybe a little looser and easier with the players.

Knight: "I don't think I talked about being easier with players. I think I talked about maybe coming from a little different direction with players. I don't think 'easier' is a word I would use. I think I said last night that, as I entertain myself sometimes in talking to the media, it wasn't always the best thing to do to maintain a good working relationship. So I think if I had to do anything over again, that is certainly something I would look at and make some changes. As far as stopping a kid in need of a lesson in manners, I'd never change that."

Q: How about your general approach to players -- will that remain the same?

Knight: "The general approach I've had with players has probably won more games in less time than anybody else in coaching. So I don't think we need any change in the general approach to players."

Q: What would you say to your former players?

Knight: "I would think that, having played under our system and under the approach I had to their playing, is an advantage to all of them in what they doing. And I would hope that all of them would always make use of the advantages created by virtue of having played basketball for us."

Q: If you had one thing to say to the fans of Indiana, what would it be?

Knight: "It would be one word, 'thanks.' The Indiana fans will always have a special place in my memory and in my heart. They were really, really good fans that didn't derive great satisfaction necessarily from the fact that we won. I think they derived satisfaction from the fact we played hard and were always a good team to watch. Their satisfaction came from what the kids got out of it, the fact that they played well, were recognized for playing well and were thought of in that vein. So the fans were just great."

Q: How long will you continue to coach?
Knight: "As long as I like it."

Time to Move On

Before leaving Lubbock, I offered this commentary.

Bloomington Herald-Times
March 26, 2001

LUBBOCK, TEXAS

As of 7:08 p.m. Indiana time Friday night, Bob Knight officially belonged to another university, thus bringing to a close a most difficult, final chapter in his 29-year reign at Indiana University.

Coupled with Wednesday's decision to make Mike Davis the Indiana coach for the next four years, the Hoosier nation now has the closure it has so desperately needed.

It has been a divided nation since last September, when the Indiana administration felt it was time for the university and Knight to go their separate ways. It was bad enough that the whole mess pressured us into choosing sides, making it an Us-against-Them proposition. In some cases you even felt required to be against Them in order to avoid accusations of being against Us.

If that doesn't make much sense, well, the entire college basketball season threw us one dead ball after another. The season was barely a week old when Dick Bennett walked away from Wisconsin, just seven months after he guided the Badgers to the Final Four. In the last week we have seen Louisville let go of Denny Crum and replace him with Rick Pitino, the former coach of Louisville's arch rival, Kentucky. And we have seen Mike Davis make the leap from assistant coach to head coach at one of the nation's most elite programs while Knight rides off into the prairie.

But it's OK because Hoosiers can now root for both Knight and Davis without feeling like they are betraying anyone. If there was ever a time for letting go of hard feelings, it is now.

"We wish everybody the best," said Indiana's retiring athletic director, Clarence Doninger. "Certainly now is the time to move forward."

Doninger and President Myles Brand have taken more than their share of heat for Knight's discharge. Granted, it probably could have been handled more delicately, but dismissals are seldom neat and tidy. In addition to the threatening phone calls, letters and e-mails, Brand and Doninger have been subject to public humiliation on occasion. In the world of sport, that kind of vehemence is extreme. This is a game, remember?

Knight also has suffered his share or ridicule, not just this year but for many years over issues often blown way out of proportion. This is not to say he was always guilt-free, but he was often a victim of his own reputation.

Now the eyes of Texas are upon him. How long will the honeymoon last? Texas Tech president David Schmidly already has served notice that men behaving badly will not fly in Lubbock.

"If the incidents that happened at Indiana were repeated at Texas Tech, I would have to terminate Coach Knight," he said. "It won't be tolerated, not for one instant, and I think he knows that."

If that doesn't sound like Zero Tolerance, it certainly is a short leash. But Knight has given every indication he intends to make it work, that he will toe the line.

For the Hoosier faithful it is time to close the book, a most compelling read, you have to admit. Players come and go, and so do coaches.

While covering the continuing saga of Bob Knight down here in Lubbock, I purchased a Texas Tech ball cap. Tech's colors are red and black, which go quite well with Indiana cream and crimson. The hat looks rather snappy with my Indiana sweatshirt. Together, they offer a sort of healing effect.

Let the healing begin.

Knight Old School at New School

When I returned to Lubbock in the fall of 2000 for Knight's first game at Tech, it was as if I was still back in Bloomington watching the Hoosiers go through their paces.

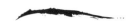

Bloomington Herald-Times
November 16, 2001

LUBBOCK, TEXAS

On the eve of his first game as coach of Texas Tech, Bob Knight talked to the media about the challenges confronting him.

"This day is very interesting because you have no more (pre-season) practices," he said. "I told our players, 'You can't come in tomorrow and correct things.' There is a tremendous amount of apprehension of how you want to play and hope you can play."

In his 29 years at Indiana, "apprehension" and Bob Knight did not belong in the same sentence. Even when his teams had legitimate question marks, the answers were rarely far away for him. But here is Knight starting over at age 61, coming off a one-year hiatus, taking over a program in a state where football rules.

As Knight explained the situation, "The degree of difficulty does not arise from making a change. The degree of difficulty arises from the experience you inherit, the players you bring in, the new ideas you are trying to do as opposed to what had been done. It's always a challenge to put a team together, but never more so than putting together a new team."

In the team's tune-up Thursday, Knight was demanding more than his players were delivering. By his standards, passes were not as crisp, cuts not as sharp, screens not as solid, block-outs not as determined. At the same time you could see the gleam in his eye as he was out there doing what he does best, teaching.

"Get up into him ... get shoulder to shoulder ... pass fake ... bounce pass ..."

A year is a long time to be away from one's passion, but Knight downplayed it.

"You are in a set of circumstances and you try to make the best of it. I probably saw only three basketball games last year."

An Indianapolis television station asked Knight what he missed about Indiana. The word "Indiana" was barely off the man's tongue when

Knight issued a terse "Nothing!" After a brief pause he added, "Except Dr. John Ryan."

In the audience was the same John Ryan, the president who brought Knight to Indiana University in 1971. He likened Ryan to Tech president David Schmidly.

"The man in the blue sweater back there is Dr. John Ryan, the guy who hired me at Indiana. Dr. Schmidly is the closest thing in this administration to John Ryan."

Knight's falling out with future IU administrations is now old news. Ryan himself was asked what had gone wrong.

"I really don't know, and if I did I wouldn't say," he replied. "I'm proud to consider Coach Knight a friend. He is one of a kind -- honest, a man of impeccable character. Texas Tech is fortunate to have him as a part of the community. The marriage is looking awful good to me.

"I never once had a situation where I thought Bob Knight would not be the man I would want to head the basketball team," Ryan went on. "A fellow Big Ten president asked, 'What sort of pressure is it that makes you keep that man on as your basketball coach?' I told him, 'I'm the only president in the Big Ten who can go to bed at night knowing there will not be a single unfavorable thing written about his basketball program the next day.' No other Big Ten president could make that statement."

The audience was full of friends from all over the country, coming to Lubbock like some sort of pilgrimage. Asked what it meant to have so many supporters, Knight said dryly, "It must mean that during my lifetime I've done some things that would kind of amaze the press in terms of friends I have accumulated over the years, people who don't confer friendship easily. I've always been proud of that."

Given a moment to rethink his answer about Indiana, Knight said, "I was being a little facetious. We had great fans at Indiana and we enjoyed the people there. I had kids I liked – the Mike Woodsons, the Calbert Cheaneys, the Joe Hillmans, the Steve Greens. What we enjoyed there we have found here. What brings you satisfaction can be found anywhere if you will let it happen."

Pat No Longer Just 'Bob's Kid'

The fresh start also was good for Knight's son, Patrick.

Bloomington Herald-Times
November 18, 2001

LUBBOCK, TEXAS

The Texas Tech players listened attentively as Coach Knight called out the various drills at practice Thursday.

Drills can be a most tedious way to spend an afternoon, and Knight is a stickler for the fundamentals of basketball.

Did I mention that this was Coach Patrick Knight? To many he is just "Bob Knight's kid," but to the players at Texas Tech, he is one of the ranking members of the staff. And when he speaks, they listen.

Since joining the staff at Tech, Pat Knight has taken on more coaching responsibilities than he did as a fledgling assistant at Indiana University. Here he is much more involved in the day-today teaching that takes place on the basketball court.

"He (Bob) wants me to take a bigger role," Pat said. "At first I didn't know what I was doing. I tended to let play go on instead of stopping it and pointing out mistakes. I was getting too caught up in just running the drills."

It almost goes without saying that coaching is in Pat's blood. As a young boy he was a gym rat in a very large gym -- Assembly Hall. He would go on to play his college ball in that same gym and spend two more years there as an assistant coach. Then came the bitter end, his dad's abrupt termination in September, 2000. As one of the casualties of that war, Pat harbors hard feelings to this day.

"I don't think I'll ever get over it," he said. "It was a learning experience. You find out who your friends are. Actually, I'm glad I had to go through it because I got to see the bad side of the business. The hardest part was saying good-bye to the kids. As an assistant coach you are almost like a brother. The head coach can't be their buddy. Telling them good-bye was tough."

Ironically, Pat landed on his feet quicker than his father did. Akron University had an opening for an assistant and hired him in October, 2000. The head coach was Dan Hipsher, a disciplinarian in the mold of Bob Knight. Pat fit right in.

"Coach Hipsher was great to me," Pat said. "He said if my dad got a job in the middle of the year, I would be free to leave."

But Bob Knight was nowhere near to being ready to coach again at that point. He came to Akron on a visit and wasn't his old self, Pat noted.

"He was really depressed," Pat said. "He wasn't any fun to be around. At that time I wasn't sure if he was going get back in it."

On an invitation from Hipsher, Knight returned for a three-day visit.

"The first day my dad was sitting up high in the stands, like he didn't want to interfere," Pat said. "The second day he was sitting by the court. By the third day he was running practice. At first the kids were a little intimidated, but after one practice they loved it. He was moving guys around, talking basketball, watching film, diagramming plays -- he was great. You could tell then he was going to come back."

Getting out of Indiana and planting new roots in West Texas has been good for his dad. The tension is gone and the old fire is back.

"I think this has added years to his life and his career," said Pat, who also has benefitted from the change of scenery -- a new identity. "If I was still at Indiana, I would still be 'Bob Knight's kid.' Here, I'm known as 'Coach Knight.' "

Not that Pat objects to being linked to Bob Knight.

"When people say, 'You're a lot like your dad,' I could not receive a better compliment," he said. "I have his temper, but I'm a little more laid back. The more I see how he does things, how organized he is, the more amazed I am."

That doesn't mean Pat isn't afraid to challenge his dad.

"We've had some brutal discussions," he said. "We can tell each other off and five minutes later go get something to eat. Like I tell the other guys, it's nothing personal."

Although he would like to make his own mark as a head coach some day, Pat is perfectly content to be Bob Knight's assistant at the moment.

"I have no timetable," said Pat, 31. "I'm in no hurry. I'm not out for the brass ring right now. I'm more worried about my dad's career than mine. I want him to finish on a good note."

*Pat Knight went from player to assistant coach under his dad. (*Herald-Times *photo by Chris Howell)*

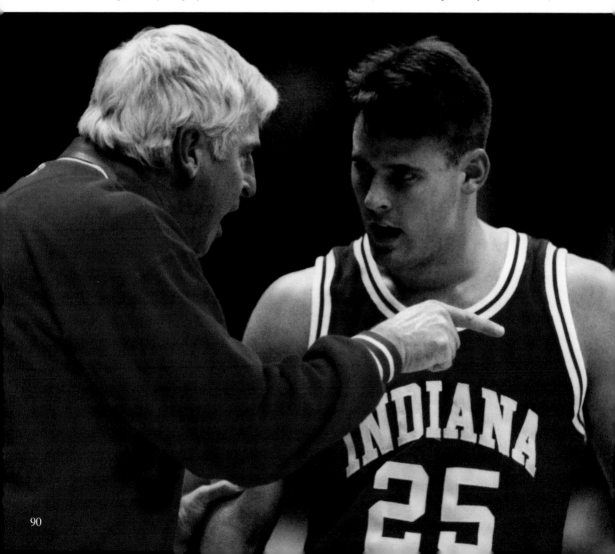

The General Marches On

Knight's official debut at Tech was a triumph for him and college basketball.

Bloomington Herald-Times
November 17, 2001

LUBBOCK, TEXAS

Old generals never die. They just fade away, Douglas McArthur said.

College basketball's "General," Bob Knight, didn't die, nor did he fade away. Like the Knight of old, he was back on the sidelines Friday night coaching a team to victory. Only this time it wasn't Indiana's sideline he patrolled. This post belonged to Texas Tech.

Knight's debut at Tech was a triumphant one, a 75-55 conquest of William and Mary in the opening game of the first Red Raider Classic. Knight became a Red Raider last March, almost a year to the day he coached his last game at Indiana. The hype leading up to his first game at Tech was enormous.

"We have been waiting a long time for this," said Tech junior Kalib Powell.

Knight downplayed the return-to-coaching angle.

"There was no doubt in my mind that if I wanted to coach again that I could coach," he said. "That was never a question. It wasn't like they found me on a barren island."

The game had a special feel to Tech's players, though.

"We wanted to make it special for him and special for us, too," said senior center Andy Ellis.

Attendance was listed at 10,444, almost 5,000 below capacity at United Spirit Arena. Actual attendance was probably around 8,000, a figure lower than some high school football crowds in Texas. The basketball game was going head-to-head with the high school football playoffs and a college football showdown with Oklahoma Saturday. On top of that, the Red Raider Classic was not included in the season ticket package.

"Frankly, I'm disappointed that we didn't have a larger crowd than we did," Knight said. "We worked awful hard on that."

The fans who showed up were into it. They even launched into a well-known barnyard chant when they felt the Red Raiders were wronged.

Knight did not try to silence them as he had done at Indiana before. He had bigger fish to fry, like getting get his team to play with some consistency. The Red Raiders were too streaky for his liking Friday night.

Just after the Red Raiders put together their best stretch of basketball, a 12-3 run near the end of the half, they gave up five points in the final 19 seconds, the last two points coming off a turnover just ahead of the buzzer. Knight was fuming as he left the floor, thinking back to the first time he brought a team into this building.

It was the United Center's grand opening in 1999, and the guest was Bob Knight and his Indiana Hoosiers. In the closing seconds of the half, IU's Jarrad Odle committed a foul that led to a 3-point play.

"I hope my team stops making bad plays at the end of the half in this building," Knight said. "When we came down to dedicate this arena, we had a kid named Odle make a really dumb play at the end of the half. He's a good kid, but I remember chewing his ass out all the way to the lockerroom."

Knight was asked if the Red Raiders played with enough patience.

"My teams never show enough patience," he said. "I've had teams that won a national championship and I would be walking into the lockerroom thinking, 'Damn, we could have slowed it down a little bit.' "

As far as William & Mary Coach Rick Boyages was concerned, it was vintage Indiana.

"Put Indiana jerseys on them and you wouldn't know the difference," he said.

Boyages had encountered Indiana eight times in the Knight era as an assistant coach to Jim O'Brien at Boston College and Ohio State. He did not expect anything less than the usual Knight trademarks -- man-to-man defense, motion offense.

"It's worked for almost 800 wins, so why change?" said Boyages, who wondered if the Tech players know what they are in for come Big 12 conference play.

"His name recognition is one of the difficulties they will have to deal with. Everybody will be ready for them. The Big 12 teams won't take Texas Tech lightly. They will be thinking, 'It's Coach Knight. We've got to beat them.' But they (Tech) will be so fundamentally sound and mentally tough that he will have them ready to deal with it."

Covering Knight Almost Like Playing for Him

Five years later, as Bob Knight was on the verge of breaking Dean Smith's record for all-time coaching wins, 879, I took a moment to reflect on the years I covered him.

Bloomington Herald-Times
December 28, 2006

In the 30 years I have been in this profession, there are two that really challenged me, 1999-2000.

In that two-year slice of life I was the IU basketball beat writer, which back then put me in direct contact with the most complex sports figure of this generation, Bob Knight.

In many ways, I felt like I was playing for the man. Like a player, I was in and out of his doghouse. One day I was the best writer since Grantland Rice. The next I couldn't write my name.

I wouldn't dare go into an interview or a game not fully prepared. Knight could sniff out an unprepared reporter like a bloodhound sniffing out an escapee. Because of that, I never worked harder in my life. And you know what? I would do it again in a heartbeat.

When I took over the beat, Knight only knew me through retired H-T sports editor Bob Hammel, one of the few members of the media Knight ever called "friend." As a frequent Hammel side kick on the IU beat, I earned Knight's confidence, which gave me a leg up as I became the "point" man.

Or so I thought. It took only a few ill-chosen questions in the first few press conferences to incur Knight's disdain and undo all those free rides I had under Hammel. For a while, it seemed like any question, no matter how well thought out, elicited a harsh answer from Knight. I felt as if he were testing me.

That first year seemed like one long final exam, one that had no end to it. A week after the season ended in the second round of the NCAA, Luke Recker bailed on the team. A month after that, Kirk Haston lost his mother to a killer tornado. It was during a crisis that you saw the other side of Knight, the compassionate side. He flew down to Tennessee to spend some time with Haston and his family.

My second season on the IU beat did not start out any smoother. At media day in October, I noticed that Knight and Iowa's new head coach, Steve Alford, never spoke to each other, even though they sat at adjoining tables. For one of his golden boys to not speak to him indicated there was an estrangement there, so I wrote about it. I even went so far as to encourage Knight to make the first move.

Knight did not see it that way. In fact, he was furious at the suggestion that he, Alford's senior and mentor, be the one to extend the olive branch instead of the other way around. Knight was hot about it that he demanded a meeting in his office. I knew it was going to be unpleasant, so I asked Hammel to come along and play the peacemaker.

But there was no peace to be had day. For a solid hour, Knight ranted and raged before "excusing" me from his office. As I started to leave Assembly Hall, it occurred to me that I might yet live to cover IU another day. Knight was known to kick players out of practice, only to ask them back within minutes. So I hung around.

Sure enough, 15 minutes later, Hammel poked his head out of Knight's office and motioned me to come back inside. Thinking the worst was behind me, I was quickly put on the defensive again when Knight picked up where he left off. Finally, having run out of ways to describe my many faults, his tone softened. With a promise that I would think first before I wrote, I was allowed to leave.

I'm still not sure what really happened in there, but I did put a lot more thought into my IU articles. And from that day on, Knight was quite cordial to me. It was like I had run the gauntlet, had survived the crucible.

Although his practices were usually closed, he allowed me to drop in on several occasions. He also allowed me to sit in on one or two film sessions. And when that season came to a controversial end, Knight included me among the seven writers he handpicked from the entire nation to hear his side of "Zero Tolerance."

That was a really sad time, the fall of Bob Knight. It seemed that each day brought a new brush fire to be put out — Neil Reed, Butch Carter, an incident in a restaurant, an encounter with a student.

Knight didn't survive it and neither did I. By the time he was formally fired, the IU beat belonged to somebody else.

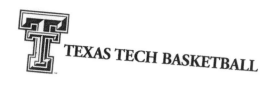

TEXAS TECH BASKETBALL

April 18, 2003

Lynn Houser
The Herald-Times
P.O. Box 909
Bloomington, IN 47402-0909

Dear Lynn:

It was really nice of you to take the time to drop me a note after our game with Nebraska in February. I appreciate very much your thoughtfulness in doing so.

I thought that Emmett would be as good a player as Cheaney was, but he just doesn't have the constant determination that Calbert had to be good on every possession. Our team really struggled this year, as we didn't have the inside game necessary to play in this league. I underestimated greatly how much we were going to miss Andy Ellis.

Again, I appreciated your note and your remarks. Best wishes to you and your family in all that you do.

Sincerely,

Bob Knight
Basketball Coach

BK:md

1701 INDIANA AVE.   BOX 42220   LUBBOCK, TX 79409-2220   806-742-7600   FAX: 806-742-0200
An EEO/Affirmative Action Institution

Even after Knight moved on to Texas Tech, he and Houser kept in touch. In this letter, written in 2003, Knight discusses his Red Raiders team.

I was actually on my way to cover a Colts game when the news of Knight's firing broke that September morning. My heart sank at the thought that the Knight era had come to such an inglorious end. A month into his unemployment, Knight was thoughtful enough to ask me to join him for a round of golf. I'll never forget what he said: "I'm mad at a lot of people, but the person I'm the most mad at is myself. I should have left five years ago."

Six months later, when he was hired by Texas Tech, the H-T sent me to Lubbock to cover the story. Knight spotted me in the mob of reporters and asked me to come back stage. He put one of his massive arms on my shoulder and promised to take me to lunch that day.

He honored that promise and also granted me an exclusive interview, an interview that went on for a good 90 minutes. Let's just say that one-on-one interviews of that length with Knight are as rare as a losing seasons for him.

I still keep in touch with him by way of short letters, and he always takes the time to respond. We are not best buddies or anything, but I think he grew to respect me. That's all a reporter can ask for.

When he becomes college basketball's all-time winningest coach tonight or some night soon, I'm going to drop him another note and tell him how much I respect him. I want to make sure he knows how much he impacted my life in that two-year window. If I wasn't a better journalist for it, I at least came out a stronger person.

Chapter 8
Out of the Blues Comes 2002

Out the despair following the firing of Knight came the wondrous 2001-02 season. Who could have foreseen Indiana's run to the Final Four? But sometimes fate, fortune and fantasy all come together in one place. That's about the only way to sum up the 2002 tournament run for Indiana. I hopped along the trail at the Sweet Sixteen in Lexington, where the Hoosiers rocked No. 1 Duke. Even now, it still seems miraculous.

Ever Leary of Duke

My press row seat for the 2002 regional finals in Lexington put me right next to Todd Leary, the former IU player and then color man for Hoosier basketball. Leary had a special disdain for Duke, having been on the Hoosiers' 1992 Final Four team that felt robbed in the semifinal by questionable officiating. Watching Leary try to maintain decorum throughout the Duke nail-biter was almost as entertaining as the game itself.

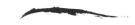

Bloomington Herald-Times
March 23, 2002

LEXINGTON, KENTUCKY

For about two hours Thursday night, Todd Leary was reliving a very bad dream.

Almost 10 years to the week, Leary was a sophomore on the Indiana basketball team that lost to Duke in the 1992 NCAA semifinals, 81-78. It was a game the Hoosiers led by double figures the first half, only to succumb to a Duke comeback aided by a series of calls that went against the Hoosiers the second half, not the least of which was a technical foul called on the IU bench.

"The thing I remember more than anything was the technical foul we got for jumping up and cheering," said Leary before taking his seat as a color man for the IU radio network. "I think we reacted to a charging foul. We didn't yell or anything. I just have never seen a call like that before, especially in a game of that magnitude. For some reason, I remember that more than anything else in the game."

Leary almost single-handedly rallied the Hoosiers to a miraculous finish with a trio of 3-pointers in the last 90 seconds, but by then the deficit was too great.

"It was just luck," he said. "The shots went in and I'm glad they did, but it didn't amount to much. It made the margin of the loss smaller than it would have been. I wish I would have hit another one to get it into overtime just to see what would happen."

It wasn't a game Leary wanted to save for his video library.

"I have only watched the game once, on ESPN Classic about two years ago," he said. "I can remember so many charging calls on us. You just don't see that many charging calls on one team in one game -- I don't care who it is, what game it is, especially in the Final Four.

"It was a tough loss because at halftime we felt we were a lot better team than they were. Everybody felt we could beat them. They had (Christian) Laettner, (Grant) Hill, (Bobby) Hurley and all those guys. Like a lot of teams when they face Indiana, they had the names you know.

"You felt like you are the underdog going into it, but at halftime we didn't. We felt we were the better team."

Four Indiana starters fouled out — Calbert Cheaney, Eric Anderson, Greg Graham and Damon Bailey. It was a somber Indiana lockerroom in the aftermath, Leary said.

"It was awful, terrible. It was silent. It was still awful after a few days because of the build-up of going into the Final Four was so great and we had so much fun. The letdown of going home after one day was a real bummer."

Leary would have liked the chances of that '92 Indiana team against the Duke team this year's Hoosiers were going up against in Thursday night's third-round game at Rupp Arena. "It's a little bit different situation," he said minutes before tip-off. "We had some All-Americans, more than one. We had a really good, talented team that played well together. This Indiana team plays really hard and plays really well together, but I'm not sure they have as much talent as we had."

Leary did paint a scenario for a Hoosier victory, though.

"Tonight, this team will have to shoot the ball well. If they shoot the ball well, it will be a basketball game. They have to cut down on their turnovers, don't allow Duke get up and down the court too much. And Indiana has to score inside. If they score inside, Duke will either have to foul them or Indiana will dominate the interior."

The first half was a recipe for an Indiana defeat. Sixteen turnovers led to 23 Duke points as the Blue Devils rolled to a 17-point lead. It was all the Hoosiers could do to get the deficit down to 13 at halftime, 42-29.

Even from his broadcaster's seat, Leary was animated from the start, experiencing some deja vu when he thought too many calls were going Duke's way.

"I hate to complain about officiating," he said on the air, "but everything seems to be leaning toward Duke."

Leary would wince, would moan, would pound his fist, would shake his head — and that was before the Hoosiers really made a game of it. As the Hoosiers crept closer and closer, Leary could hardly control himself.

"I can't talk, Don," he said on the air to play-by-play man Don Fischer. "I've got chills. This is college basketball at its best."

When Tom Coverdale hit a baseline jumper to put the Hoosiers ahead in the final minute, Leary abandoned all decorum.

"Don, I can't sit," he said. "I don't care if they throw me off press row, I've got to stand."

Leary's angst was justified when IU's Dane Fife fouled Duke's Jason Williams as Williams was making a 3-pointer with the Hoosiers nursing a four-point lead in the final seconds.

"I can't believe what I just saw," Leary wailed.

Fortunately for Fife, Williams missed the tying free throw and the Hoosiers survived, 74-73. By this time, Leary was on standing on his chair, waving a clenched fist.

"We're here to Saturday, boys," he beamed, delighting in the fact that the Hoosiers were still playing while the Dukies were going home.

In the bedlam on the court, Fife came over to the radio booth and playfully exchanged punches with Leary. As Fife recalled the exchange, "Leary said, 'What the heck were you thinking?' I took a swing at Leary, and he took a swing at me. We almost got in a brawl."

Leary worded it a little differently. "We made eye contact and Fife grinned. I said, 'You dumb---, I ought to hit you in the mouth.' He knew he had escaped death. If they had lost he could not have gone back to Bloomington. He would have had to finish his classes through correspondence courses."

When some calm had been restored, Leary put his head set back on and rejoined Fischer, who was still trying to put the game in perspective.

"Don, why don't you get off the air so you can enjoy this?" Leary said. "You are the biggest professional I've ever seen, and I am the biggest rookie in the world."

Editor's Note: In 2009, Leary was arrested for real estate fraud and wound up serving some jail time. However, since his release he has spoken openly about his mistakes and is now getting his life back together in Carmel.

The (Blue) Devil Made Fife Do It

Only the hand of God – first on a missed free throw, then on a missed putback -- prevented guard Dane Fife from being the ultimate goat in IU's quest to beat Duke.

Bloomington Herald-Times
March 22, 2002

LEXINGTON, KENTUCKY

If Dane Fife was not a God-fearing man before, he is now.

Fife was looking as if he had just been condemned to eternal fire after committing basketball's mortal sin — fouling a 3-point shooter with a four-point lead.

Against No. 1 Duke, yet.

With a date in the regional final beckoning.

But sure enough, there was Fife getting too close to Duke's Jason Williams as the latter sank a 3-pointer with the Hoosiers clinging to a four-point lead in the last five seconds of Thursday's NCAA white-knuckler.

Of course Fife, forever in denial, argued that Williams took a flop, but that was beside the point. College basketball's player of the year was going to the line to shoot a potential tying free throw with 4.2 seconds left.

"He (Williams) did a very good job of drawing attention to make it look like a foul," Fife claimed. "That's what any smart player would do. I've seen that stuff happen before. I didn't think it would happen to me, but I should not have even went for it. He just fell down."

To Fife's momentary relief, Williams missed the free throw, but that wasn't the end of it. Duke's other All-American, forward Carlos Boozer, collared the rebound and had a very makeable putback. Boozer also missed and, after a couple of wild swipes at the ball, IU's Jeff Newton came down with it rebound as time ran out on the defending national champions.

"There is a 99 out of a 100 percent chance Williams is going to make that shot," Fife said. "I hate to credit God, but I think he was on our side. And then he helped us again when Boozer missed."

Indiana 74, Duke 73.

Does that score ring a bell? How about Indiana 74, Syracuse 73 — the final score when Indiana won its last national championship 15 years ago. In many ways this felt like an NCAA title game.

"This is a history-making game," said Jarrad Odle, IU's senior forward. "Any time you can be a part of that, it is amazing."

One person who could really appreciate it was assistant coach Jim Thomas, who played on IU's 1981 national champions.

"For this group here, this is a very proud moment," Thomas said. "We had lost a valuable scorer in Kirk Haston (who left early for the NBA). We weren't sure how they would respond. Each month they would get better and better. It was a proud achievement to see our guys play against one of the best teams in the nation and come out with a victory."

Fife credited the coaches with "selling" them on the idea they could beat Duke by just playing their game.

"We were a little skeptical because it was Duke," he said. "They (coaches) made us believers right when we found out we were going to play them."

"It kind of made us mad that we were 12 1/2-point underdogs," said Tom Coverdale, IU's junior guard. "We knew they were a great basketball team, but that was a slap in the face. They can keep slapping us in the face as much as we want."

However, there were plenty of doubts after the Blue Devils pounced all over the Hoosiers and led by as much as 17 points the first half. Asked if the Hoosiers were playing scared, Fife answered, "I don't think we were scared at all. We were just so fired up, had so much adrenaline, we weren't thinking. We weren't concentrating. It had nothing to do with being scared. We were just too fired up. I mean, it's Duke, guys."

The Hoosiers felt fortunate to be down by just 13 at halftime, 42-29.

"We took their best shot and were only down 13," Newton said.

"Certainly, when you're down 13 at halftime, you are wondering what the heck is going on," Fife said. "We felt we took their best shot, particularly in the first five minutes. What we had to do was just go out and lay it on the line. We were just too hyped up."

Moye, Newton Heading Home

Riding a wave of momentum following the enormous upset of Duke, Indiana hit Kent State with a barrage of 3-pointers in the regional final and went on to punch their ticket to the Final Four in Atlanta.

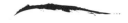

Bloomington Herald-Times
March 24, 2002

LEXINGTON, KENTUCKY

Who says you can't go home again? Tell that to Indiana's Jeff Newton and A.J. Moye.

They are homeward bound to Atlanta for the Final Four after helping the Hoosiers defeat Kent State in the regional finals Saturday, 81-69.

"It hasn't sank in yet, man," said Newton, a junior forward out of Mays High in Atlanta. "I'm going to the 'house.' I just can't wait to get there."

"Me and Newt — that's my brother," said Moye, a sophomore guard who followed Newton to IU from Atlanta Westlake. "I love him. That's why I came here, right after him. I get to go home. Everybody can't come to the game — I'm telling you guys now. It's going to be ticket hell, but I'm going to get so much love. I'm probably going to go down to the radio station, tell everybody to come out and support me. There are so many faces I miss, so many faces who helped me become the man I am today."

Making the Final Four was in the back of Hoosier minds from the very beginning, Moye recalled.

"It was pre-season conditioning. Coach (John) Treloar stopped it and said he was never more excited about basketball than he was this year. We put a plan in motion right there."

"Nobody believed in us but us," said senior forward Jarrad Odle, who prepped at Oak Hill. "We were the ones who knew we could get it done. Making the Final Four, you can't imagine that. It's such a great feeling. To be able to look up to your parents, the ones that took you to AAU practice to get you better at basketball, that's what makes it the best."

Odle was a part of an early 3-point assault that vaulted the Hoosiers to a 12-3 lead, a lead that would never dip under seven points. By halftime the Hoosiers were 9-for-11 from the arc and by game's end they were an amazing 15-for-19. Against Duke Thursday night they were just 2-for-10.

"Our plan was to go inside," Odle said. "That kind of hit the wall when we hit our first couple 3s. When I stepped out and knocked one down, you knew something was going to happen. Our guards really stepped up and shot the ball. They didn't have a lot of opportunities against Duke, but tonight they stepped up and did it."

As Moye observed, "I guess Kent State thought they had to shut down (Jared) Jeffries first and they paid. I thought, 'What are they doing?' They were leaving everybody open. We probably got six, seven guys who hit for 20 this year. They found out tonight."

We are not a fluke. We're in the Final Four. We did not have the easy road. We beat Duke, 'lottery heaven.' If you let us shoot, it's Russian Roulette. You're putting yourself on the crap table and they crapped out."

Even with the incredible 3-point shooting, the Hoosiers still had to weather a furious charge by the Flashes, who scored 13 straight points to cut a 20-point deficit down to seven with 6:38 left. In the eye of the storm was Indiana freshman Donald Perry, who had to come in for Tom Coverdale when the junior guard went down with an ankle sprain at the 9:35 mark.

"At first I was just trying to protect the lead instead of attack," he said. "I was nervous because they were making a run. We knew they were going to make a run. Coach told us before the game, 'If you going to be a champion, you've got to be able to take their best shot and keep going.' They were trying to get me rattled. Once we called a timeout and got situated, we started breaking it pretty easy."

Perry scored one basket and set up two others as the Hoosiers held on.

"We all know what Don can do," Newton said. "We knew we would withstand their best shot, as long as we kept playing, kept playing. They had to come to us."

"These games come down to playing with heart," Odle said.

By George, by Donald

A couple of roll players, Donald Perry and George Leach, came up big in the win over Oklahoma in the NCAA semifinals.

Bloomington Herald-Times
March 31, 2002

ATLANTA, GEORGIA

It is safe to say that Indiana would not have beaten Oklahoma if it weren't for the play off the bench of sophomore George Leach and freshman Donald Perry. Both played pivotal minutes — Leach in the first half, Perry the second half.

Perry came in for Tom Coverdale when the injured guard had finally hit empty with just over three minutes left. In the previous minute, Coverdale had just committed his fourth and fifth turnovers of the game. The ankle he sprained a week ago was about to blow.

"Tom gutted it out and did his best," said assistant coach John Treloar. "Tom is a competitor. He wanted to be out there, but injury-wise, he had given all he could give. He was gone."

Thrust into hot seat was Perry, who had the benefit of a week's preparation with the first unit while Coverdale rested his badly sprained ankle.

"I had more 'reps' in practice, got a little more confidence and got a little more used to the system," said Perry, who was ready to answer the call from Coach Mike Davis. Perry already had contributed five points and one assist in eight minutes of play earlier in the game.

"Coach saw I wasn't playing scared," he said.

Perry came in and delivered one of the game's biggest baskets. With just over two minutes to play and the Hoosiers leading, 62-60, Perry came down on a 2-and-1 break with Jared Jeffries and took it all the way to the house.

"Jared kind of picked his man. All I had to do was beat one man," he said.

Said Jeffries, "I always tell Donald, 'If you're on a break with me, go ahead and drive to my side because I'll hold my guy up.' Donald recognized that and got a layup."

Perry then sank five of six free throws in the remaining time to send Indiana into Monday night's title game against Maryland.

"Down the stretch, Donald Perry stepped up big for us," Treloar said. "He had to bring it home for us.

"Basketball is basketball no matter what age you are," said Perry, who was expecting Coverdale to start. "I saw that he was running pretty well. I just came out more aggressive. Coach just told me to go with my instincts. I was under control. Whether there are 5,000 people out there or 50,000, it's still basketball."

"Without Donald, we probably wouldn't have won the game tonight," said Coverdale, who probably would have pulled himself had he been a coach.

"It was more about me being stupid out there," Coverdale said. "I made some stupid plays. They took me out to settle me down and Donald made two great plays. Why take him out when I was hurting the team? There was no reason for me to be in the game at the end. I'd like to say I did that for my team, but this team has been fighting like that all year long. It just wasn't me out there. That's just what makes this team so great."

In addition to some poor decisions, Coverdale said it was a weakening ankle, not stamina, which forced him to the sideline.

"My conditioning was fine," he said. "At the beginning of the game my ankle felt fine, but close to halftime it started hurting. "

At halftime, Coverdale stayed on his feet to keep the ankle from stiffening up.

"I just walked around the whole time, trying to keep it loose. They wouldn't let me sit down because it could tighten up. Toward the end of the game, it was hurting pretty bad. But that is no excuse for the mistakes I made. I'm just glad my teammates picked me up and we got a win. I'll try to do better on Monday. The main thing I need to work on is my jump shot — get my timing back."

Coverdale played 29 minutes and scored just one basket, a 3-pointer. His real value was leadership.

"He gave us a great lift because he gave us regularity," Jeffries said. "He was there to get us into our offense."

Leach played only six minutes, but they were very solid ones. He spelled Jeffries after the Hoosier forward picked up his second foul. Leach made an immediate impact on the defensive end, sending an Aaron McGhee shot into the IU pep band. For the rest of the half he had McGhee and the other Sooner forwards looking over their shoulders.

"I changed some shot selection," said Leach, who averages about nine minutes a game.

Moments later he brought the IU bench and the Hoosier fans to their feet with a thunderous dunk. He finished his six-minute stint with three points, two rebounds and two blocks. He was 1-for-3 from the free throw line.

"I was nervous. That's why I missed those free throws. I don't care who you are, Cov' (Coverdale) or Dane (Fife), you're going to be nervous. I played about four or five minutes, but it felt like forever."

"They better give George a drug test or something," Jeffries joked. "The whole bench was jumping up and down, waving towels. He just played unbelievable."

Leach went in with the Hoosiers in danger of falling behind by double figures and helped them close the gap to four by halftime. Had Leach succumbed to nerves, Jeffries was prepared to go back into the game despite his two fouls.

"The coaches said, 'If we get too far down, we will have to put you back in.' But they (the entire team) just played great. I did not have to go back in."

Jeffries was more than willing to let George do it.

"You've got to understand," he said. "This was the biggest day of George's life. He gets my MVP vote for the game."

Hoosiers Walk Away with Heads Held High

The 2002 run came up one win short of an improbable title. Maryland ended the dream season with a 64-52 decision in the title game. Fifteen years earlier, I had been in the Syracuse lockerroom after the Orangemen lost a 74-73 heartbreaker to IU in the championship game. This time I was in IU lockerroom, observing how the Hoosiers handled a devastating defeat. Like the Orangemen of 1987, the 2002 Hoosiers demonstrated lots of class.

Bloomington Herald-Times
April 2, 2002

ATLANTA, GEORGIA

Having never lost an NCAA title game in five previous tries, Indiana is not about moral victories or second-place finishes, but these Hoosiers had every reason to hold their heads high after Monday's 64-52 loss to Maryland.

For a program of such tradition to go a decade between trips to the Final Four, the 2001-2002 Hoosiers brought it back to where they felt it belonged.

"We just made a lot of Indiana fans happy and surprised a lot of people," said Dane Fife, one of two seniors on the team along with Jarrad Odle. "It was very exciting up to this point. It was a great atmosphere to be in, an amazing situation. I was proud, but I was angry because we lost. I thought we could beat Maryland. They were just awesome tonight, especially down the stretch."

It was a subdued Indiana lockerroom — quiet enough to hear the Terrapin fans still celebrating out in the arena.

"We would like to be still out there on the court, but you have to give Maryland credit," junior guard Tom Coverdale said. "They made the plays champions make down the stretch and we didn't."

Coverdale was forced to labor on his injured ankle by the constant pressure of Maryland guard Steve Blake.

"Blake kept me fullcourt the whole time, so I had to work," Coverdale said. "Their defense in general was great. It (the ankle) bothered me, but it didn't force any mistakes on my part. I can't use that as an excuse at all. I thought I had too many turnovers (4) for a point guard."

"Coverdale had no explosiveness because of the ankle, and Blake is tough, is quick, and he guarded him," assistant coach John Treloar said. "I think another thing they tried to do was get their guys out on Fife and (Kyle) Hornsby at all costs, take away their 3s and make them drivers. They did a good job."

"I could hear Coach Williams saying, 'Don't let 'em shoot 3s. Make 'em drive,' " Hornsby said. "We tried to force some things — everybody did. Whether it was them trying to force some things and we went with it, but I felt we tried to force some things early and maybe late."

Indiana suffered through a similar start against Duke but was able to overcome a 17-point deficit. Although Maryland's biggest lead was only 11 points the first half, the Terps had more answers in the second half.

"This was a totally different game (than Duke)," Hornsby said. "They (Maryland) were never up that much. They had much more of an inside presence than Duke. That was the biggest part of this game. Their inside game was really good."

The Hoosiers were able to exploit Duke's weak interior, but the Terps had too many wide bodies. Forwards Jared Jeffries, Jeff Newton and Odle could hardly get close to the basket because of Maryland's sheer mass.

"Everything we put up got blocked because their big guys are so athletic," Hornsby said.

"They wore us down," Newton said. "It showed at the end of the game. They had four big guys and they were all skilled. We made one move and another guy was there to help them."

"They've got five big bodies that they rotate in out and out," Treloar said. "Jared probably gives up 60 pounds to those guys. They're big, they're strong and they're good. Jared was working, trying to get the shots, but they weren't coming easy. They defended him."

It was all Jeffries could do to manage eight points and seven rebounds.

"Jared is such an unselfish guy," Hornsby said. "That's what makes this team so good. If he would force some things, I'm sure he would do better, but the team wouldn't be as good. They had guys there every time he tried to make a move. I thought he did a pretty good job considering the circumstances."

The Hoosiers did not want to get in a track meet with the Terps and succeeded in making it a halfcourt game.

"We were at the pace we wanted to be, a low-scoring, tempo game," Treloar said. "But they were able to just get a little ahead and we just couldn't catch them."

"Legacy is an awful big word, but I hope these guys get a taste of what we did this year and will be back next year fighting for the same thing," Odle said. "I think we put Indiana basketball back to where people are used to seeing it. I think that was a very big for me and Dane as the season went on."

"It's hard to enjoy right now, but after we look back, I think we will be proud of ourselves," Coverdale said. "We got Indiana back to competing for national championships."

"People know us now. People know we are back on the map," Newton said.

"We brought a resurgence back to the name of Indiana," sophomore A.J. Moye said.

"To play with these guys was a tremendous experience, an honor," Hornsby said. "It was just so fun. Everybody liked each other and were happy for each other. Never have I played on a team like this. There are much worse things in life than losing basketball games. This hurts a lot. To have it end like this feels badly, but there are many more important things to look forward to."

Flashbacks of a Final Four Run

The same after-glow that followed IU's 1987 Final Four run spilled over into another look-back column a few days after the Hoosiers settled for second.

Bloomington Herald-Times
April 5, 2002

No, it still hasn't sunk in, this most unexpected, unbelievable, unthinkable, unfathomable tournament run by the Indiana basketball team.

But I've been saying that for 15 years, ever since I had the privilege of witnessing Indiana's last run to NCAA glory.

With all respect to the 1992 Hoosiers, who advanced to the Final Four but no further, their success was not all that startling because they were a strong team from the first tip-off. The same can be said of the '87 Hoosiers, who went the distance.

But this year's Hoosiers ... well, 'fess up. How many of you had them advancing past the first round? For a team that was mediocre in December, a team that sputtered to the Big Ten finish line in February, a team that was smarting from an Iowa-Luke Recker dagger in the Big Ten Tournament, for such a team to reach college basketball's ultimate game is the stuff of legend.

For me, it comes back like this:

* Jared Jeffries dominating the second halves of the UNC-Wilmington and Duke games.

* Jarrad Odle almost single-handedly keeping IU in the game against Duke with five buckets in the first five minutes of the second half.

* The electricity in Rupp Arena, home of rival Kentucky, as a pro-Indiana crowd sensed a Hoosier upset if they could only get Duke's lead down to a single digit.

* Sitting next to the IU radio team of Don Fischer and Todd Leary as the urgency and expectancy of their voices buoyed you for another chapter in Indiana's grand history.

* The looks on the faces of the Blue Devils as IU's relentlessness began to break their will.

* Seeing the Indiana bench standing and reacting to every play down the stretch.

* The look of absolute anguish on the face of Dane Fife after his foul gave Duke's Jason Williams a chance to tie the game with a 4-point play with four seconds left.

* The audible groan of Leary as Carlos Boozer rebounded Williams's missed free throw and went up for a winning putback.

* The look of utter relief on Fife's face after Boozer missed, Jeff Newton rebounded and Indiana had its astounding upset.

* The look on the face of Duke coach Mike Krzyzewski as he realized his defending champions had just been dethroned by an Indiana team not coached by Bob Knight.

* IU coach Mike Davis running around looking for somebody to hug like North Carolina State's Jim Valvano in 1983.

* Jeffries high-fiving his way toward the IU locker room while proclaiming, "Those are all men in there."

* The collective moans of the Kent State section each time a Hoosier sharpshooter loaded up for a 3-point shot during a 15-for-19 binge from the arc.

* The sickening feeling when replays showed how severely Tom Coverdale rolled his ankle in the second half against Kent State.

* The panic when Indiana's 20-point lead melted away in minutes after Coverdale went down.

* The relief when Fife stopped the bleeding with the biggest 3-point shot of his career.

* The hustle of Kyle Hornsby, going horizontal to keep a ball from going out of bounds and flipping it to Fife for a clinching lay-up.

* Jeffries parading Coverdale around in a wheelchair as the Hoosiers celebrated a regional title.

* The anxiety of seeing Coverdale on crutches in the days leading up to the Final Four.

* The feeling that all was right with the world when Coverdale trotted out for the opening tip against Oklahoma.

* The chants of "A.J. Moye" reverberating around the Georgia Dome in his native Atlanta.

* Seeing Jeff Newton, IU's other Atlanta native, celebrate his homecoming with the highest scoring game of his career, 19 points.

* Watching Donald Perry grow up in a month, from a shaky freshman to a player Davis trusted with the game on the line against Kent State and Oklahoma.

* Seeing Hornsby go from a reluctant shooter to a player calling for the ball at big moments -- and delivering.

* Seeing George Leach's "game" face after he sent an Oklahoma shot into orbit.

* The look in Fife's eyes as he locked in on Oklahoma's Hollis Price and Maryland's Juan Dixon.

* The look in the eyes of those defensive targets as they realized Fife was not going to go away.

* The emptiness that settled in when it became apparent that Indiana was going to come up short of a national championship.

* The class the Hoosiers showed in defeat -- no excuses, no grumbling, no pointing fingers.

* Seeing Jeffries consoling Odle as they left the court, heads held high.

* Seeing Moye withdraw into the solace of his locker, unable to put into words the emotions he felt.

* Seeing Coverdale handle tough questions, with his swollen ankle submerged in a tub of ice water.

* Hearing Hornsby talk about the "honor" of playing with so many selfless young men.

* Feeling the love from one end of the lockerroom to the other.

They say it takes awhile for such moments to really sink in, that it takes the passage of time for you to really appreciate them. Although second place leaves Indiana followers somewhat unfulfilled, this is one time where second almost feels like first. The Hoosiers may not be champions, but without question they are winners.

Give yourself a little time to think about it, to let it sink in. That empty feeling will surely go away.

Fife One of Dane's Toughest Foes

One of the things you had to like about Dane Fife was his candidness. In this interview in the summer following his graduation, he talked about the demons he had to confront in his playing days at IU.

Bloomington Herald-Times
August 25, 2002

For four years Dane Fife gave the impression of a supremely confident basketball player -- one who gave maximum effort, one who exuded toughness, one who walked with a swagger.

That was what you saw on the outside. On the inside was a boiling cauldron of insecurities. No matter how many ways Fife made Indiana a better basketball team, his struggles on offense tormented him. It got to the point where he sought medical help.

Fife came to Indiana with the expectations of being a college star. He had every right to think that after averaging over 23 points a game his last three years of high school and winning Michigan's Mr. Basketball honors in 1998. He also was named a McDonald's All-American.

But somewhere in his first two years at IU, Fife lost faith in his abilities. Even though he immediately became a regular on Bob Knight's 1998-99 team, Fife was on the floor because of his defense, not his offense. Fife certainly wasn't the first freshman to struggle on the offensive end, but he remained in that state for three years. Although his coaches and teammates could count on him for defense and effort, his offensive game was anything but reliable.

"I was a very good scorer in high school because I could get into the lane," Fife said. "I could always outsmart guys and usually out-work them, too. College was a different game. I came in thinking I was a much better shooter than I was."

Fife would get his share of points in practice, but when the bright lights came on, his confidence dimmed.

"I was very narrow-minded on the basketball floor," he said. "I wasn't creative."

With the likes of A.J. Guyton, Luke Recker and Kirk Haston on the floor with him, Fife tended to look for their shots first and his shot as an afterthought. When the time did come for him to pull the trigger, it wasn't with a confident hand. Although he appeared in all 33 games his freshman year, starting 11 of them, he took only 80 shots. He made 45 percent from the field and 24 percent from the 3-point line. He averaged 3.3 points, hitting double figures just twice and topping out at 13 points.

Fife's sophomore year wasn't much better, even though the transfer of Recker theoretically opened up more offensive opportunities. Fife started 22 of 27 games and took just 101 shots, hitting 45 percent again. He took 15 fewer 3-pointers and connected at a poorer rate, 23 percent. He averaged 4.9 points with five double-digit games. He could only match his modest personal high of 13.

At the insistence of coach Mike Davis, Fife started taking more shots his junior year, but his field goal percentage dipped to a career-low 37 percent. He did score 15 points in one game but reached double figures only three times.

Fife was keenly aware these were not the numbers of a high school All-American, and he finally sought the help of his family doctor in Clarkston, Mich., Dr. Larry Bayless. Bayless suggested the anti-depressant, Zoloft.

"I don't think I was depressed," Fife said, "but before games and during games I would get so worked up that I couldn't perform. Zoloft also is anti-anxiety."

At the same time Fife sought the counseling of a Bloomington sports psychologist, Dr. Steve Curtis, who specializes in performance skills and has worked with many an IU athlete.

"The college level always comes with a lot more pressure," Curtis says. "Every college athlete needs to know how to manage that stress and the expectations of high performance. Shooting a basketball is a fine motor skill. Dane had lost confidence in his shooting. For a couple of years he didn't look for his shot because he believed he couldn't put it in."

"I was basically dealing with the 'choke' mechanism," Fife said. "All I could think about was, 'I play against those guys in practice, I know I can get around them, I know I could do things, but it's just not happening.' I could make a lay-up in the seventh grade better than I could my first couple of years in college. I'm speaking the truth."

Once Fife lost his self-esteem, he also started to lose the belief he could play professional ball.

"The larger picture for Dane was more complicated," Curtis said. "His performance the first couple years here caused him to conclude he had no chance of playing at the next level. When he lost those larger expectations, he lost his vision for the future in regards to basketball. I find when people don't have a clear next step in their life, they show signs of anxiety and depression. There is grief over the loss of the dream and the failure to have another one in its place."

Curtis recommended a diet of physical and mental exercise. The physical exercises were designed to strengthen his legs, a vital component in any jump shot.

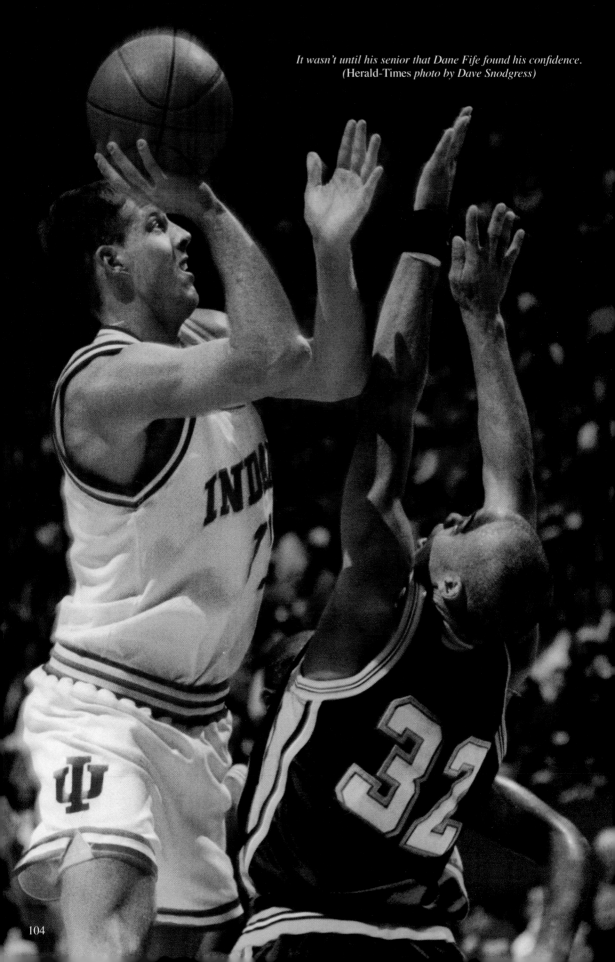

It wasn't until his senior that Dane Fife found his confidence.
(Herald-Times *photo by Dave Snodgress)*

"The first couple of years I remember Dane falling down a lot," Curtis noted. "Kids that are anxious and nervous often lose their balance. With confidence you play with a more stable base, which allows you to be a better shooter."

To build up his legs, Fife took to the hills, running up and down the local slopes. The mental exercises involved positive thinking.

"We talked about calming down and 'feeling' the basketball, stop feeding people and start working on your own skills," Curtis said.

"Dr. Curtis taught me how to relax, how to re-train my mind during games," Fife said. "He told me to 'Feel your feet touching the floor, feel your hands touching the ball, feel your hand grabbing the guy's jersey.' My floor vision came back."

Between the anti-depressant and the power of positive thinking, Fife was a new man his senior year.

"I was almost too calm," he said. "Before this season, and the guys will tell you this, I would be jumping around, could not sit down. Before games this year, I was just sitting there, chilling. I call Zoloft the 'Jump Shot Pill.' I still take it."

And what a difference a year made. Fife shot 46 percent from the field and even better from the 3-point line, 48 percent. He averaged 8.1 points and scored in double figures 17 times, with a single-game high of 23. In one 20-point explosion against Illinois, Fife nailed five of six 3-pointers.

"I was in a zone against Illinois," he said. "I had never been in the zone before."

Fife was not the least bit afraid to shoot critical times. He made perhaps the biggest shot of the post-season when the Hoosiers were caving in to a furious Kent State rally in the regional final.

With a 20-point lead having dwindled to seven and the basket starting to shrink for Indiana, Fife stepped forward and delivered the 3-pointer that averted the collapse. Would he have had the nerve to take that shot back when he was struggling?

"I wouldn't have even been on the floor in that situation," he said. "The first three years was a personal struggle. It was hard for me to focus on winning and losing because I was having an inner battle. This year should have been my freshman year."

"It all came down to the vision and the hard work follows," Curtis said. "Dane had been a great performer in high school. It was just a matter of getting his head back on straight, realizing how good a player he was. I just gave him a road map. He did the work. He had the guts to confront this thing."

'The Block' Made Moye a Big Man on Campus

As the Year 2002 came to a close, the Herald-Times *assigned each of its reporters to capture a unique moment in that calendar year. I chose A.J. Moye's memorable block in the Duke game.*

Bloomington Herald-Times
December 31, 2002

If ever there was a moment frozen in time for A.J. Moye, it occurred on the evening of March 21, 2002, in Lexington, Kentucky.

It was the night Indiana took on mighty Duke in the NCAA South Regional at Kentucky's Rupp Arena. After trailing by as many as 17 points, Indiana had clawed back to within one with a little more than five minutes left.

Duke was trying to add to that lead when its future NBA forward, Carlos Boozer, had the ball on the right baseline, about three feet from the basket. Up went Boozer, all 6-foot-9 and 235 pounds of him. Rising up to challenge him was Moye, generously listed at 6-3, 215 pounds.

But Moye kept going up and up and up — until he was eye-to-eye with Boozer and his left hand was squarely on top of the ball. Boozer stopped abruptly, like an elevator that had run out of floors. Whistles blew as Boozer and Moye descended back to earth.

Jump ball, it was ruled, with the possession arrow pointing in Indiana's direction.

Courtside announcers and writers gasped in disbelief while 22,435 fans — most of them jumping on Indiana's bandwagon by this time — howled with glee. Chants of "A.J. Moye ... A.J. Moye ..." echoed throughout the area.

Hindsight showed this play to be as significant as any in Indiana's 74-73 shocker. Although Moye contributed 14 points, including the free throws that turned out to be the margin of victory, it is that block that made him into the cult hero is on campus today.

"I get asked about that by 90 percent of the people who approach me," said Moye, now a junior on an Indiana squad striving to make some memories of its own.

"It was kind of a David-and-Goliath thing. Like David pulling out the sling shot and taking out Goliath, little ol' me jumped up and blocked that shot."

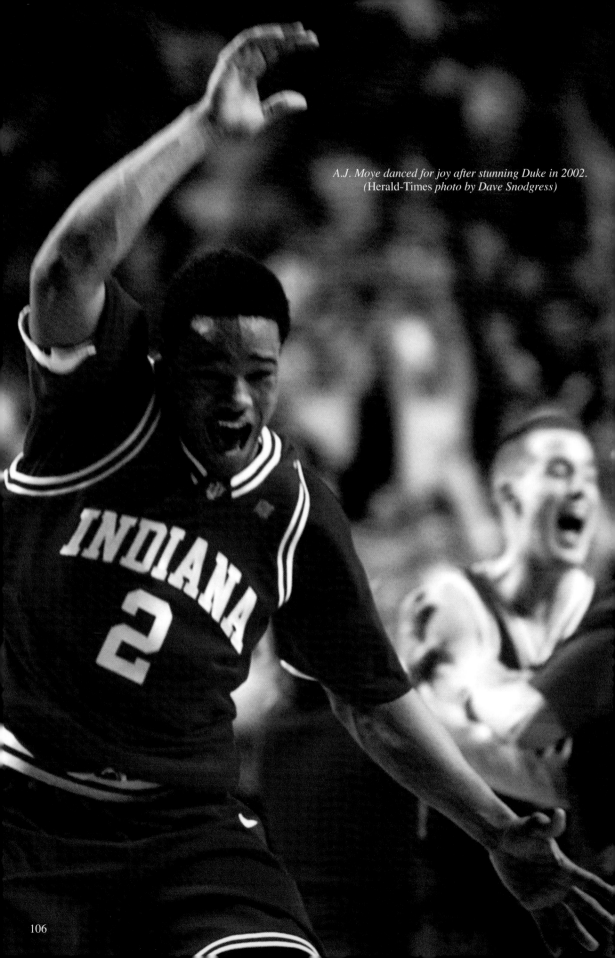

*A.J. Moye danced for joy after stunning Duke in 2002.
(*Herald-Times *photo by Dave Snodgress)*

Two nights later, Moye was homeward bound after Indiana shot down Kent State for a ticket to the Final Four in Atlanta, Moye's home town.

"It was every kid's dream come true, to play in a game of that magnitude, and to play in one's own back yard made it even sweeter," he said.

Moye scored nine points in the 81-69 win over Kent State and contributed nine more in the 73-64 semifinal win over Oklahoma, sending the Hoosiers to the title game against Maryland. That was where the joyride ended, 64-52. In the locker-room after the defeat, Moye could not summon up the words to express his disappointment.

"I didn't want to talk," he said. "I was pretty hurt."

In time Moye was able to appreciate what he and his Hoosier teammates had accomplished. A visit to his old Atlanta neighborhood, East Point, picked his spirits up.

"A lot of people are proud of me, mainly my church," he said. "Where I'm from, it is like they say, 'It takes a whole village to raise a kid.' Everybody was so proud of me, not just my mother (Beverly). People like to be associated with something positive."

But that is old news, Moye said. With the current Hoosiers breaking out to a fast start, it is time to forget the past and focus on the present. "You have to put last year out of your mind and work toward this year," he said. "That run is over. It was a great part of my life, but you've got to move on."

2002: Fortune or Destiny?

After Indiana lost in the second round of the 2003 NCAA tournament, you had to wonder how much good fortune had them going all the way to the title game the year before. For that reason, the magical 2002 run was worth revisiting. The print was barely dry when IU coach Mike Davis called to express his disappointment with this column, claiming IU's run had nothing to do with luck. Read on and judge for yourself.

Bloomington Herald-Times
March 26, 2003

In the aftermath of Indiana's early exit from the 2003 NCAA Tournament, some of the talking heads are wondering if last year's Hoosiers were more lucky than good.

Long before the Hoosiers made this year's field, they were claiming they were a legitimate Final Four team in 2002.

"It couldn't have been a fluke," said junior guard A.J. Moye, one of last year's tournament heroes. "If you watch the games, see the way we rebounded the ball, our spacing on offense ... you can see it was no fluke."

If Indiana's dash to the 2002 Final Four wasn't a freak of nature, it was at least charmed. The "evidence:"

Exhibit A: The opening game against Utah. Having lost its best post player, Duke transfer Chris Burgess, to a season-ending injury, the Utes are no match for Indiana's inside trio of Jared Jeffries, Jeff Newton and Jarrad Odle, who outscore Utah's front line 35-10.

Exhibit B: The Hoosiers are spared a second-round match against fourth-seeded Southern Cal when North Carolina-Wilmington spills the Trojans in overtime, 93-89.

Exhibit C: In the epic game against top-seeded Duke, Jason Williams (college basketball's Player of the Year) fails to take advantage of Hoosier generosity by missing a potential tying free throw with four seconds left.

Exhibit D: Duke's Carlos Boozer, a future NBA draftee, rebounds Williams' errant free throw but can't convert the putback.

Exhibit E: Kent State defeats Pittsburgh, setting up a regional final with Indiana that gives the Hoosiers an emotional edge, a first-round loss to Kent State the year before. Indiana comes out blazing from the 3-point line and wins, 81-69.

Exhibit F: In the NCAA semifinal against Oklahoma, Indiana takes its first lead of the second half on a 3-point shot by Jeffries, a straightaway brick that banks in hard off the glass.

Exhibit G:: Oklahoma forward Aaron McGhee is having his way inside against Indiana until he fouls out on a marginal call with 4:40 to go.

Exhibit H: With the score tied at 60-60, Oklahoma's Daryan Selvy goes to the line with a chance to put the Sooners ahead. Selvy misses the front end of the one-and-one, Newton rebounds and 12 seconds later scores the basket that sends Indiana on its way to a 73-64 victory.

"Man, it's still unbelievable," Newton said in hindsight.

It is said you have to make your breaks in sport, and the Hoosiers did a lot of things to swing those games in their favor.

The biggest thing they did was hit shots. The Hoosiers shot .553 from the field in those five games leading up to the title game, including .529 from the 3-point line. Their 15-for-19 3-point shooting against Kent State would be hard to duplicate in a shootaround, let alone with a hand in the face.

But Indiana had shown earlier in the year that it was capable of going off from the 3-point line. The Hoosiers went 17-for-27 from the arc against Illinois, 16-for-24 against Alaska-Anchorage, 14-for-26 against Michigan State, 11-for-21 against Texas, 11-for-23 against Iowa and 10-for-16 against Eastern Washington. They also hit eight of 13 against Oklahoma.

"We did that (3-point onslaught) a lot," Moye said. "The fact that we did it in the tournament made it seem more significant."

In the tournament the Hoosiers also hit their free throws when they absolutely had to. Before Williams ever missed that potentially tying free throw, the Hoosiers hit their last six attempts from the line in the final three minutes — all coming after reach-in fouls by Duke. And before Boozer could break Hoosier hearts with a rebound basket, Jeffries got enough of the ball to make Boozer put it up too hard. It glanced off the glass and into the hands of Newton as time ran out. Speaking of rebounds, Indiana dominated the boards against Duke, 47-32.

Indiana's defense was there throughout the five-game run, holding the opposition to less than 40 percent shooting (.399).

So, for every bounce or break the Hoosiers got, there also was solid play behind it.

"You can't get to the national championship game being a fluke," senior guard Tom Coverdale said.

Neither can one forget that the Hoosiers also had some obstacles to overcome, particularly a pair of Coverdale ankle injuries. Coverdale injured one ankle in the tournament opener against Utah, then suffered a more severe injury in the second half of the Kent State game.

"Just from the pain I knew I wasn't going to be able to play the rest of the game," said Coverdale, thinking back to the regional final. "I couldn't put any pressure on it. The first thing I said to (trainer) Tim Garl was, 'Am I going to be able to play next week?' He said, 'We'll see.' I had heard him say that too many times. I was scared."

Coverdale played but wasn't up to form. Even though the Hoosiers got by Oklahoma with the help of reserve guard Donald Perry, they ran out of answers against Maryland in the title game.

"Coverdale ran out of gas the second half because (Steve) Blake was really guarding him and, conditioning-wise, he wasn't where he had been," Indiana assistant coach John Treloar noted.

Getting that far was no accident, though, Treloar insisted.

"A lot of hard work went into it. The guys continued to get better from day one. It is an example of what a group of guys can do if everybody is unselfish and pulling in the same direction. That is what those kids did. For the fans it was probably a magical time, but for the players there was the determination to win a national championship."

Chapter 9
Gamers

Ask any sports writer about memorable games he has covered and will be happy to share his favorites. Here are some of mine.

Were You There When Harry Met Destiny?

One of the biggest perks of my days as the Kendallville News-Sun *sports editor was an annual press pass to Notre Dame games. On this particular day, I had a field pass, putting me right there on the sideline for one of the most epic moments in the history of Notre Dame Stadium. It was voted No. 2 on ND's all-time list of greatest home victories, second only to the 31-30 thriller over No. 1 Miami in 1988. The hero for Notre Dame that day was unheralded placekicker Harry Oliver. As you will note, I got a little carried away with hyperbole, but it felt that sensational at the time.*

Kendallville News-Sun
September 22, 1980

SOUTH BEND, INDIANA

You had to be there.

You HAD to be there – South Bend, Ind., September 20, 1980.

At 4:32 p.m., junior Harry Oliver added his name to the long list of Notre Dame legends by booming a 51-yard field goal with time running out to shock Michigan in one of the epic college battles of all time, 29-27.

Instantly, a tidal wave of humanity poured onto the field, mobbing Oliver and the rest of the jubilant Notre Dame players. It was a celebration not seen in South Bend since the Gipper galloped up and down the Irish gridiron.

Only seconds before, victory seemed remote for the Irish. Michigan had rallied from a 26-21 deficit to take a 27-26 lead on a deflected touchdown pass with 41 seconds left.

The Wolverines had methodically driven the length of the field after Phil Carter had given the Irish the lead on a 4-yard run with just over three minutes to play.

The tension grew with every play until Michigan quarterback John Wangler rolled to his right on a third down play and forced a pass into a crowded corner of the end zone. Luckily for him and the Wolverines, Butch Woolfolk got his hand on the ball first, tipping it in the direction of tight end Craig Dunaway. Dunaway dove and caught the ball inches off the ground before rolling out of the end zone.

Six points, Michigan. Heartbreak, Notre Dame.

But wait, there's freshman quarterback Blair Kiel of Columbus coming in for his first varsity test at Notre Dame, and what a test it will be.

He must drive the Irish 80 yards into a stiff wind and a proven Michigan defense. His first pass is nothing to write home about, a floating duck of a throw that receiver Tony Hunter has to wait on for what seems like an eternity.

However, Hunter is bumped by a Wolverine defender, resulting in a pass interference call at the Michigan 48.

Two incomplete passes later, the Irish face a third-and-10 situation. Kiel hits Carter for nine yards to the Michigan 39 with seconds remaining. Facing a fourth-and-one play with no time-outs left, the Irish must make a crucial decision. Do they gamble for six or do they go for a first down and try to get as close as possible for Oliver to try a field goal?

The Irish opt for the latter and get their first down on a 5-yard wing pass to Hunter, who almost does not get out of bounds.

Four seconds showed on the clock as Oliver lines up the ball on the right hash mark, 51 yards away from the south goal post.

With the wind blowing in from the south, a hush falls over the crowd as if Oliver is facing a firing squad.

But this is Notre Dame, where miracles are seemingly manufactured on the gridiron. Can Oliver pull off the possible?

Oliver keeps his head down and booms a line drive that hooks inside the upright for a heart-stopping finish. He never sees it go through himself, thanks to an onrushing Michigan lineman who flattens him while desperately trying to block the kick.

What a sight it was to see the spontaneous eruption of hysterical fans pouring out of the stands! It took almost 10 minutes for the police to escort Notre Dame coach Dan Devine off the playing field, and the band waited long after that to perform its post-game show. Even then, the band had lots of company on the field as the crowd lingered for a half hour.

For Michigan, it was a bitter defeat – with a twist of irony to it. A similar sight was seen at Michigan last year when Anthony Carter caught a 50-yard touchdown pass from Wangler on the final play of the game to stun Indiana, 27-21.

This time, the Wolverines were the victims. Many of the Michigan players milled around the field in a state of shock after Oliver's heroics.

Also ironic was the fact that Michigan lost to Notre Dame on a last-second field goal attempt last year at Ann Arbor. Only then it was the Wolverines who were trying to win it with a three-pointer. Trailing 12-10, Michigan lined up for a 37-yarder, but Bob Crable smothered the kick to ensure the win for Notre Dame.

You had to feel some compassion for the Wolverines, who stormed back from a 14-0 deficit with three touchdowns in an eight-minute span over the second and third quarters to take a 21-14 advantage.

They completely turned the game around and almost tucked it away when Wangler made a crucial mistake, a pass interception that John Krimm ran back 49 yards for a Notre Dame touchdown. Even though Oliver missed the extra point – with the wind at his back yet – the momentum was back on Notre Dame's side.

But the Irish still needed a little luck and got it when Michigan fumbled away a scoring chance at the Notre Dame 26 midway through the fourth quarter.

A flea-flicker pass from Hunter to Plymouth's Pete Buchanan moved the ball into Michigan territory on the first play following the turnover.

Carter eventually climaxed the drive with a 4-yard dive to give Notre Dame its five-point lead. A field goal would do Michigan no good at that point.

Undaunted, the Wolverines then put together an 81-yard drive against the Irish "prevent" defense, with the big play being a 39-yard draw play by Woolfolk on third-and-10 at the Irish 41.

From the Notre Dame 2-yard line, the Wolverines tried two unsuccessful line plunges, which forced Wangler to go to the air on third down. His pass easily could have been intercepted had not Woolfolk gotten to it first.

That would have been a fitting finish in itself for this classic struggle, but one more miracle awaited the 59,075 fans.

Years from now, those same fans will be talking of this game in the same breath as Notre Dame's great come-from-behind win over Ohio State in 1934 and the monumental 10-10 tie against Michigan State in 1966. It was that kind of game.

You had to be there.

Editor's Note: Cancer claimed Harry Oliver in August, 2007. He was just 47.

Take That, Pilgrim

The closest thing Indiana had to a small school repeating Milan's 1954 conquest of Muncie Central took place 28 years later when Plymouth outlasted Gary Roosevelt in the 1982 championship game. The game thrilled fans for all of regulation and two overtimes. Milan had its Bobby Plump. Plymouth had its Scott Skiles.

INDIANAPOLIS, INDIANA

Do you believe in miracles?

The city of Plymouth does after Plymouth High School completed a story book season with a pulsating 75-74 double-overtime win over Gary Roosevelt in the state championship game Saturday night at Market Square Arena.

It was the first state title for Plymouth, the smallest school to win it since Milan's memorable 32-30 triumph over Muncie Central in 1954.

But right up there with the "Miracle of Milan" is Saturday's championship game – a game that will be remembered for its human drama more than anything else.

There was Plymouth, a school with an enrollment of 894 students, against Gary Roosevelt, a perennial power with an enrollment of 2,360.

Plymouth was a finesse team that relied on precision passing, team defense and self-discipline. Roosevelt was a power team that employed superior physical ability, blazing speed and a mental toughness that only a school from "The Region" could understand.

Although Plymouth was all-white and Roosevelt mostly black, there were no racial overtones. It was just two schools from northern Indiana going for the most coveted prize in the state.

The end result was one of the greatest championship games of all time, one that lasted longer than any other since 1913. That was the year Wingate upended South Bend in overtime, 15-14.

Save, Skiles!

What made this game unlike any other in recent years was a stubby, 6-foot-2 senior from Plymouth, Scott Skiles.

It was Skiles who saved the Pilgrims time and again with a near-record 39 points, including a dramatic 22-footer at the end of regulation which knotted the score at 60-60.

A free throw by Anthony Stewart with four seconds to go gave the Panthers some insurance at 60-58, but the Pilgrims miraculously worked a play they perfected in practice.

The play called for Skiles to take the inbounds pass and thread his way into an opening for the final shot. In the event Skiles was covered, another teammate would take the inbounds pass and look for Skiles after that.

Skiles was covered, indeed, by two Panther defenders, forcing junior Todd Samuelson to take the pass instead. Samuelson, according to plan, immediately relayed the ball to Skiles on the right sideline.

Skiles got the ball near halfcourt, dribbled straight down the side and drilled the qualizer from inside the NBA 3-point line with a hand in his face.

Plymouth's "impossible dream" was still a possibility, but it took six more minutes before it became a reality.

Working Overtime

In the first three-minute overtime, the Pilgrims quickly fell behind by four points before rallying again.

A short bank shot by sophomore James Johnson cut the deficit to 64-62, and a reverse move by Skiles tied it at 64-all. A free throw by senior Ron Sissel put Plymouth on top with 19 seconds left, but Roosevelt's Renaldo Thomas hit one of two free throws with three seconds left to force a second overtime.

This time it was Plymouth who seized the early lead on a baseline jumper by Skiles and another field goal by Mark Stukenborg.

Roosevelt hung tough on five points by Darryl Scott sandwiched around a pair of free throws by Skiles.

Skiles then hit a double-pumper on a fast break to up Plymouth's lead to 73-70 before Stewart hit from outside to bring the Panthers back within one at the 1:12 mark.

Both teams then missed opportunities from the free throw line in the next minute until Skiles rolled in a couple of charity tosses to give Plymouth a 75-72 advantage with 16 seconds left.

Thomas, the hero of Roosevelt's afternoon upset of No. 1 Evansville Bosse, drove the length of the court and scored, but Plymouth was able to run of the final seven seconds.

Skiles believed the Pilgrims could do it all along.

"It doesn't make any difference if you are a big school or a small school," he said. "The big schools may have more players, but the little schools always have the hope of getting there."

Skiles also felt he would make the game-tying shot. According to Coach Jack Edison, during the time-out preceding Skiles' historic shot, Skiles told the team, "I'm going to hit it."

Then came "Scott's Shot," and Plymouth went on to capture the hearts to small-town Indiana.

Jones-to-Edwards to Victory

As key members of Marion's three-time state champions from 1985-87, Lyndon Jones and Jay Edwards continued their success at Indiana University, helping the Hoosiers to a Big Ten championship in the 1988-89 season. The pivotal games in that title run were one-point victories over a Michigan team that would go on to win the NCAA championship. After squeaking out a 71-70 win in Ann Arbor in January, the Hoosiers were about to fall at home to Michigan until Jones and Edwards combined for a last-second game-winner.

Bloomington Herald-Times
February 20, 1989

It was a situation Marion high school fans felt right at home with: one-point game, time running out, Lyndon Jones with the basketball, looking for his long-time teammate, Jay Edwards.

It is a situation Indiana opponents are beginning to dread. Only a week ago, Purdue felt the pain of an Edwards deuce at 0:04 that sent the Boilers home 64-62 losers.

Sunday, Edwards waited four more seconds to stun Michigan with a trey as time expired, 76-75.

Edwards almost didn't get the ball in time to do anything with it as Jones nearly dribbled away Indiana's chances while looking for his favorite target. With most of the 17,311 fans in attendance were urging Jones to shoot, he spotted Edwards open on the left wing. Edwards got the ball with a fraction under two seconds left and released a 25-foot fallaway jumper that was airborne as the horn sounded.

Edwards never saw the finish of his storybook shot.

"I didn't know if it was going in because I was falling back and (Michigan's) Sean Higgins was in front of me," he said. "Then I heard the crowd screaming. I'm just now realizing it happened."

Michigan's hearts momentarily fluttered when referee Ted Valentine began to wave off the basket, only to be emphatically overruled by fellow official Gary Muncy, who signaled "good" with both arms repeatedly.

The shot might have been the final dagger in Michigan's Big Ten hopes. The Wolverines are now 7-5 in the league, four full games behind the 11-1 Hoosiers. The irony of Sunday's shocker was

the fact that the Wolverines missed two shots in the final five seconds of last month's 71-70 loss to Indiana in Ann Arbor.

Edwards was on the floor when the ball swished through, soon to be joined by delirious teammates, coaches and fans.

"This is the biggest basket of my life," said Edwards, who had a career of them in teaming with Jones to lead Marion to three straight Indiana state championships. "I heard the horn while the ball was in the air. I wouldn't say it was a Hail Mary, but ... Lyndon and I have been through this situation before."

Just 54 seconds earlier, Edwards was at the free throw line with the Hoosiers trailing by four, 75-71. A miss there and the Hoosiers would have needed an even greater miracle to avoid losing at home for the first time this year.

But Edwards converted both ends of the one-and-one to draw the Hoosiers within a single basket. With the 45-second clock due to run out on the Wolverines at 0:09, all the Hoosiers needed was one last defensive stand.

The Wolverines used all 45 seconds before Glen Rice missed a short jumper and Eric Anderson rebounded for Indiana. Anderson lost almost three seconds before locating Jones on the left sideline.

Jones carefully worked the ball up court and stopped at the top of the key with about three seconds left. Ignoring orders from all angles to shoot, Jones passed up a chance to pull the trigger himself.

"It took me about three seconds to get the ball up the court, and I got it to him (Edwards) with about two seconds left," Jones said. "I couldn't hear him, but I saw him coming. He got the shot up, and we won."

Jones admitted he wasn't aware how close he came to dribbling out the clock.

"I wasn't aware of the time," he said, "but after I passed the ball to Jay I looked at the clock, and it had '1' as he was shooting the ball."

Edwards was Jones' first option, Joe Hillman his second and himself his third.

"I was looking for Jay or Joe or to take the ball to the basket," the 6-foot-2 sophomore guard said. "I don't always look for Jay, but I'm glad I did today."

Hillman was in the right corner, screened from Jones' view by a Michigan defender. Hillman wanted the ball as soon as Anderson rebounded Rice's miss.

"I was on the right side of Eric, and he probably should have given the ball to me," Hillman said. "I took off down the right side, but a guy got between him (Jones) and myself."

By this time Edwards was frantically calling for the ball.

"I was screaming at Lyndon, but I don't think he could hear me," Edwards said.

Asked if he enjoys taking the big shot, Edwards replied, "Who wouldn't?"

Put Your Hands Up for Kirk Haston

Following Jay Edwards' heroics against Michigan in 1989, it would be 12 years before Indiana would go from defeat to victory as time expired. (Lynn Washington's buzzer-beater against Michigan State in 2000, covered in Chapter 5, came with the score tied).

On January 7, 2001, Kirk Haston, a 6-foot-10 forward, stepped behind the 3-point line with time running out and hit a shot that is still replayed over and over in the popular Indiana video, "This is Indiana." At the end of that clip, as Haston raises his hands in victory, the viewer is urged to "Put your hands up! Now put your hands up!"

Haston already had become one of my all-time favorites for the inner strength he showed following the unthinkable loss of his mother, Patti Haston, to a killer tornado in 1999 (also covered in Chapter 5). Watching Haston make the improbable 3-pointer to beat Michigan State, I had to wonder if Patti wasn't steering it directly toward the basket.

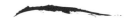

Bloomington Herald-Times
January 8, 2001

The first team other than Indiana to swagger into Assembly Hall ranked No. 1 left the arena Sunday with its ranking surely to fall.

Top-ranked Michigan State was a blink of an eye away from preserving its ranking and unbeaten status, but IU's Kirk Haston swung victory to defeat with a single stroke.

It was Haston, a junior center, who delivered a 3-point dagger at the final buzzer to deal the Spartans a numbing defeat, 59-58.

With the Hoosiers trailing by two and with time running out, Haston took a pass from Kyle Hornsby and pulled the trigger with about 1.4

seconds. By the time the ball splashed through the net, the clock showed all zeroes and the Hoosiers went delirious.

"It's a standard play we run for Hornsby," explained Haston. "I'm kind of the back-up option. It's Hornsby's choice. He might have hit a 2, but I'm glad he made the choice he did."

Zach Randolph, the 6-foot-9 wunderkind out of Marion, rushed over to challenge the shot, making Haston apply more than the usual arch. But having hit Indiana's only other 3-pointers in the game, the 6-10 junior already had a feel for the range.

It put the finishing touches on a 27-point afternoon, easily making him the leading scorer in a defensive grinder that saw no more than six points separate the two rivals. There were 14 ties and 16 lead-changes.

Michigan State twice enjoyed the six-point advantage, the last at 46-40 with 12 minutes left. From there Hoosiers fashioned their best run of the game, scoring the next nine points to take a three-point lead, their biggest.

Haston's second of three 3-pointers pushed the Hoosiers on top, 47-46. His layup off a feed by Jared Jeffries brought the sell-out crowd of 17,128 to its noisiest — until the final delirium.

But there was going to be no pulling away from the nation's No. 1 team. Two baskets by Randolph put MSU in front, 55-53, with 4:13 left. Two free throws by Jeffries tied it at the 3:07 mark. A jumper by Charlie Bell with 2:50 left broke the tie and was to be the last field goal until Haston connected.

The only scoring in the meantime were free throws by Jeffries and Randolph. The Spartans had more free throw chances, however. With the Hoosier fans shaking the building with noise, Jason Richardson twice missed the front ends of bonus opportunities inside the final minute. Randolph rebounded the latter and drew a foul at 11.3 seconds. Assured of two shots, Randolph opened a door by making only one.

"Our fans played a big role," junior guard Dane Fife said. "I'm sure they helped make Michigan State miss those free throws."

The Hoosiers worked the ball to halfcourt and called time with 8.3 seconds remaining. Hornsby, the team leader in 3-pointers, was inserted with the thought of going for the win right there. He had a similar look at a tying 3-pointer against Missouri two weeks ago but missed. Haston was option No. 2.

"I had a good look against Missouri but Kirk had a better one," Hornsby said.

Even with the help of a double-screen, Hornsby couldn't shake Bell, the State's best defender.

"Bell is a good defensive player. You're not going to lose him," Hornsby said. "I thought Kirk was open, but it turned out that Randolph was right on him. He hit a great shot."

"It was the same play we ran against Missouri, but Coach (Mike Davis) got on him a little bit because I was more open," Haston said.

"Coach Davis did a great job of recognizing that they wouldn't be guarding Kirk that closely out on the perimeter," said Tom Coverdale, who made the initial pass to Hornsby. Haston was barely behind the 3-point line as he caught, turned and released.

"From under the basket it looked left to me, but it went right through," said Fife, who was jockeying for a possible putback. "I sprinted out to the 3-point line and passed out on my back. Then I looked up and here came the students, so I had to jump back up. From then on it was one big party."

"I thought I was dreaming," said A.J. Moye, IU's freshman guard. "I had to look up at the clock to see if it was real. Then I was jumping on as many backs as I could."

It was the first time in 12 years that the Hoosiers went from defeat to victory with no time left on the clock. In 1989 Jay Edwards stunned Michigan with a 3-pointer at the gun for another one-point Hoosier win.

Sunday's shocker also was the first win over a No. 1 team since Indiana spilled Kentucky in the 1993-94 season. But that game was played at the RCA Dome, not Assembly Hall.

After Haston came through, the floor was swarmed by students fresh from their semester break. It was the first time this season that Assembly Hall was filled to its capacity.

"Their crowd was awesome," said Michigan State coach Tom Izzo. "They did a great job of rallying their troops. Maybe they should take a page from their own book and make sure they get 17,123 in here every game. That's what belongs in this arena, what this place is all about."

Izzo wasn't pleased with the composure of his veteran team, the defending national champions. "I'm not going to speculate that we were fat and sassy, but we lost our focus sometimes," he said. "We've got five seniors who played in every hostile arena in America. They have played in hostile environments, but this is as good as it gets."

Michigan State's last loss was to none other than Indiana on February 26, an 81-79 thriller decided on a putback by Lynn Washington just ahead of the overtime buzzer. The Spartans then won their last 11 games of the season en route to the NCAA title and picked up where they left off by winning their first 12 games this season, giving them the nation's longest win streak, 23 games.

"We played a great team today," Izzo said. "We got what we deserved. There's your headline."

Pacers Go 'Dutch'

Memorial Day, 1995 ... NBA conference finals .... Shaq,' Reggie, The Big Dutchman ... four lead-changes in the last 13 seconds ... What more could you ask for?

Bloomington Herald-Times
May 30, 1995

INDIANAPOLIS, INDIANA

Down a point with 1.3 seconds left, the Indiana Pacers were about to join the list of endangered species in the NBA playoffs.

Anfernee Hardaway's 3-pointer had just given the Orlando Magic a 93-92 lead with 1.3 seconds left. Already leading 2-1 in the NBA Eastern Conference final, the Magic were about to take a 3-1 lead back to friendly Orlando for Game 5.

The Pacers, who had taken a 92-90 lead on Reggie Miller's 3-pointer with 5.2 seconds left, were reeling after Hardaway's sword thrust.

But 1.3 seconds would turn out to be enough time for yet another Pacer playoff miracle. To the rescue this time was 7-foot-4 Rik Smits. The "Big Dutchman" took the inbounds pass from Derrick McKey, drew Tree Rollins past him with a pump fake, then sent a 15-footer goalward.

The Memorial Day crowd of 16,477 was hushed as the horn sounded with ball in flight. The ball found the bottom of the net, touching off a gleeful explosion.

And now the Pacers are alive and well, all tied at 2-2 following the chilling 94-93 triumph.

"1.3 seconds is enough time to do a little fake, see what he would do -- draw a foul or get him up in the air," Smits said. "It (the fake) was in my mind when I came out of the timeout. I was on the low post, on the low block on the ball side. I was supposed to get Byron Scott open. I turned back and asked for the ball, then turned and hit the shot. I just felt really good. There was never a doubt in my mind."

"We knew Smits was the last option," said Orlando coach Brian Hill. "Unfortunately, we left our feet on the play instead of bodying up. In going to block the shot, you give him a clear look at the basket."

"Coming out of the timeout, Vern (Fleming) told Rik to ball-fake because he (Rollins) would try to block it," said Indiana coach Larry Brown. "He would have time to shoot it."

Rollins, the 39-year-old reserve center, was on the floor because starting center Shaquille O'Neal and forward Horace Grant had fouled out, depriving the Magic of their two best interior defenders.

"We felt that it was a lost opportunity if we didn't pull this one out," said Indiana guard Mark Jackson. "We had Shaq and Grant on the bench and we needed to take this one."

Both teams got off the deck several times to get Game 4 to its dramatic finish. The Magic stormed back from a 12-point deficit late in the third quarter to take an 83-77 lead. The Pacers, scoreless for the first five minutes of the fourth quarter, clawed back to tie the game at 87 when Grant fouled out with 1:41 left. When O'Neal followed 14 seconds later, it looked as though the Pacers would ease their way to the finish.

Hardly.

The Magic, trailing 89-87 with less than 28 seconds left, worked the ball to Brian Shaw behind the 3-point line. Shaw swished it for a 90-89 Magic lead with at 13.3 seconds.

That was plenty of time for Miller Time. Miller the hero of Game 1 in New York, looked as though he would be the man again when he drilled a 3 from deep on the left wing to put the Pacers up, 92-90.

There were still 5.2 seconds left, and, as Miller said later, "As we saw in New York, that's a lifetime in this league."

The Pacers had a one-point lead in Game 5 at New York, ready to close out the Knicks, only to watch Patrick Ewing score with 1.8 seconds left to beat them.

The Magic inbounded to Hardaway, who lost the 6-foot-10 McKey on a screen and found 6-3 Haywoode Workman in his place. The 6-7 Hardaway drifted to his left and hit a fallaway 3-pointer to send the Pacers and the crowd into shock.

"When I saw Penny catch the ball with Haywoode on him, I knew he could get the shot off," Miller said.

"We put our best defensive team out there and Penny just dumped it over Haywoode," Brown said.

It should have been the game-winner, but the Pacers have a way of winning in improbable fashion.

"I guess if we could have had one more possession, we could have changed the outcome," said Hill. "It was one of those games where whoever had the ball last was going to win."

"I've never seen 28 seconds like that, especially when you consider they (Orlando) hit every shot they needed to," Brown said. "Nobody lost this game. Our pulse is just beating. We've got a heartbeat." The Magic threatened to run the Pacers out of Market Square Arena with a 15-3 start.

"The way it started, I thought it was going to be the biggest blowout in history," said Brown.

The Pacers, thanks to foul trouble on O'Neal, caught up by the end of the quarter (26-26) and scored the last seven points of the half for a 53-47 lead. The lead would grow to a dozen, 69-57, before the Magic went on a 24-8 tear to take their biggest lead, 83-77.

The Pacer offense was spinning its wheels at that point. In fact, the only Pacer to score a field goal over that 8-1/2-minute stretch was McKey. Smits ended the famine for the rest of the Pacers with a field goal at the 4:36 mark, bringing his team to within one, 83-82.

It was anyone's game after that. There were 13 lead-changes in all, four in the last 13.3 seconds. It wasn't only foul trouble that hurt the Magic. Their inability to hit free throws (11-for-21) was just as costly. Eight of those misses came from O'Neal, who failed to make a single free throw.

O'Neal still had 16 points and 10 rebounds. Hardaway topped all scorers with 26 points and Dennis Scott added 22. Miller had 23 for the Pacers and Smits finished with 21. McKey added 14 and Mark Jackson 13.

"I have never been involved in a game like this one, shot after shot," Jackson said.

"I'm proud of our guys -- they played through adversity," Hill said. "We will bounce back from this. The Pacers haven't won a game in our place. The percentages are with us. We've played 82 games for the home court advantage."

"We shouldn't feel bad or ashamed," Shaw said. "It's a game of wills."

"It's a whole new series," Smits said. "Now it's the best-of-three. We still have to go there and win a road game."

Editor's Note: The series went seven games before the Magic successfully defended their home court in the decisive game.

This Game Was Hell-Bent

When Indiana went to class basketball in 1998, ending 85 years of hallowed, single-class tradition, it took me seven years to buy into it. What finally made a believer out of me was the 2005 Class 3A sectional championship game at Greencastle's McAnally Center. Matching bitter rivals Edgewood and Owen Valley, the game went three overtimes and featured amazing individual performances by Edgewood senior Kyle McGlone and Owen Valley sophomore Jared Maners. After tying the McAnally scoring record with 41 points, McGlone provided one of the best quotes I ever heard from a high school player: "I was bent on hell." Not bad for a kid who averaged a modest 15 points a game. And to think the game probably wouldn't have happened under the old format because Edgewood and Owen Valley took different tournament paths back then.

Bloomington Herald-Times
March 6, 2005

GREENCASTLE, INDIANA

Edgewood and Owen Valley have tangled on the basketball court almost 50 times over the years, but no game was ever more thrilling or ever more meaningful than the epic they staged Saturday night.

Meeting for the first time ever with a sectional championship on the line, they went toe-to-toe for 32 minutes of regulation and three overtimes before Edgewood triumphed, 80-75.

The sectional title was the third in Edgewood's 40-year history, and the second Class 3A title in three years. The Mustangs (12-10), a .500 team entering the sectional, now head to the Washington Regional play Class 3A's No. 1 team next week, the Washington Hatchets.

But the Mustangs and their fans really aren't thinking that far ahead right now. They are all too busy changing their undershirts.

There were so many swings of momentum, so many swings of emotion, that nobody left the gym with much energy left.

"This is the most exciting, agonizing game I've ever been a part of," said Edgewood coach Jay Brown, who has invested 18 years of coaching on top of three years of playing at Edgewood.

The man of the hour was senior guard Kyle McGlone, who averaged a point for each minute he played, all 41 of them.

"I was bent on hell," McGlone said with his jaw still locked after the game.

Beginning with the final minute of regulation and the first overtime, McGlone scored all 15 of Edgewood's points, 12 of them coming on four old-fashioned 3-point plays.

But the game's decisive basket came off the hands of sophomore Daniel Lowers. With the scored tied at 75-75 in the third overtime, Lowers deflected a pass, ran it down and laid it in at the other end.

After an Owen Valley misfire, junior forward Mike Lay rebounded for Edgewood and was fouled. A 72 percent free throw shooter, Lay made both with 13.9 seconds left. A quick 3-pointer by Owen Valley came up short, and Edgewood sophomore Scott Pedersen applied the finishing touch with a free throw at 8.0 seconds.

It was a bitter ending for Owen Valley (16-7), which played so gallantly in defeat, especially Jared Maners. In a classic, individual duel, the sophomore guard matched McGlone basket-for-basket in the first two overtimes. Maners wound up playing all 44 minutes and scoring 30 points.

"Where did that kid come from?" McGlone asked afterward in disbelief. "He didn't even play varsity last year, and this year he averages 18 points a game. He is going to break some records."

McGlone put his name into the record books by tying the McAnally Center scoring record with 41 points, a record set by Greencastle's Brett Hecko 17 years ago. McGlone fell one shy of the Edgewood scoring record of 42, set my Clarence Figg against Martinsville in 1969.

McGlone didn't waste any time getting into the fray. He went to the basket early and often, launching Edgewood to a 22-14 lead at the end of the first quarter, a quarter in which the Mustangs played error-free basketball.

With McGlone sandwiching two baskets around a jumper by Lowers, the Mustangs had the Patriots doubled up on the scoreboard midway through the second quarter, 28-14.

But the Patriots chipped the deficit down to eight at halftime, 29-21, and to four by the end of the third quarter, 38-34. However, they were already in some foul trouble, including the other half of their talented backcourt, Harry Marshall.

It was Marshall going to the offensive glass for three putbacks that helped the Patriots close the deficit entirely. They took a 48-47 lead when senior forward Jake Zeunik intercepted a pass and scored. Zeunik then set up Nick Taylor for a two-pointer and broke Edgewood press for a basket that gave the Patriots a 53-48 lead with 41.8 seconds left.

Coming to Edgewood's rescue was McGlone, first with a 3-point play that cut the deficit to two. Then, after Zeunik hit one of two free throws, McGlone swished a tying 3-pointer with 14.6 seconds left. After Maners missed a jumper just ahead of the horn, the two rivals were headed for overtime, all tied at 54.

Seeing the way McGlone was taking over the game, Brown kept calling his number. The 5-foot-10 playmaker scored all nine of Edgewood's points in the first overtime.

"Coach put the game on my shoulders," McGlone said. "I've worked my butt off. I wanted it for myself and everybody else on my team."

Zeunik got the Patriots off to a good start in the first overtime with a 3, but two McGlone drives yielded three points and fouled out Marshall. McGlone had a chance to win it at the end of each of the first two overtimes, but missed a 17-footer on the first opportunity and lost his footing before getting off a shot on the second.

Edgewood had the advantage in most of the second overtime, thanks to Daniel Lindsey's first basket of the game, a 3-pointer, followed by a McGlone 3-pointer. But Maners kept the Patriots alive by scoring all seven OV points as they went to the third overtime tied at 70-70.

The start of the final overtime saw Maners convert a fast break into a 3-point play, then hit Jake Lester underneath to give the Patriots a 75-71 lead. However, they failed to score the last three minutes.

Four points by McGlone tied the score, and Lowers's grand theft put the Mustangs ahead to stay.

"I pulled up and missed from about the same spot earlier," Lowers said. "This time decided to go all the way to the basket."

"This was just an unbelievable basketball game," Brown said. "Truly, there was no loser."

"Nothing personal against Owen Valley, but I did not want to end my high school career against them," said McGlone, who was 0-3 against the Patriots until Saturday night.

"Kyle's individual effort was one for the history books," Brown said. "We set our game plan completely around him. We felt he could get Maners and Marshall in some foul trouble and he did.

He fouled two kids out. I told him not to be afraid to win the basketball game. He practically willed us to victory."

Editor's Note: Edgewood lost in the regional to a Washington team that would go on to win the Class 3A state title, but not without an amazing finish. Read about that next.

Zeller Was Stellar

Twenty-three years after Scott Skiles led Plymouth to a state title, the Pilgrims were on the other side of a dagger. This time it was Washington's Luke Zeller bombing in a 40-foot 3-pointer as time expired to shock the Pilgrims, 74-72. Zeller was the first of three brothers, all 7-footers, who combined for four Class 3A titles for Washington from 2005-2011. Joining him were Tyler and Cody. All three went on to receive Indiana's highest high school honor, Mr. Basketball. All three also went on collegiate stardom – Luke at Notre Dame, Tyler at North Carolina, Cody at Indiana. All three also went on to play in the NBA. No other family in Indiana history can claim all that.

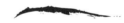

Bloomington Herald-Times
March 27, 2005

INDIANAPOLIS, INDIANA

Washington's Luke Zeller leaped into Indiana high school basketball lore Saturday night, taking his place right next to Bobby Plump, Scott Skiles, Stacey Toran and all the other authors of last-second heroics in the state finals.

With his team trailing 72-71 with 1.8 seconds left in overtime, the 6-foot-11 Zeller hauled in a pass at halfcourt, whirled to his left, dribbled once and let fly. With the Class 3A championship hanging in the air, Zeller's 40-footer zeroed in on the basket and ripped through as 18,000 fans gasped in disbelief. When they finally exhaled, the roof nearly came off Conseco Fieldhouse as the Hatchets pulled out the 74-72 win.

"I took a dribble, let it go and God did the rest," Zeller said. "God is good, let me tell ya."

The miraculous finish brought Washington its first state title since 1942 and sent retiring coach Dave Omer out a winner.

"This is a situation that won't sink in for a while," said Omer, almost lost for words after a 40-year career without a state finals appearance.

"Maybe this makes up for all the years of getting beat on shots like that," he said.

The loss denied Plymouth coach Jack Edison a second state title and his 500th coaching victory. His first came in 1982, thanks to a game-saving 20-footer by Skiles that got his Plymouth club into overtime against Gary Roosevelt.

"In 20 years, this will be the greatest shot ever," Edison said with a little tongue in cheek. "Skiles's shot is now up to 40 feet. Zeller did what champions do, rise to the occasion. You knew it was close, knew it was going to be there. It wasn't like Skiles', which curved in."

What made the finish even more dramatic was the fact that Plymouth had just taken a one-point lead thanks to a smaller miracle worker, 5-9 freshman Randy Davis. With two regulars having already fouled out, Davis was on the floor out of necessity.

"Randy was our third option, behind Kyle Benge and Geoff Scheetz," said Edison, referring to his two best 3-point threats. "I did tell Randy before he left the huddle to be ready."

With Benge in possession of the ball and heavily guarded, he bounced a pass to Davis at the top of the key. Davis guard saw an opening down the lane and set his course for the basket. Awaiting him was 6-8 Bryan Bouchie, Washington's sophomore forward. Davis hesitated, then executed a perfect up-and-under move to score the go-ahead basket.

By the time the Hatchets got the clock stopped, they had less than two seconds to work with.

"We had just enough time to take no more than one dribble," Omer said. "We didn't want somebody just catching the ball and wheeling it down the floor in 'Hail Mary' fashion.

During the timeout, Zeller begged for the ball.

"I didn't want anybody else on the team to have that on their shoulders," he said. "I wanted to be the one who was going to hit it or miss it."

"We were going to Luke the whole time," Omer said. "He said, 'Get the ball to me. I'll score.' Luke making the basket doesn't surprise me. The time he had to do it in surprises me."

Edison chose not to guard the inbounds passer, Washington guard Joel McDonald.

"We wanted to keep three guys back. The gym has such a high ceiling that you could still lob it up. Luke had to go his left with a guy guarding

him hard on his right side. You've got to feel like we made him take a tough shot."

The Plymouth players collapsed on the court in shock. The turnaround wiped out a gallant comeback that saw them rally from 11 points down with four minutes left in regulation. Two free throws by Kyle Plumlee tie the score at 64 with 21.6 seconds left. The Pilgrims nearly won it in the final seconds of regulation when Plumlee stole the ball and got off two shots under the basket, only to have each attempt roll off the rim.

The first half, nine of Plymouth's first 10 field goals were 3-pointers. They were 10-for-20 from the arc in the first half alone.

Scheetz, the smallest player on the court at 5-foot-8, was 5-for-9 from 3-point range the first half for 15 points. However, Scheetz went scoreless the rest of the way as Washington's 6-4 Isaac Stoll clamped down on him.

Washington wasn't quite as 3-point happy, but the Hatchets did sink four from beyond the arc to stay within two at the half, 36-34.

Triple-teamed, the entire half, Zeller stepped out to hit one of those 3s along the way to 11 first-half points, but his biggest contribution came as a passer, where he dished out six assists. The Notre Dame recruit finished the game one rebound shy of a triple-double — 27 points, 11 assists, nine rebounds.

"We were just as concerned with Zeller's passing as his shooting," Edison said.

"It's the perfect ending," Zeller said. "I told someone that is like the 'Amen' on a great season. It's a great way to go out."

Editor's Note: Two years later, Edison's 28th and final year as head coach, the Pilgrims sent him out a winner by capturing the 2007 Class 3A state title.

A Proper Hoosier Thanksgiving

This is a game story of a different kind – more of a "day-in-the-life" story.

The 2007 Old Oaken Bucket Game was an emotional one for Indiana. There was a lot on the line as Indiana braced for Purdue. Not only did the Hoosiers want to end a five-game losing streak to Purdue, they needed a win to become bowl eligible. And on top of that, it was the first Bucket game played since the death of Indiana coach Terry Hoeppner, who passed away the previous summer.

You could sense Hoeppner's presence all day long, especially in the eyes of his widow, Jane Hoeppner. After IU pulled out a 27-24 victory on Austin Starr's last-minute field goal, I replayed the day from my perspective for the H-T's Thanksgiving issue.

Bloomington Herald-Times
November 22, 2007

We've all had our days, days where nothing seems to go right. Those days seem to linger in our memories at the expense of the really good days, days where everything seems to fall into place, days where you catch yourself thinking, "It's great to be alive." Thanksgiving is a good time to remind yourself of that.

I had one those truly marvelous days Saturday, a day that could have gone either way. As an IU alumnus who had covered 18 Old Oaken Bucket Games over the years, I knew going in that the chances of it being a winning day for Indiana were one in three. Purdue was 12-6 in the games I had witnessed.

But Hoosier expectations were higher this time. All week long you could feel the momentum building toward the 3:30 kickoff. At Tuesday's press conference, coach Bill Lynch unveiled the uniform to be worn for the occasion, a retro look in honor of the 40th anniversary of IU's epic 19-14 win over Purdue in 1967, a victory that gave the Hoosiers their last Big Ten title and only trip to the Rose Bowl. The members of the '67 club were going to be the day's honored guests.

Thursday night, a reception at the convention center honored IU great Anthony Thompson, who will be inducted into the College Football Hall of Fame in December. In addition to the good feelings for Thompson in the room that night, there was an uncommonly large buzz about the upcoming Bucket Game.

So that brings us to Saturday. Allow me to take you through my day.

12:15 - More than three hours before kickoff, all roads to the stadium are clogging up, but I find a back-way that allows me to beat most of the traffic, a good start to the day already. Others aren't so lucky. Many of the would-be spectators, including media, miss the entire first quarter because of the congestion.

1:15 - Members of the '67 team join ranks with the current team members to make "The Walk" to Stadium. The path is lined by fans at least six deep. One player after another accepts a high-five from a spectator. Their eyes are as wide as hub caps. You can feel the electricity.

I catch up to Jane Hoeppner. I have known her since 1979, when I was the sports editor of the *Kendallville News-Sun* and her husband, Terry, was the coach of East Noble there. This is going to be a day of extreme emotions for Jane, watching the Hoosiers finish the season without their coach and her husband, who died in June. And the fans know it. So many of them come up to her and wish her well. She graciously thanks each one.

1:30 - I stick around for the pre-game show of the IU Marching Hundred. I had forgotten how wildly entertaining they are. When they march into the stadium to a war-like drum beat, the blood begins to boil.

2:00 - I go to the "I" Association tent to hang with the '67 team. I meet Harry Gonso, Doug Crusan, Al Gage, Jim Sniadecki, Ken Kaczmarek and coach John Pont. Their presence really makes for a lot of good vibes.

3:25 - Five minutes before kickoff, I am invited to the Memorial Stadium rooftop by Jeff Keag, IU's assistant sports information director. "You've got to see this view," he insists. He isn't kidding. From up high you can see not only the entire field, but the entire landscape — the campus, downtown Bloomington and the beautiful fall colors on the horizon. Better yet, you can hear the crowd and soak in the atmosphere. When IU kicker Austin Starr puts his foot onto the ball at 3:30, the stadium is almost filled to capacity, a rarity at IU these days.

3:30-7:00 - This part of the game is a blur. I am busy doing a quarter-by-quarter analysis for Sunday's H-T. The Hoosiers are dominating the game in many ways but are allowing the Boilermakers to hang around. When Purdue comes all the way back from a 21-point deficit to tie the score at 24 with 3 1/2 minutes to go, you can see Hoosier spirits sinking.

7:06 - Starr boots perhaps the most important field goal in IU history, a 49-yarder with 30 seconds left to break the tie. The stadium quakes.

7:12 – A desperation play by Purdue fails and the Hoosiers have the Bucket and probable bowl bid. Fans stream onto the field, lifting the players on their shoulders while chanting, "Terry Hoeppner ... Terry Hoeppner."

7:45 – After covering the post-game press conference of Purdue coach Joe Tiller, I see a young Hoosier fan decked out in red come up to Tiller and say, "Great game, coach." The scowl on Tiller's face gives way to a warm smile. "Thanks, kid, and congratulations to your guys," he replies.

7:55 – I catch up to Jane Hoeppner outside the Hoosiers' lockerroom. We share an emotional hug. In the next 10 minutes she answers reporters' questions with a poise and eloquence that is downright queen-like. On this occasion, she is Bloomington's queen for a day.

10:30 – I catch up with the '67 team for a post-game reception at the IU Foundation. The Bucket is there. You can see it needs some attention, some spit and polish. Marty Clark, the IU equipment manager, promises it will receive lots of tender loving care over the next 12 months.

11:15 – After everybody else has left, I am gazing lovingly at the Bucket with Clark and Mark Deal, assistant director of the Varsity Club.

"Do you mind?" I say, nodding in the Bucket's direction. They give their wholehearted consent.

I cradle it as if it were the Holy Grail. At that moment, I think, "It doesn't get any better than this."

Too often, we let little things ruin our days while forgetting our many blessings. This was a good day. No, make that a GREAT day.

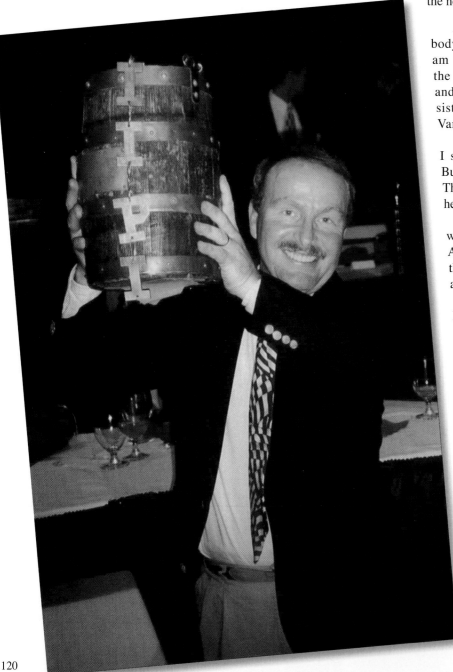

Hoisting the Old Oaken Bucket is about as good as it gets. (Courtesy photo)

120

Chapter 10
The Long Haul

Some of the most time consuming projects also are some of the most satisfying ones. Each of these pieces took several weeks and, in some cases, even months to complete. Looking back, they were all well worth it.

MYSTERY MAN

In 1997, a photo came across my desk that aroused my curiosity to the point I couldn't let go. To find the ultimate answer, I had to go all the way to Akron, Ohio. The story was later picked up by IU Alumni Magazine.

Bloomington Herald-Times
May 11, 1997

It was the face, a black face peering out of a field of white faces on a faded photograph from 1906, a picture of the Indiana University track and field relay team.

A black man, mind you, in 1906. This country was barely 40 years removed from slavery.

He is the only man of color in the picture, the only one pictured in an I-Man's sweater, proudly wearing it, it appears.

On the border of the picture are four surnames -- Johnson, Williamson, Thompson and Seward.

By the positioning of the names, the man in question figures to be Thompson.

Who is this man, I wonder, already hooked.

A quick check of Indiana University "I-Men's Directory" lists a "G.W." Thompson as a two-time award winner in 1905 and '06. Was this the same Thompson? Where did he come from? Was he the first black man to run track at IU? What sort of man was he? What obstacles did he encounter? Where did he go after college?

Little did I know at the time, these questions would consume me for the next month. They would lead me on a manhunt which would keep me on the phone for hours, draw me deep into the history sections of public libraries, take me into the homes of some of Bloomington's most senior citizens and ultimately send me on a journey 350 miles away.

The questions would not let go until I could put it all on paper. This then is the mystery that was G. W. Thompson.

Digging for Clues

The immediate task was to put a first name and middle name behind the initials "G" and "W." A call to the Registrar's Office located a "George William" Thompson who attended IU from 1903-07 and again from 1914-15. His home town was listed as Covington, Ind., which was surprising because Covington and Fountain County have not been known to have much of a black population.

A call to Covington High School athletic director Randy Tolley caught him by surprise. He was not aware of any Covington athlete by that name and certainly no black athlete. He, too, was intrigued and promised to look into it.

The next call went to a Covington geneologist, Miriam Luke. The only black family Luke was aware of went by the name "Richey." She recommended checking the census of 1900.

In the public records section of the IU library, I scrolled through so much microfilm I was physically dizzy. I came across a George W. Thompson, age 16, Covington. That would have put him at the right age to be attending IU in the early 1900s. There was one snag, however. The census designated the young man's race as "W" for "white."

I continued to scroll until I had gone through every Thompson listed in Indiana in the 1900 census. Not finding another George W. from Covington, I went back to the one listed as "white." My hopes soared when I noted that Thompson was listed as a nephew of a Malinda L. Richey. Another call to Miriam Luke confirmed that this was indeed the Richey family she had mentioned. But that nagging "W" remained.

Tolley called back to verify that there was a George William Thompson, son of Charles W. Thompson, who attended Covington from 1899 to 1903 and ran track, quite well in fact. Tolley even had a copy of a newspaper article from the *Covington Republican* dated April 25, 1902. It told of how Thompson dominated a track meet against Danville (Ill.) by winning the 220, 440, 880, mile and pole vault. Shades of Jim Thorpe, I thought.

Thompson would go on to dominate college meets as well, especially in the 440 and relays, I learned. According to the Indiana *Daily Student*, he set the school record in the 440 at 51.8 seconds. There was one reference to Thompson in the IDS as the "Cuban Indian."

Doris Seward

Walking up the path toward the stately brick house on Bloomington's east side, I didn't know whether to thank Doris Seward or to curse her. It was Doris who forwarded the photograph that had started all this. The Seward pictured on Thompson's left is Fred Seward, Doris's deceased father.

Doris meets me at the door and welcomes me into her parlor, which is tastefully Victorian. A plate of fresh, dried dates is positioned on the table next to my chair.

"I am so glad somebody is looking into this," she said, offering me a date. Doris is just as fascinated by the black man in the photo as I am. She remembers how her father talked fondly of the man.

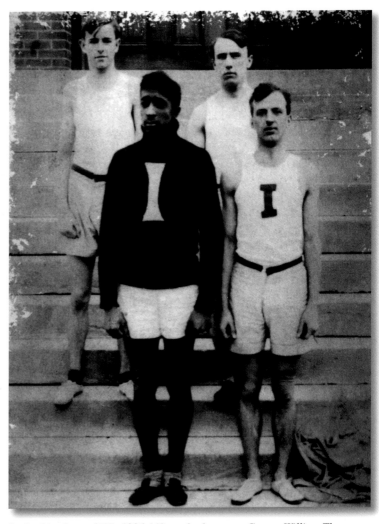

In the this photo of IU's 1906 440-yard relay team, George William Thompson is front row, left. Next to him is Fred Seward, the father of Doris Seward, who donated the photo. In back are Johnson and Williamson. (Courtesy photo)

"My father was proud to have the young man on the team. He was a team member. There was never any question."

Doris recalled an anecdote Fred told her about the time the team went to Cincinnati. The clerk at the registration desk looked in the direction of Thompson and said, "How about him?" knowing that blacks were not permitted to stay at the hotel.

"He's from Hawaii," Fred Seward said. The clerk waved Thompson through with a suspicious look and mumbled, "Last year he was from Cuba."

Doris suggested a few contacts, one of them being another one of Bloomington's most respected senior citizens.

Elizabeth Bridgewaters

From the well-to-do east side of Bloomington I go to the poorer west side, to the home of 88-year-old Elizabeth Bridgewaters. Although her modest home is half as much house as Seward's, it is every bit as neat and well-preserved.

"My mother started buying this house when I was 12 years old," said Bridgewaters, who has now spent 76 years in the house on West Seventh.

Also known as "The Hill," the Bloomington west side has been home to many a black family over the years. It was here that George Thompson was supposed to have resided during his college days at IU.

Through a long and interesting life, Bridgewaters has become a sort of unofficial historian for Bloomington's black community. She is the daughter of Preston Eagleson, who while attending Indiana in the mid-1890s, became the first black to play intercollegiate sports at IU (football, baseball). He thus preceded Thompson by 10 years.

Elizabeth takes one glance at the photo and instantly recognizes Thompson.

"That's him," she says. "He was very slender, very tall, copper-brown. He came here to visit my mother (Ollie) when I was a senior in high school. She knew him and his wife when he was in school. He lived with one of the families down the street, the Profit family, I think.

"Blacks couldn't stay on campus. They would stay with one of the local black families. The Profits trained most of the black barbers around town. I think he married one of the Profits. They're all gone now."

Elizabeth seemed to think Thompson was from Crawfordsville, but it was Covington, I said. He had some ties to Crawfordsville, she insisted, recalling a story she heard.

"I think it was Crawfordsville where he went to a track meet and was told, 'A black man can't run here.' The coach said, 'He's an Indian.' He ran."

There's that Indian connection again, I thought.

"George Thompson was proud of his ancestry," Bridgewaters continued. "He was very polished. He was an adult when I knew him. He was no child. He was in his 40s. I think he lived in Akron, Ohio and worked for one of the big rubber companies there.

"You should talk to Maurice Evans. He lives in one of those nursing homes on the west side. I think he might have been a neighbor of the Profits."

Maurice Evans

Maurice Evans is enjoying an afternoon nap when I step into his room in the Hospitality House, a Bloomington retirement home. A man of his age, 103 years, is entitled to a nap now and then.

Maurice isn't exactly thrilled to have his slumber interrupted by a strange white man thrusting a dated photo in his face, but perks right up when he realizes who's in the picture.

"Thompson, George Thompson," he says. "Lived with the Profits, right down the street from us. Married a Profit girl -- Lotta, her name was."

Maurice is fighting a cold and strains to speak, which comes out in a whisper. It reminds me of a scene out of the 1970 movie, *Little Big Man*, where a journalist tries to pry information out of a 121-year-old man played by Dustin Hoffman.

However, there is still plenty of spark in Maurice's eyes, not to mention sparkling fragments of memory. I ask him about Thompson's heritage.

"Full-blooded Indian," he claims.

That could explain why Thompson's race was listed as "white" on the census form, I think to myself.

Maurice goes on to talk about the occasions he saw Thompson run.

"Ran so fast they would stretch out a blanket to slow him down."

As for the kind of person Thompson was, Maurice could only answer, "Nice man, very nice man."

With that, Maurice closes his eyes and resumes his nap.

Striking the Mother Lode

Although the pieces were coming together, the portfolio on Thompson was still sketchy at best. On a whim I dialed the public library in Akron. Sylvia Leddon of the Historical Records Section ran a quick trace. Within minutes she came back with a small folder on a George W. Thompson.

Black man? Yes.

Educated at IU? Yes.

Star athlete? Yes.

Wife named Lotta? Bingo! We had a match.

Leddon not only had an obituary on the man -- he died in 1944 -- she also had a newspaper article detailing his contributions as a prominent black leader in Akron. It was obvious the real story of G.W. Thompson was just beginning.

Leddon forwarded a packet of information containing three items of immense importance: the obituary which appeared in the Akron *Beacon Journal*; a final tribute which appeared on the editorial page the day after Thompson's death; and a 1985 newspaper column remembering Thompson 40 years after his death.

The small obituary read:

"Thompson, George W., 1303 Murray Ave., passed away Tuesday morning. Survived by wife, Lotta; three cousins, two aunts, one uncle. Burial at Mt. Peace Cemetery."

The editorial was much more substantial, calling Thompson's death a "grievous loss to the community." It also went on to say, "Yet among his many friends, there must be a feeling of satisfaction that they let him know before he died just how highly respected he was by men and women of all colors and creeds.

"Almost a year ago, upon the occasion of his 25 years of service in Akron, a civic banquet was held in his honor. At that time, the *Beacon Journal* said, editorially: 'More than any other one individual, George W. Thompson is responsible for the understanding and mutual trust which prevails between the white and negro populations of the city of Akron.'

"That understanding will remain, we hope, as a monument to Mr. Thompson's diligent and intelligent labors. It is not to say that he was a credit to his race. George Thompson was a credit to mankind and was a living example of the fact that whites and negroes can get along with mutual respect and confidence."

By the time I had read those paragraphs, it was clear I had just encountered the rest of the iceberg known as George William Thompson.

I read on.

In 1985, James S. Jackson, the late black columnist, compared Thompson to a more recent black leader, Opie Evans, a TV personality who knew Thompson. Jackson described them both as "well educated and of unusual ability and personal charm ... dedicated to the welfare of not only blacks but all humanity."

Jackson also mentioned that Thompson and Evans were criticized by some members of the black community for realizing that "to make progress on behalf of the blacks, it is absolutely necessary to deal with the whites -- particularly the white power structure."

"A tall, handsome man and fluent speaker, Thompson addressed white groups, including service clubs and the Akron Real Estate Board. He became the personal friend of many of the city's white leaders."

The article went on to describe how Thompson came to Akron after World War I and was put in charge of the YMCA. With the help of a $10,000 gift from Harvey S. Firestone (of Firestone Rubber), Thompson later founded the Association for Colored Community Work (ACCW) to provide employment opportunities for blacks. It was an affiliate of the National Urban League.

It was evident by now that all roads led to Akron, Ohio.

Road Trip

Sports columnist Jim Murray, king of the metaphor, once put Akron, Ohio and Munich, Germany in the same sentence by calling Munich "Akron with a crew cut."

That was Murray's way of painting Akron as one of those tough, industrial, mid-sized Midwestern towns such as Gary, Fort Wayne or Toledo.

Once the home of nation's major tire companies, Akron proudly proclaimed itself the "Rubber Capital of the World." Although most of the tire companies have since relocated to other cities, Akron still produces enough rubber to maintain its title.

When the tire industry first took off in the 1920s and '30s, the prospect of factory jobs lured blacks from the South at a rate of over 100 per week. Not all of them could find work, or homes for that matter. That is where George Thompson came in.

On East Market Street is the 47-year-old Akron Community Center, built in 1950 to replace the one on Perkins Street which served the city so well under Thompson.

In the library of the ACC is a stack of dusty old pictures, portraits of past leaders. One appears to be Thompson in his later years. I pull it from the stack and prop it up on a pile of books on the shelf. The man responsible for all this deserves to be seen.

After rummaging through the library's archives, I come across a progress report authored by Thompson in 1942, two years before his death.

Under the heading, "We Too Are Americans," it said, "The chief responsibility of all American citizens in this year, 1942, is to concentrate on winning the war. Negroes take this as their first MUST... Victory abroad and victory at home is our motto."

Under the heading, "Some of the Things We Did in 1941," it listed:

* 446 job placements by the employment department, an increase of 226 percent over 1940;

* initiating employment for 150 blacks at Goodyear Aircraft;

* helping 400 blacks find jobs at Atlas Power Co.;

* establishing a Civil Service training program;

* establishing six scholarships for black students;

* working with the Tuberculosis Association to set up a Patch Test for blacks throughout the county.

There was a personal angle to the latter. Thompson contracted Tuberculosis in the late 1930s and never fully recovered.

Shirla Robinson McClain

Shirla McClain, a teacher at Kent University, is recognized around Akron as a local expert on the city's black history. In fact, she wrote a dissertation on the subject entitled, "The Contributions of Blacks in Akron, 1825-1975." The name George Thompson dominates the piece, just like the man dominated track meets.

On page 101 is a most interesting nugget on Thompson. It says he participated in the 1904 Olympics in St. Louis and "ran the quarter mile in 49 and 2/5 seconds."

Thompson, an Olympian? The Indiana Track & Field Media Guides does not list Thompson as a Hoosier Olympian, but it was quite possible he still competed at St. Louis because it was a loosely structured, mostly American meet which welcomed all-comers. The U.S. Olympic Headquarters in Colorado Springs had no record of an Olympian by the name George Thompson, but a spokesman said the records from that time are not comprehensive.

McClain's dissertation also revealed that, before coming to Akron, Thompson served as a principal for a colored school in Crawfordsville, Ind. In checking with Mary Johnson at the Crawfordsville Public Library, Thompson indeed was the principal at Lincoln Colored School in Crawfordsville from 1914-15. Lotta Thompson also taught there, Johnson noted. Elizabeth Bridgewaters was right about that Crawfordsville connection.

From Crawfordsville, Thompson was called to military duty in World War I and worked with the YMCA while stationed in France. After the war, he was invited to Akron to open up a YMCA for blacks. The Akron YMCA, under Thompson, became a temporary home to many of the blacks migrating from the South.

According to McClain, Thompson emerged as a major voice in the black community, speaking frequently to civic groups and becoming one of the earliest blacks in Akron to hold an official position when Judge H.C. Spicer named him as Deputy Probation Officer of the Summit County Juvenile Court.

As McClain wrote, "The leadership which the (ACCW) provided in getting negroes accepted to a greater degree as community citizens was considered as possibly their greatest achievement."

Raymond Brown

McClain suggested I put in a call to Raymond Brown, who served under Thompson at the ACCW in the 1930s. Brown, who will be 90 later this month, was eager to talk about his mentor.

"He was tall with Indian features," Brown said. "He had some Indian heritage. He came to Akron at the request of the YMCA to open up a negro branch. The rubber companies were importing a lot of blacks. George tried to find them employment. After a while, the 'Y' said that wasn't his job, so he affiliated himself with the Urban League.

"He had a very good mind and an excellent facility for public speaking, so he made an excellent impression on the rubber companies. George got them to hire blacks in production, not just the dirty jobs. C.W. Seiberling (of Seiberling Rubber) bought the idea and Thompson found the people with the necessary qualifications.

"He made very good contacts and was well accepted. He was able to sell the idea of more employment opportunities for blacks, as well as housing and education. It was just a matter of getting people to give blacks a break. He got me my first job at a rubber factory.

"George was also very good about going around to churches, Lions Clubs, Rotary Clubs and speaking up for equal opportunity. He didn't want handouts, just equal opportunities."

Brown said Thompson took his position as probation officer seriously. "Any problems with the police or the courts, he was there."

Brown could not help me with the whereabouts of Lotta after Thompson's death but remembered her as a "charming lady, very quiet, didn't interfere at all. She was the kind of person you'd like to have as a wife to give you support."

A City Says Thanks

On Thompson's 60th birthday, November 9, 1943, the city of Akron put World War II on the back burner and threw quite a party in his honor. The reservations numbered 200, the Akron *Beacon Journal* said. On hand were representatives from all the major rubber companies -- Goodyear, Goodrich, Seiberling -- as well as representatives from the United Auto Workers, Ohio Edison and the Red Cross.

Thompson was presented with a diamond ring and also received personal telegraphs from all over the country.

"The tall, soft-spoken Thompson heard himself eulogized by both races," the *Beacon Journal* said. "In his testimonial, Thompson disclaimed credit for himself and said the praise rightfully belonged to the understanding men and women of both races who have worked with him."

Accompanying the article was a picture of Mr. and Mrs. George Thompson, with George looking gaunt and Lotta looking worried. George did not live to see his 61st birthday. He died of complications from his long battle with Tuberculosis in October, 1944.

George William Thompson

Lot 79, Section 25, in Mount Peace Cemetery is Thompson's final resting place.

When I ask the groundskeeper for directions, he surprises me by answering, "George Thompson," before I had even mentioned the man's name. Apparently George has had a visitor or two over the years.

It is an isolated plot, however, with no other Thompson buried nearby. A small American flag provides company, a sign a visitor has stopped by. The gravestone is nothing more than a flat, two-foot long slab of marble with the inscription, "George W. Thompson, 1883-1944."

Simple and unassuming, not the grave of a rich man.

Next to the flag I place a tube containing two carnations -- one red, one white, for old IU. After a moment of silence, I find myself talking to the deceased.

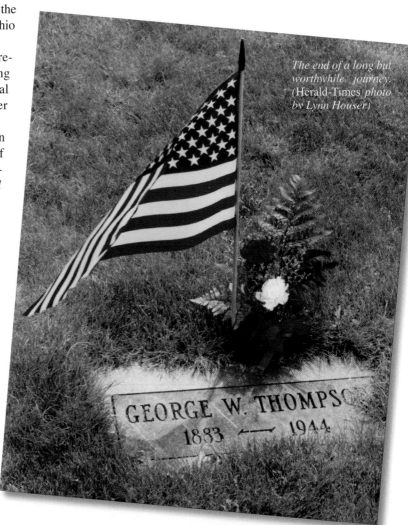

The end of a long but worthwhile journey. (Herald-Times photo by Lynn Houser)

126

"George, you don't know me, but I feel I know you. If you only knew how many hours I spent getting to know you. I even drove all the way from Indiana for some answers, yet so many questions remain.

"I mean, did you really have some Indian blood in you? Did you really run in the 1904 Olympics? What was it like to be the first black man to run track at IU? Were those fond memories or painful ones? Did those racial barriers you encountered drive you to breaking them down through your lifelong work?

"That race thing -- it's still out there -- but thanks to people like you, we've come a long, long way. Before there was a Martin Luther King, there were pioneers like you blazing a trail.

"You will be pleased to know that the organization you founded is still going strong. They moved into a new building on Market Street in 1950 and it's still thriving today. In 1996, the organization found jobs for 800 blacks. It also provided Thanksgiving dinners and Christmas toys for 200 families.

"All because of you, George. You made a difference. The world was a better place when you left it.

"Rest in peace, George William Thompson."

'Coach' Thorpe

It was a little known fact that the great Jim Thorpe was an IU assistant football coach in the early 1900s. I didn't know about it until I received a tip in 2002. Right away I had to learn more about the circumstances that brought Thorpe to Bloomington, and what it was like to have him on campus at the height of his glory. To my astonishment, I discovered Indiana could have landed Knute Rockne as well. It was quite a find almost 90 years later. The Rockne nugget was packaged in a side bar.

Bloomington Herald-Times
January 19, 2003

Imagine having Tiger Woods on your college campus to assist with the golf team. Or Michael Jordan around to work with the basketball team. Or Barry Bonds sharing batting tips with the baseball team.

In the fall of 1915, the Indiana University football team had an assistant of that caliber, Jim Thorpe. That is the one and only Jim Thorpe, considered the greatest athlete of his time and still hailed as the "Athlete of the Century" by the United States Senate as the 20th Century came to a close.

So how was it that a fledgling football program such as Indiana's lured the great Jim Thorpe, and what was it like to have him as a Bloomington guest? Pull up a chair and take a trip back to the days when Jim Thorpe roamed Jordan Field.

Help Is on the Way

In the fall of 1915, Thorpe was a legend. He was just three years removed from the 1912 Olympics at Stockholm, Sweden, where he shattered world records in sweeping the pentathlon and decathlon. That came on the heels of an All-American football career at Carlisle Indian Industrial School in Pennsylvania.

In one of his many extraordinary football games, the opponent was Army, a perennial power. Thorpe rambled 92 yards for a touchdown, only to have the play called back because of a penalty. On the next play he dashed 97 yards for a touchdown.

Feats of that magnitude made Thorpe a champion of the underdog. You must remember that Thorpe was an American Indian in an era when minorities were still rendered second-class status. For an Indian to dominate the American sports scene was unheard of. If the Heisman Trophy had existed back then, Thorpe surely would have won it.

In September, 1915, football coach C.C. Childs was in his second year at Indiana and looking to augment his staff at a time when young men were facing the possibility of being drafted into military service. America's neutrality in World War I was about to end.

Childs came to Indiana in 1914 and guided the Hoosiers to a 3-4-1 record. Two years earlier he won a bronze medal in the hammer throw at Stockholm. It was there he came to know Thorpe.

It didn't matter to Childs that Thorpe had been engaged in an international scandal following the Olympics. Before Thorpe could find a place for his medals, he had to return them. The Olympic Committee learned that he had played summer baseball for a small amount of money, thereby making him a "professional." Despite a public outcry for leniency, the Olympic Committee stripped Thorpe of his honors.

There was outrage, according to author Nicholas Leeman: "For being guileless, for being an Indian above his station, Thorpe was singled out for humiliation."

Childs could have cared less about Thorpe's troubles when he sought to fill the opening on his staff. As Thorpe was winding up the baseball season with John McGraw's New York Giants, Childs was hoping Bloomington would appeal to Thorpe because it was only a short train ride from Lafayette, the hub of a semi-professional football league known as the Wabash Athletic Association.

Thorpe was interested in playing professional football, and the Indiana job afforded him an opportunity to both coach and play. Thorpe's asking price from Indiana was $1,000 plus a room for his family at a Bloomington hotel.

On September 2, Childs telegrammed the terms to IU administrator Ulysses H. Smith:

> "Jim Thorpe can assist in football ... One thousand and hotel. Believe many desire extra coach ... Satisfied either way ... Advise attitude."

Smith wired back his approval and Childs fired off another telegram to IU President William Lowe Bryan:

> "Positive to have James Thorpe, world's greatest athletic, assist in football ... Your position is mine ... Kindly advise."

Bryan gave his consent and the deal was struck.

"World's Greatest Athlete will Arrive When Big Leagues Close," the headline beamed in the September 28, 1915, issue of the Indiana *Daily Student*.

"James F. Thorpe, the famous Carlisle Indian athlete, reputed the world's greatest athlete, will arrive here in a few days to assist Coach Childs in football," the article said. "Thorpe will take charge of the backfield upon his arrival and will, no doubt, be able to turn out a strong offense from the material on hand."

The Indiana yearbook, *Arbutus*, would later state: "When it was learned that the great Jim Thorpe, the best all-'round athlete in the world, was to be added to Indiana's coaching staff, the wildest enthusiasm prevailed in the Crimson camp. His coming to town was a greater event than Foundation Day is to a freshman, and the Bloomington schoolboys were more in their glory than when a circus comes to town."

Thorpe's obligation to the Giants would keep him another 10 days. When he arrived on October 7, he told the *Daily Student*, "I regret I could not come to Bloomington sooner than I have, but now that I am here, I will make every effort to develop the backfield men and kickers to the best of my ability."

His arrival also made the front page of October 8 edition of the Bloomington *Weekly Courier*, sharing space with news from the war front: "After some weeks of anxious waiting, McGraw's national pastimers turn over to the university football coaching staff one of the greatest athletes the world has ever known, James Thorpe. Students, alumni and, in fact, the entire college world look forward to the coming of this great athlete, with real eagerness to know exactly how his coaching will compare with his known ability as a player. In fact, foremost in the minds of these men is, can this All-American star teach the Indiana backfield men the tricks that made him so famous at Carlisle?"

A Warrior's Mentality

With Thorpe now coaching Indiana's running backs, expectations were high when the Hoosiers journeyed to the University of Chicago for a Western Conference clash against the highly regarded Maroons of Amos Alonzo Stagg. An estimated 15,000 Indiana fans made the trip to Chicago's Stagg Field and witnessed a classic contest. Indiana outplayed the host Maroons the entire second half but lost, 13-7.

"Indiana Deserved To Win Game," the headline read in the October 19 issue of the Bloomington *Weekly Courier*.

Using the metaphorical style of this wartime era, G.W. Axelson of the *Chicago Herald* wrote: "Taking a leaf out of Balkan unpleasantness, Chicago and Indiana went into grip at Stagg Field yesterday. Meat axes were not used, but that was about the only implement of warfare not employed by the contending forces, and before the fracas ended, the sidelines were littered with the wounded."

Axelson credited Thorpe for helping with the halftime adjustments.

"In the second half, the visitors had apparently been handed some extra information by Childs and Thorpe, as they took the ball on their own side of the center line and pushed it to the Maroons' 5-yard line ... Indiana presented a mystifying lineup, with a set of silent signals, which had the Maroons up in the air at the start, the team lining up in an L-shaped formation, with Whitaker (quarterback Frank Whitaker) slugging the code in the deaf and dumb language."

Silent signals and the "L" formation were innovations Childs brought to Indiana the year before, but equally surprising to the Maroons was Indiana's newly acquired toughness.

Thorpe had a reputation for being brutal on the gridiron. George Halas, the Chicago Bears great, recalled an encounter with Thorpe in the pros: "He blocked with his shoulder and it felt like he hit you with a 4-by-4 ... He never tackled with his arms and shoulders. He would leg-whip the ball carrier (an illegal method now). If he hit you from behind, he would throw that big body across your back and damn near break you in two."

Axelson noted Indiana's rough play that day at Chicago: "Penalties were frequent, but a lot of rough work escaped the officials, as a few full arm swings were noticed, not to mention gouging and strangle holds. The visitors had the advantage until the Maroons discovered that it did not pay to turn the other cheek."

Back in Bloomington, Thorpe became the big man on campus, according to the *Arbutus*: "Jim won a place in the heart of every player and every rooter before the week was out. His hearty smile livened up the gloom that reigned often on Jordan Field, and his occasional exhibitions of running or kicking inspired Indiana's kicking staff and back-field men to emulate him."

A Marvel in the Midst

Thorpe was his own halftime show back then -- a veritable Punt, Pass and Kick Contest.

The late John E. Stempel, former head of the IU School of Journalism, recalled: "Those of my generation remember Thorpe's kicking exhibitions between halves of IU games. There were not great band shows in those days, and he provided excellent entertainment."

"Men came from distances to see Jim's exhibitions of punting between halves," the *Arbutus* wrote. "It was nothing for him to dodge a dozen tacklers, or to punt 75 yards with an easy nonchalance that seemed almost uncanny. One evening he drop-kicked from the 60-yard line and when asked about it later retorted that he was "just foolin' around and never drop-kicked any.' "

Years later, in one of his "Looking Back" columns, former Bloomington *Daily Telephone* editor Herbert H. Skirvin recalled a Thorpe feat that left him and his two older brothers "bug-eyed with astonishment and talking about it for years."

The three of them were in a crowd observing some kicking tryouts at Jordan Field when they noticed a "big, dark stranger" conducting a demonstration.

"He punted four balls, all of them sailing downfield 45 to 55 yards in the air (still a good

boot today)," Skirvin wrote. "Several gridders came over for a closer look and we asked one, 'Who is that guy?' The player replied, 'That's the great Jim Thorpe. He's one of our assistant coaches now.' The name didn't mean anything to us then, but having heard the word 'great,' seeing the man kick and noticing he looked like an Indian, we edged in as near as possible.

"From this vantage point we heard one of the backfielders ask Thorpe, 'What was the longest punt you ever got off, Coach?' In so many words Thorpe answered, 'I'll try to show you,' and he told the center to heave him another ball. Catching the ball on the goal line, he took a couple of strides forward and gave the pigskin a terrific smash with his foot. As the 'plunk' reverberated over the area, the ball soared through the air, landing 75 yards away, then bouncing and rolling over the far goal line.

"Everyone watching, except me, gasped. I was only six. I didn't understand what had happened. My oldest brother, nine, explained, 'He kicked the ball 100 yards!' "It was almost unbelievable, as I fully realized several years later. Perhaps, over the years, one or more other kickers have matched that distance. I don't know. I do know Thorpe's punt that day was the longest one I've ever seen, and I've watched a lot of football."

Thorpe the Man

Outside of the football field, information on Thorpe's days in Bloomington is sketchy at best.

He brought with him his wife, Iva, and their toddler son, Jimmy. They lodged at the Hotel Bowles, located on the corner of Sixth and College, where Graham Plaza now stands.

On Sundays, Jim would take the train to Lafayette to play in the Wabash Athletic Association football games as a member of Pine Village Athletic Club. Other players came from Purdue, Wabash, DePauw and even Notre Dame, although many used assumed names to protect their "amateur" status.

When Thorpe was not playing or coaching football, his favorite pastime was sleep. "Sleep, to him, was the most important point in training," Wilbur J. Gobrecht wrote in his 1972 biography, *Jim Thorpe, Carlisle Indian.*

Thorpe, whose Indian name was Bright Path, also was part Irish and raised a Roman Catholic. If he wished to attend Mass, St. Charles Catholic Church was two blocks away at the corner of Fourth and Madison.

When it came to eating, Thorpe was a meat-and-potatoes guy. The Thanksgiving fare served at the Hotel Bowles in 1915 was right up his alley. The menu, as listed in the November 25 issue of the *Weekly Courier*, consisted of "Hoosier" turkey, sweet potatoes, dumplings, scrambled calf brains, wild rabbit and, get this, "braised o'possum."

Thorpe also liked a good whiskey and a good game of billiards, so he probably dropped into the Greek Pool Room on the east side of the square or into one of the many establishments in an area known as The Levee, located a couple of blocks north of the square approximately where the Showers Building is now. If he drank too much, Thorpe could stumble home to the Bowles.

Thorpe's weakness for alcohol would be a problem for life.

"The wild sprees that followed his drinking bouts are legion," Gobrecht wrote. His stay in Bloomington was free of any such incidents, perhaps because he had a wife and baby with him. When sober, Thorpe had a magnanimity about him.

As Gobrecht discovered in the recollections of those who knew him, "There is a grandeur about Jim when he talks to a crowd. With quiet dignity, the simple, homespun Indian speaks the only way he knows, with plainness and truthfulness."

It was this demeanor that spared Thorpe much of the indignities suffered by native Americans of that era. There were no reports of racial unpleasantries during Thorpe's time in Bloomington.

"During their stay here, Mr. and Mrs. Thorpe made many friends," the *Weekly Courier* wrote.

Moving On

For all of the hype about Thorpe's influence on the Indiana football team, the Hoosiers had only one win and a tie to show for the five games he served as an assistant. The victory came at Northwestern's expense, 14-6. The tie came against Washington and Lee, 7-7. The other losses came at the hands of Ohio State, 10-9, and Purdue, 7-0.

In early December, 1915, Thorpe's days in Bloomington came to an end. Football season was over and baseball season was around the corner. The December 3 issue of the *Weekly Courier* noted his departure: "Assistant coach Jim Thorpe, wife and son, Jimmy Jr., departed today for Yale, Okla., where they spend most of the winter on Mr. Thorpe's farm. It is said that Thorpe received $1,000 for his seven weeks of services here and that he picked up $500 more after the Purdue game playing with Pine Village and Canton, Ohio (another

pro team). Mr. Thorpe will begin training with the New York Giants baseball team at Marlin, Texas during the early spring."

Thorpe would go on to play six seasons of professional baseball with the Giants, Reds and Braves. He also continued to play professional football for the Canton Bulldogs and was elected president of the American Professional Football Association in 1920.

In 1917, his son Jimmy would die at the age of four from infantile paralysis. The Thorpes would later adopt a son, William Thourlby, who would become the Marlboro Man of cigarette fame.

Thorpe would eventually divorce Iva and marry two more times. He would father six more children. His problems with alcohol would keep him drifting from job to job -- everything from a sideshow to a movie extra to a bouncer. He was nearly destitute when a heart attack took him in 1953.

Thorpe was buried in Tulsa, Okla. and later moved to Mauch Chunk, Pa., not far from where he rose to fame at Carlisle. Mauch Chunk, which means "Sleeping Bear" in the Indian tongue of that area, was later renamed Jim Thorpe, Pa.

In 1983, over seven decades after stripping Thorpe of his gold medals, the international Olympic Committee saw fit to return them. In 1999, a resolution was put forth in the U.S. Senate proclaiming Thorpe "Athlete of the Century."

And while the great Jim Thorpe now belongs to the ages, for seven weeks in 1915 he belonged to Indiana University.

Hoosiers Drop-Kick Rockne

Bloomington Herald-Times
January 19, 2003 (side bar)

Before C.C. Childs welcomed Jim Thorpe as an assistant coach in 1915, he considered other candidates.

One of the applicants was a recent Notre Dame graduate, Knute Rockne -- yes, **the** Knute Rockne.

Hoosiers, 10 Years After

While the movie Hoosiers *was being filmed in Indiana in 1985, there were several local connections, beginning with the screenwriter, Angelo Pizzo, a Bloomington native and Indiana University grad. I started following the story back then and continued to write about it following its astonishing success. When the 10th anniversary of the film arrived in 1996, it was time to examine what made it one of the best sports movies ever. With that in mind, I tracked down the principal architects and most of the cast. Although Gene Hackman did not return my call, one of the film's biggest fans did – George Steinbrenner. This was published in the* Herald-Times *and later in* Indianapolis Monthly Magazine.

Bloomington Herald-Times
September 15, 1996

They came from the heartland and found their way into our hearts, all-American boys with all- American names like Merle and Buddy and Ollie and Rade.

They would become perhaps the most celebrated champions in the illustrious history of Indiana high school basketball, and the wonder of it all is that they are merely figments of our collective imaginations.

They are the Hickory Huskers, the fictional heroes of the movie *Hoosiers,* which is 10 years old this fall. Has it really been a decade since the ball left the hands of Jimmy Chitwood and proceeded on its inevitable goalward route, lifting Hickory over mighty South Bend Central in the Indiana state championship game?

It has.

Forget all the sports movies that have come out since – *Blue Chips, Rudy, The Babe* and all the *Hoosiers* wannabees. None of them has endured like *Hoosiers,* which continues to amaze its creators with its longevity.

"I've had so many people over the years tell me they love the story for all kinds of reasons, obviously because it was so inspirational," director David Anspaugh said. "It reminded them of where they came from, and the people. One lawyer called to tell me the movie made him weep because his children will never find that kind of life."

Following his brilliant playing career at Notre Dame, Rockne hoped to go into medicine. He applied to St. Louis University but was turned down. At the time Rockne was engaged to Bonnie Guendolen Skiles. With a bride to look out for in the near future, Rockne needed some employment. Coaching was an option.

Childs was in his first year at Indiana and looking for some help. But Childs, a former Ivy Leaguer out of Yale, did not think Rockne was suited for Indiana, despite the latter's All-American credentials.

In a letter dated June 28, 1914, a letter reeking of Ivy League arrogance, Childs expressed his feelings to president William L. Bryan: "It has been suggested to me that a Mr. Rockne of Notre Dame assist in football next year. For several reasons I am not in favor of this plan. It has been my intention to interest the alumni as far as possible this coming season, and I am sure that the methods of Notre Dame are quite different than those of Indiana or Yale. If you think that this particular third system will be beneficial to the athletic life at Indiana next year, I will be glad to assist in carrying out your judgment."

Bryan deferred to the judgment of his new coach, and Rockne was passed over. Hired in his stead was Arthur Cotton Berndt, a three-sport star at Indiana from 1908-11 and future mayor of Bloomington (1935-38). Berndt was later inducted into the Indiana Athletic Hall of Fame.

Rockne returned to Notre Dame, where he taught chemistry and served as an assistant to Jesse Harper. Rockne replaced Harper in 1918 and led Notre Dame to unprecedented glory the next 13 years before perishing in a plane crash in 1931.

To think that Indiana considered Rockne unsuited for its mediocre program only makes the decision all the more staggering. Looking back at a century of losing tradition, Hoosier followers now are left to wonder, "What if ..." '

For those who have not had the opportunity to see *Hoosiers*, it is a story which has its base deep in the roots of Indiana basketball, little Milan High's upset of vaunted Muncie Central in the 1954 state championship game.

The movie takes you back into that innocent time when "basketball was the only game in town," said Bobby Plump, the real Jimmy Chitwood of Milan fame. "It was a period of maybe the best time for athletics and tranquility in the United States in this century."

It was Plump who sank the last-second jumper to beat Muncie Central in '54, and Plump who was on the set in '86 to make sure the *Hoosiers* version was authentic.

"It was identical," he said proudly.

The movie was the brainchild of Anspaugh and screenwriter/producer Angelo Pizzo, who longed to make such a movie from their Sigma Nu fraternity days at Indiana University. As Hoosier natives, they wanted to make the quintessential movie on Indiana high school basketball.

"We had a love, a passion, an understanding of Indiana high school basketball," said Pizzo, who grew up in Bloomington and was determined to make Indiana more a part of the movie than Steve Tesich's 1979 film, *Breaking Away*, based on Indiana University's renowned bicycle race, the Little 500.

To give the movie its true flavor, the creators decided to shoot the film off the beaten path in Indiana at such remote locations as New Richmond, Nineveh and Knightstown.

Initially, the creators tried to find California actors who could play basketball. That experiment failed.

There was a shortage of basketball ability and an intangible that Pizzo called a "regional quality about them, which is not so easily defined ... There is no question that there are differences between someone who grew up in San Fernando Valley and someone who grew up in Brownsburg, Ind. It shows in the way they walk, the way they look, the way they talk."

Searching for Hoosier Hoopsters

Pizzo and Anspaugh auditioned more than 700 young men on the courts of Indiana University-Purdue University at Indianapolis in the fall of 1985. They were looking for two things: basketball ability and that 1950s Midwestern look. They not only wanted the characters to be authentic, they wanted the basketball to be authentic.

"You can't fake playing basketball," Pizzo said. "To be a good basketball player, you have to start playing when you're six years old. There are so many kinds of skills. It is not just dribbling and shooting. It is a second sense that you only get by playing basketball for years and years. We decided we had to cast guys who were good basketball players, and hope they could act."

From out of this mix came seven of the eight Hickory Huskers:

* Steve Hollar: 18, a member of Warsaw's 1984 state championship team. He would play the headstrong Rade Butcher.

* Scott Summers: 18, a former high school player at Bethesda Christian; cast as Strap, the religious son of a preacher.

* Brad Boyle: 18, prepped at Bellmont and cast as the slow-minded Whit.

* Brad Long: 22, son of former IU player, Gary Long; played high school ball at Greenwood and cast as the rebellious Buddy.

* Kent Poole: 20, prepped at Western Boone and cast as the scrappy Merle.

* Wade Schenck: 17, the youngest Husker, still playing high school ball at L&M at the time of the filming. He played Ollie McPike, the unassuming manager who saves Hickory in the semifinals.

* Maris Valainis: 21, attended Indianapolis Chatard but never played organized basketball. He was 5-foot-8 in high school and sprouted to 6-2. He showed enough skill in the auditions to land the part of Chitwood, the ultimate hero.

The only Husker chosen from out of state was a 22-year-old California actor, David Neidorf. He would be cast as Everett, the son of the alcoholic assistant coach, Shooter, played by Dennis Hopper. What Pizzo saw in Neidorf was the "perfect marriage of a character with an actor. He has a rural quality about him. He fits right in. You can't tell he grew up in California, and he plays a good game of basketball."

The others basically played themselves. From the very beginning the men were told to call each other by their (stage) names, Pizzo said.

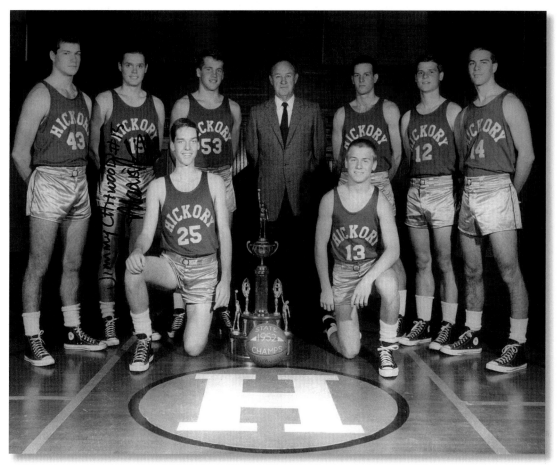

The Hickory Huskers of Hoosiers *lore. Front row: "Rade Butcher" (Steve Hollar), "Ollie McPike" (Wade Schenck). Back row: "Whit Butcher" (Brad Boyle), "Jimmy Chitwood" (Maris Valainis), "Strap Purl" (Scott Summers), Coach "Norman Dale" (Gene Hackman), "Everett Flatch" (David Neidorf), "Merle Webb" (Kent Poole), "Buddy Walker" (Brad Long). Autographed by "Jimmy Chitwood" at 10-year reunion, 1996. (Photo courtesy of Orion Pictures)*

"Friends would tell me, `Merle, that character is you,' " said Poole, who now coaches junior varsity girls' basketball at Western Boone. "It truly fit my personality. When I played ball, I always played with the attitude of trying to help the team. There is a scene in the state finals where I'm diving on the floor. That wasn't scripted. That's the type of thing I try to teach my kids."

As the wise guy, Buddy, Long is kicked off the team early in the movie but works his way back.

"I acted awful early but redeemed myself and was captain of the team," said Long, who now enjoys giving motivational speeches. "That is what the movie is all about, redeeming yourself, like Shooter (Hopper) and Norman Dale (Gene Hackman). I use that in some of my speaking engagements."

Boyle felt comfortable playing the soft-spoken Whit because "I'm pretty quiet," he said.

"Whit is a play on words, like `dimwit.' I was supposed to play a slow character. I acted dumb-founded, not quite with it. I thought I did a good job until some people told me I didn't have to act."

The guys got a crash course in acting right on the set, sometimes from Hackman, the leading man.

"They are all very enthusiastic and professional in terms of attitudes," said Hackman during the filming. "They are quite talented. They were cast as ballplayers, but then they had readings to do and were quite good."

Neidorf found himself blending right in with the Hoosier natives.

"I was the only person from California and they were super nice to me," he said. "I stayed at Wade's farm and at Kent's house."

Even though Neidorf went on to play prominent roles in *Empire of the Sun*, *Platoon* and *Bull*

Durham, his role as Everett in *Hoosiers* "seems to be the one people remember me by. In later movies, there were a lot of jealousies, people trying to grab the spotlight. Here there was a sense of togetherness. Their value system is a lot different. I grew up on the West Coast where rebellion was normal. In the Midwest, there is more of a sense of value and duty."

Rolling the Dice

Upon completion of the filming, there were some lingering doubts.

"We had no idea whether people would walk out of the movie, whether they would get it, whether anybody but our family would buy tickets to see it," Pizzo said.

The first screening was at a mall in Los Angeles. The reception was lukewarm.

"I didn't sleep because I felt David and I had no career," Pizzo said. "This was our one shot."

Pizzo and Anspaugh decided to take the film to its inception, figuring "If it didn't make it in Indiana, it wasn't going to be released," Pizzo said. The Indiana reception was much more encouraging, so Pizzo and Anspaugh went from one motion picture company to another making their pitch.

"We went to all the studios with various presentations, sometimes with Gene Hackman and sometimes without him," Pizzo said. "Nobody believed in its commercial potential. They just thought of it as a regional film. Nobody had made a film about basketball before and made money.

"How do you make a pitch and reduce it to one sentence, one paragraph and not make it sound banal: `A coach goes to a small town to coach a basketball team ...' If you can pitch it in one sentence, you have a chance. If you cannot communicate the essence in one sentence, you're in trouble. I never felt in a million years I could pitch this to an exec' and he would want to buy it. If I sent the script in right now, no one would buy it."

Finally, Orion Pictures took the leap of faith. The film cost $6 million to make. It cleared over $35 million at the box office and much more in video sales. In addition to frequent appearances on Home Box Office or Cinemax, *Hoosiers* has other indicators of its enduring quality:

* A major phone company using it as a motivational tool.

* A movement in New Richmond to rename the town New Hickory.

* A losing high school basketball team in Ohio watching it before each game and advancing all the way to the state finals.

"I still meet people out there who say they play it before their volleyball tournaments and other sports," said Valainis. "They come up to me and say, `You're the reason we won this championship.' "

Even 'the Big Guy' Liked It

George Steinbrenner, owner of the New York Yankees, has seen the movie over 40 times.

From his business office in Tampa, Steinbrenner was delighted to talk about one of his favorite subjects. Steinbrenner has Indiana ties from his days as a student at Culver Military and later as an assistant football coach under Jack Mollenkopf at Purdue.

"The movie brought back so many memories of Indiana," he said. "One time Lee Iacocca (the former CEO of Chrysler) and I were flying to Europe. I said I would bring a movie. Lee didn't want to watch a movie, but I put on *Hoosiers* anyway. By the end of the film he was sitting there with tears welling up in his eyes, just like I do every time. I can recite all the lines. I use it for self-motivation whenever I'm feeling bad, like whenever something goes wrong with my team."

"It transcends languages and countries," Plump said.

There was the time Anspaugh was attending a screening in Russia. Throughout the movie, the audience sat in stone silence. Anspaugh was wondering if it message was lost on the Russians. It wasn't until the final credits appeared that the audience arose in unison and gave a standing ovation that lasted 10 minutes.

The ingredients were there all along, hindsight has showed.

"It is a good movie, a good story and well told," said Anspaugh. "Everything, starting with Angelo's words, right down to the performances, down to the crew, down to the people of New Richmond. We even got lucky with the weather -- overcast, gray, powerful. So when we went into the gyms, it was bright and dreamy. The movies that are made today are mostly special effects. When you leave the theater, nothing stays with you. That's not the case with *Hoosiers*."

The Fallen Hoosier

Ten years later, as the 20th anniversary of Hoosiers *neared, I was inspired to write a much more sobering story. In 2003, I saw a small AP wire story noting the sad death of Kent Poole, who played "Merle" in the movie. The more I looked into the story, the sadder it got. The* Herald-Times *gave "The Fallen Hoosier" front-page play over two days in June, 2006. It also was picked up by* Indianapolis Monthly. *I now look back on it as one of my finest works, worthy of honorable mention in the 2007 edition of* Best American Sports Writing.

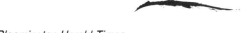

Bloomington Herald-Times
June 25-26, 2006

There was something in the man's voice that left Angelo Pizzo with an uneasy feeling that September night.

As a Hollywood screenwriter, Pizzo is tuned into people's inner feelings and emotions, and there definitely was emotion in the voice on that answering machine. It was the voice of Kent Poole, the steely "Merle" of *Hoosiers* movie fame, a movie scripted by Pizzo.

Thinking back to a chance encounter at the 2002 Final Four more than a year earlier, Pizzo recalled Poole requesting his address so he could send him something -- something important, Poole said. And there was that same request on the answering machine, but in a much more serious tone this time.

Pizzo always had a soft spot in his heart for Poole, the kid who took a small part in *Hoosiers* and helped it become one of the most endearing films of the last 20 years. It was Poole/Merle uttering one of the film's most inspirational lines, "Let's win this for all the small schools that never had a chance to get here."

It also was Merle getting the fictional Hickory Huskers to clap in unison before their regional fi-

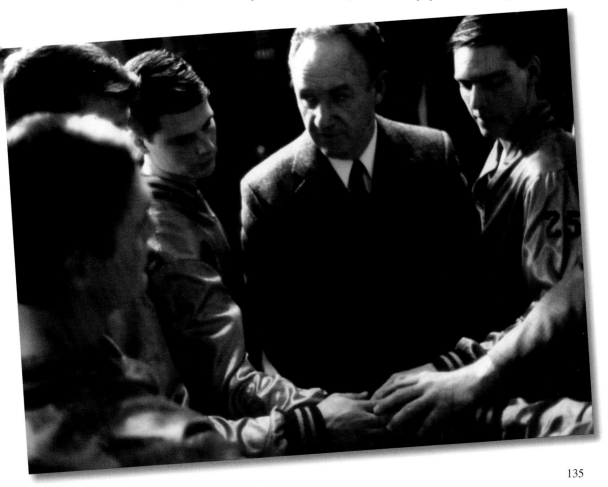

Although Kent Poole (third from left) will forever be remembered as "Merle Webb" in the 1986 movie classic, Hoosiers, *his life was all too short. (Photo courtesy of Orion Pictures)*

nal, and it was Merle who, at the end of that game, patted Ollie on the butt and convinced the lad he could make the game-winning free throws.

But the voice on the answering machine lacked the conviction and confidence of years past.

"There seemed to be a strain in his voice," Pizzo would say later. "Kent said, 'It's really important. I want to send you something, but I lost your address. I need your address again.' I thought, 'This doesn't sound well,' so I called him up hoping he would answer."

But Poole was not there and did not return the call. Three days later, Pizzo received a call from another former Hickory Husker, Brad Long ("Buddy"). It was the worst of all possible news: Kent Poole was dead -- by his own hand. He was only 39.

For the next month, Pizzo went to his mail box every day yearning for something from Poole, something that would offer insight into the man's troubled last days. Nothing ever came.

'Merle'

When Pizzo and director David Anspaugh were trying to assemble a cast to play the Hickory Huskers, they were looking for somebody who could really play basketball and who could be coached into making a limited number of lines believable. More than 1,000 young men auditioned for the eight parts. A kid who helped lead Western Boone High to within a basket of the Indiana state finals in 1982 was one of those elite eight.

He was Kent Poole, a 21-year-old farm boy with a square jaw, an honest face and a serious disposition.

"We chose Kent because of the combination of three things," Pizzo recalled last month over lunch in Bloomington, where he now makes his home. "He looked like an Indiana high school player and really was a good basketball player. The third thing we looked for was sincerity. He was a deeply sincere person."

As one of the older members of a group ranging in age from 17 to 23, Poole became one of the enforcers.

"When you get guys of that age together, it's like 'Animal House,'" Pizzo said. "Kent was always the one who said, 'All right guys, let's get back to work.' He took it more seriously than anybody. You could see it in the expression in his face. He was a very responsible guy."

"Kent was the anchor of that group," said Bloomington's Don "Strats" Stratigos, who had a

small part in the movie and also acted as one of the film's advisers. "Kent came to work every day with his lunch pail. He was a rock."

"Kent and I were roommates," said Long, who kept in touch with Poole. "We got along well. You can imagine getting eight boys together between the ages of 18 to 23. There were a lot of shenanigans. Whenever we did the scenes, Kent was methodical -- worried something might go wrong."

"Kent and Brad were over 21 and hung out together," said Greene County's Wade Schenck, who played the part of Ollie. "They were like the older brothers of the group. They watched over us and made sure we stayed in line."

"Kent was the glue that held everybody together," said Maris Valainis, who played the team's star, Jimmy Chitwood. "He was a good person -- upbeat, positive."

"There wasn't a cynical bone in his body," Pizzo said. "He didn't lobby for extra lines or try to make any more out of his part than what was asked. He was the most mature in terms of his ability to adapt as a nonactor to some really difficult demands for someone who has never been in front of a camera before."

In a 1996 interview with the *Herald-Times*, Poole said, "I've been told, 'That (Merle) character is you.' It truly fit my personality. When I played ball, I always played with the attitude of trying to help the team."

When called to make his "win-one-for-the-small-schools" line, Poole delivered it straight from the heart, Pizzo said.

"Nobody could have said that line better -- out of all our guys. We could have given it to anybody, but it was a tough line. If it was said wrong, it was going to come out as corny as can be. It had to be authentic and sincere in a truthful way, not an acted way. That was the way Kent was."

Little did Pizzo, Poole or anybody else know at the time, the movie was going to change their lives.

Glory Days

Thanks to the movie's enormous success, the guys who played the Hickory Huskers became overnight sensations.

"We just didn't realize what we were a part of," Poole said in that H-T interview from '96. "We never dreamt the movie would be what it is."

Poole and two other Huskers, Valainis and David Neidorf ("Everett Flatch"), garnered other movie offers out of it. Poole's second go-around came in the 1988 film, "Fresh Horses," shot in Ohio and directed by Anspaugh. It was Anspaugh who thought Poole was the right fit for a small part as Molly Ringwald's boyfriend.

"We were looking for the clean-cut, all-American boy," Anspaugh said. "The part wasn't big enough to fly in somebody from L.A., so I thought of Kent."

It was just enough of a tease to make Poole wonder if he shouldn't leave the farm for Hollywood.

"Farming was his love, but I think he did question whether he should look into that," recalled his wife, Judi.

Kent Poole and Judi Johnson met in their sophomore year at Western Boone. They became high school sweethearts and continued to date when she went off to Purdue and he went off to film *Hoosiers*. They got married the year the movie was released, 1986. She went into education and he came back to tend the family farm.

"After the movie, people wanted to be around him," Judi said. "He didn't know a stranger. He was friendly to all types of people, rich or poor, educated or non-educated. It didn't matter."

The second taste of acting made it harder to put *Hoosiers* behind him, Judi said. "I don't think *Hoosiers* changed him, but I think it did probably make him question what his purpose was. He was told after the movie, 'Maybe you should go out there (Hollywood). You have a knack for this.' But he was married and loved farming. He thought at the time, 'Yeah, right,' but I think he probably always wondered whether he should have pursued something."

Poole continued to keep the movie flames burning by offering his services at speaking engagements around the state.

"I think the movie had more impact on him than anybody," said Schenck, who wound up living not far from the Pooles in Hendricks County. "I think it was hard for him to come down from that spotlight. Once all the glitz and glamour was over, it was like, 'Now I have to go sit on a tractor for eight hours?' It didn't hit me like that. I just went back to high school."

"Kent loved to talk about the movie and loved to be interviewed about it," said longtime friend and short-time business partner, Kim Demaree. "The movie was such a rise for a kid from a small town. That publicity set the stage for everything else. From then on, everything in life that wasn't grand was a disappointment to him."

Downward Spiral

By the late 1990s, the movie was well into its second decade and growing in stature. Kent Poole's life was going the other direction. His farming partnership with Demaree was on its way toward being dissolved, and his marriage also was headed that way after he admitted to an affair.

"When I found out Kent was in an affair, I hit a brick wall," Judi said. "I thought I was in a happy marriage. I knew we weren't spending as much time together, but never in a million years did I sense that. I guess there is no such thing as a safe marriage."

Living in a small community, Kent's public image took a major hit.

"Put us in Indianapolis, and only your neighbors know," Judi said. "Put us out here, and everybody knows. Kent wanted to have a good image. That was important. After he went through that mess, it was hard for him to hold his head high because he knew the community knew. He had been the star basketball player, the *Hoosiers* star, the good father, had three beautiful kids. After that he really struggled with his reputation."

Although the Pooles continued to have marital difficulties, Kent never shrank from his duties as the father of two daughters and one son. Kassi was born in 1988, followed by Trevor in 1990 and Paige in 1996.

"He was a great dad," Judi said. "He was a part of their life in every shape and form. He would quit work in the field to catch a game of theirs. Then he would go right back out there and get started as soon as the game was over. At home, he would be in the front yard playing pitch and catch. He would even give the kids their baths and read them stories at night. He did all the things a dad should do."

Poole also volunteered his time as an assistant coach for the Western Boone girls' freshman team. At that point, however, he might have been spreading himself too thin.

Inner Torment

For all Poole had going for him, he could not find happiness, Judi said.

"I can remember him saying, 'I don't know why I can't be happy. I know this is what I want, what is inside this house -- you, these kids, this house. Why can't this be enough?' Kent knew he had to get some issues straightened out."

They tried marriage counseling, but Kent still couldn't find any inner peace. Near the end, he was supposedly getting some therapy, but his friends questioned how earnest he was about it.

"He just wasn't happy with himself," said Demaree, who remained friends with him after the partnership was dissolved. "He was always looking for something to take away that eternal pain. I don't know if it was depression or what, but it was an illness. I think he was hurting so bad, he would do anything to feel better."

Kent and Judi tried for three years to resolve their differences before she filed for divorce in November 2002.

"We both fought to keep that marriage together," she said. "Neither one of us could leave. We tried several times to leave or end it and couldn't. That probably showed the deep commitment and love we had for each other. Neither could walk away."

Once the divorce papers were served, their paths did not cross much. They both started seeing other people and trying to move forward with their lives. But for Kent, the reality that his marriage was truly over didn't sink in until the 10th of September, 2003.

Down and Troubled

The last day of Kent Poole's life started badly, with an unsettling visit to his wife's office. As the assistant superintendent of Western Boone Schools, Judi Poole was well into a busy September school day when her estranged husband showed up about 10 a.m.

Kent wanted to resolve some issues in their pending divorce, a divorce that was taking its toll on both of them. After the discussion became heated, Judi hurriedly left the office, got into her car and headed toward nearby Thorntown. In her rearview mirror, she could see Kent tailing her in his 2003 Silverado pickup.

Once she got to Thorntown, she pulled over on Main Street and waited for Kent to climb in.

"He got into the car and was very agitated," she said earlier this month from behind the same office desk where that ill-fated day began three years ago. As the argument in the car began to heat up again, Judi resigned herself and yielded to Kent's demands. Her sudden concession seemed to catch him off guard, she noted from the startled look on his face. Kent left quietly.

About 6 p.m. that night, he called her at home. As she recalled, the conversation started off with him asking, "Why is it so easy for you to just give up?"

"I just told him I was tired of arguing," she responded.

"That's all? Don't you want to talk about it?"

But the time for talk had long since passed in Judi's book, much to Kent's dismay.

"As I think back on it, that (settlement issues) was the one thing keeping us together, our only communication," she said. "And when I conceded he realized, 'We're done.'"

Last Call

Later that night, Poole dropped in to one of his favorite watering holes, the Good Ol' Boys Sports Bar in Jamestown, a community of less than 1,000 on the Boone-Hendricks county line.

It was Wednesday night, karaoke night at this popular spot. Already there were Demaree and the bar's owner, Randy Eck, a mutual friend. Recalling the events at a Hendricks County diner three years later, Demaree remembers it all too well.

"Kent came through the front door and it was typical Kent. He just threw his arms up and said, 'Whoa, am I glad today's over.' He sat down there with us. We had some dinner, a few beers and even went up there to sing."

The karaoke song Poole chose fills Demaree with melancholy now. It was James Taylor's version of "You've Got a Friend."

> "When you're down and troubled, And you need a helping hand, And nothing, nothing is going right ..."

Demaree estimates he left Poole at the bar around 11:30. Ahead of Poole was a 20-minute drive to his cottage on Lake Holiday, a quiet spot south of Crawfordsville. Sometime around 1:30 a.m., Poole turned onto County Road 400 West in Montgomery County, less than a mile from the cottage. However, with an alcohol content later measured at almost 2.5 times the legal limit, Poole turned too sharply and hung his truck up on a culvert.

Shortly after that, the phone roused Demaree from a deep sleep. On the other end was Judi, informing him that Kent was in need of a tow. A few minutes later, Kent got through to Demaree.

"He was sobbing because he ran his truck off the road," Demaree said. "He told me specifically what I needed to bring to get his truck unstuck — a hoist and some chains. It was stuff that somebody who was going to commit suicide would not have cared about."

Demaree called Eck and asked for his help, and Eck obliged. They weren't overly concerned because Poole was an easy 15-minute walk from the cottage. On the way to the lake house, Kent called Judi a second time. There was something in his voice again that set off an alarm, probably the same tone Pizzo detected in a phone call a few days before.

"I had a sense of nervousness about it, although Kent really didn't give me any reason to be worried," Judi said.

Judi's intuition was dead-on, because somewhere on the walk down that dark county road, it all caught up with Kent — the guilt from the affair, the loss of self-esteem, the long descent into depression, the reality the marriage was over and now this, wrecking his new truck while under the influence.

Said Demaree, "He probably looked at it as one more thing to explain, one more embarrassment."

While hastening her drive to the cottage, Judi kept dialing Kent's cell phone, but the signal around the Lake Holiday area was faint. About 10 minutes from the cottage, she finally reached him. It was an even more foreboding conversation.

"Tell the kids I love them," he said. "Please, they have to know."

A cold chill swept over Judi as the phone went dead. She nervously continued to dial but could not get through.

Her Worst Fears Confirmed

When Judi pulled into the driveway, it was pitch black and deathly quiet. The headlights from the truck caught something over by the trees in the front yard. She turned the truck and aimed the lights in that direction. From a distance, it looked like Kent was leaning against a tree. She got out of the truck and cautiously approached.

"I kept saying, 'Kent, turn around. Turn around, Kent.'"

But as Judi got closer, she could see his feet weren't touching the ground. And then she looked up and saw an orange extension cord — one end looped around a branch tree, the other around Kent's neck. Terrified, she ran back to her car and frantically dialed Demaree. He and Eck were down at the crash site trying to figure out how to free the truck. At the sound of Judi hysterical voice, they rushed to the house and saw the grisly scene for themselves.

"When we got there, Judi was sitting there with her lights pointing toward the yard,"

Demaree said. "It looked like Kent was leaning against the tree, but it seemed a little peculiar he would be out there like that. I was trying to talk to him but getting no response. As we got out there, I could see something in the tree.

"At that point, I was trying to put all this together," Demaree continued. "I was still trying to talk to him when I realized his feet weren't on the ground. Then it all made sense. Randy and I took off running at the same time."

Eck lifted Poole up while Demaree unfastened the cord. A former EMT, Demaree immediately attempted to resuscitate the victim but knew it was futile.

Kent Poole, still Merle to many, was gone.

After Shock

Revisiting it all three years later, Demaree had to fight back tears and choke out the sentence, "He was … a good friend."

It still doesn't make sense to him.

"Never did I dream Kent would do anything like that because he loved life. He lived to have a good time, just everyday fun stuff like boating, fishing and snowmobiling. But Kent was also one of those guys who would do something and then raise his hands and say, 'What was I thinking?' I guarantee before he died he was already thinking, 'What have I done?' "

Three days after his death, Poole was laid to rest near the Old Union Church in Boone County. The man who thought he was no longer respected drew 1,300 to his memorial service. Most of them never saw it coming.

"I never even considered it," Long said. "Kent was always larger than life. I was sitting in my office when my minister called me. When you first hear news like that, a kind of storm comes over your head like, 'Why? When? Where?' I had just talked to him two weeks ago. That's when I started putting the puzzle together."

Long now finds it difficult to watch the movie or even look at the Huskers' team photo.

"When I look at (the photo), I can't help but be drawn to Kent," he said. "It's still hard to believe, even three years later. I still think about him almost every day."

The tragedy has given Valainis perspective.

"It crosses your mind how precious everything is, how something can change from minute to minute," Valainis said. "You look at your kids and your wife and everything important, and it makes you prioritize."

Schenck, a father himself, is not so forgiving.

"When you leave behind three little kids, it's hard for me to respect that," he said.

Judi has chosen to let the anger go. She has since remarried and is savoring that second chance.

"The only time I get angry is when I think of the kids not having their dad," she said, dabbing her eyes with a tissue. "I knew him better than anybody and that's not what he wanted. That's where the sadness comes from, to know the man was tortured that much."

Anspaugh speaks from experience when he says people should not be too hard on Poole. Anspaugh had his own demons to wrestle with when he went through an agonizing divorce with actress Roma Downey, star of TV's "Touched By An Angel."

"I went through a pretty dark period in my life, too," Anspaugh said. "I know what depression is about. I dealt with it for years. When Roma pulled the plug, I went to some very dark places."

If there is a lesson here, Judi said, it is that the Kent Pooles of the world are not alone.

"In the first few months after Kent's death, I bet I had a half-dozen men come into my office and break down in front of me saying, 'I know exactly how he felt.' Even during our counseling, Kent would say, 'It's not about you, Judi. It's what is inside of me.'"

Pizzo continues to get a queasy feeling when he goes to his mail box, still longing for some clue from the grave, something that would reveal what Poole wanted to mail to him just days before his death.

"It was a blow under any circumstance," Pizzo said, "but the fact I had this voice message three days prior … I couldn't sleep that night. I was haunted by it, haunted for some time afterward. I've speculated about a lot of things. With me being a writer, I'm guessing it was something he had written. That's the only thing I can figure out."

Having kept in closer contact with Poole than the other cast members, Long also heard something disturbing in Poole's voice in a phone conversation two weeks before his death.

"At the time of the conversation, there was something that bothered me," Long said. "It was the first time he had been short with me. Was he sad and didn't want to talk? Was he too embarrassed? It just wasn't the same Kent."

"I wish it were me Kent called," Anspaugh said when he learned of the calls to Pizzo and Long. "Maybe things would have been different.

Maybe Kent would have shared how much pain he was in. I know where Kent went, but he went deeper than I did. I checked into a hospital. That's the tragic thing about Kent. He felt there was no other alternative.

"Hopefully, this story will change the life of other Kent Pooles, male and female alike," Anspaugh concluded. "Maybe more people will be aware of this disease and realize it is nothing to be ashamed of. It is universal, shared by everyone in every walk of life."

The Spirit of '76

On the 25th anniversary of IU's 1976 national championship season, the last perfect season in college basketball, I was summoned to do a look-back piece. The editors didn't have to twist my arm for this assignment. Although I found the players more than happy to talk about it, I wasn't counting on much input from Bob Knight. Knight isn't big on revisiting the past, but on one of my visits to Lubbock he agreed to talk about his first championship team at Indiana. This article was the meat of an entire section devoted to that historical season.

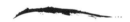

Bloomington Herald-Times
April 1, 2001

Every once in a while a team comes along that commands your admiration, a team whose members become household names, a team whose deeds become legend, a team whose memory refuses to fade. The basketball season of 1975-76 saw such a team, Indiana.

You want Hoosier household names?

How about May, Benson, Buckner, Wilkerson and Abernethy.

How about Bob Knight.

You want deeds?

How about going wire-to-wire as the No. 1 team in the polls. How about beating the reigning Olympic champions, the reigning collegiate champions and every other team in its path, all 32 of them. How rare is that?

Well, no other college basketball team has gone undefeated since, 25 years and counting.

This being the silver anniversary of that celebrated Hoosier team, the time is right to look back at that memorable season. In the last month we caught up with many of the players and even Knight himself. You would think their memories would be a little bit rusty by now, but, as Kent Benson said, "It seems like it happened yesterday, the reason being is that not a day goes by that someone doesn't come up and talk about it."

Unfinished Business

As the 1975-76 college season was about to tip off, times were pretty good around the land. Although the Cold War was still very much an issue, the climate in America was upbeat. Vietnam, Watergate and the civil unrest of the 1960s and early 1970s were in the rear view mirror as America entered its Bicentennial year. You could buy a gallon of gas for 50 cents. You could go see a matinee for a dollar. You could buy a compact car for less than $3,000 and a middle-income house for $30,000.

On the sports front, it was an era of dynasties. Cincinnati's Big Red Machine was dominating Major League baseball. Pittsburgh's Steel Curtain was ruling the National Football League. The Boston Celtics were on their way to their 12th NBA championship. The Montreal Canadiens were on their way to four straight Stanley Cup titles. The Oklahoma Sooners were coming off back-to-back college football titles. The UCLA Bruins were coming off their 10th NCAA championship in 12 years.

Title No. 10 for the Bruins sent John Wooden off to a happy retirement. And by returning the nucleus of that team -- Marques Johnson, Richard Washington, David Greenwood, Andre McCarter and Ralph Drollinger -- the Bruins once again figured to be a force in 1975-76. They were ranked No. 2 in pre-season. Ahead of them was Indiana.

The Hoosiers were returning four starters from a team that went 31-1 in '74-75, beating the opposition by an average margin of 23 points. The returning starters included Player of the Year candidate Scott May, a 6-7 senior forward; Benson, a 6-11 junior center; Quinn Buckner, a 6-3 point guard and a natural leader; and Bob Wilkerson, a 6-7 senior guard who jumped center.

Other seniors included 6-7 Tom Abernethy, a solid forward, and 6-3 Jim Crews, who started on IU's 1973 Final Four team before giving up his starting spot to Wilkerson.

May, Benson, Buckner and Wilkerson would go on to become first-round NBA draft picks. Abernethy was the 43rd picking of the '76 draft. And the Hoosiers were guided by one of college basketball's rising stars, Knight, who at the age of 35

already had directed Indiana to three Big Ten titles and one Final Four appearance in his first four years in Bloomington.

The previous season saw the Hoosiers mow down every team in their way until May broke his arm at Purdue in February.

"The team we developed in 1975 was as good a basketball team that ever played in the Big Ten," Knight said just last week. "They were not as good defensively as the team we had in '76 but better offensively because there were more guys who could score."

The '74-75 season came to a crashing halt in the regional finals at Dayton when Kentucky, a 24-point loser to a healthy Indiana team in December, jolted the Hoosiers, 92-90. The mood in the Indiana lockerroom was one of total despair.

"That might have been the lowest I ever saw our team," said May, who tried to play with a soft cast in that game but was ineffective. "Mentally and physically we were drained. In the lockerroom guys were crying. You could see how much the year, the season, all the things we had gone through, how much it meant to us."

"We were all devastated because we felt we had the team in place to win it all," said Benson, who was magnificent in defeat with 33 points and 22 rebounds against a bruising Kentucky front line.

As the Hoosiers left the lockerroom that day, their mood shifted from despair to resolve.

"We made a vow to work over the summer to improve our individual games so that when we got back together in the fall, we would work collectively toward a national championship," Benson said.

"That time period was the beginning of the national championship season," May added. Knight recalled a meeting he had the day before practice began the following October.

"I told them, 'The only thing that equates to total fulfillment is to go undefeated this year. There is no reason we should lose a game.' "

Meet Me in St. Louie

Some time during the summer, Knight summoned May and Buckner, his two co-captains. It was a short meeting, Buckner recalled.

"Coach said, 'We've got a chance to play UCLA in St. Louis.' Both of us said, 'Let's do it.' "

Knight and his seniors had a score to settle with UCLA. His second Indiana team ran into UCLA in the 1973 Final Four, at St. Louis, and had the Bruins reeling until a Steve Downing-Bill Walton collision resulted in Downing's fourth foul when it easily could have been Walton's fifth. Downing fouled out seconds later, and UCLA pulled away to a 70-59 decision on the way to title No. 9 under John Wooden.

But first up for Indiana was a pre-season test against the Soviet Olympic team, the team that ended America's string of Olympic triumphs in stunning and controversial fashion at Munich in 1972.

The big question for Indiana was May, whether he would be his old formidable self. The arm bone he fractured at Purdue now had a steel rod in it. A summer's worth of rehabilitation had yet to remove all the doubts in May's mind. Those uncertainties were put to rest when he hit 13 of 15 shots and scored 34 points as the Hoosiers conquered the Soviets, 94-78.

Said May, "I remember walking off the court and Coach coming up to me saying, 'You're back.'"

From there it was off to St. Louis, where a crowd of 19,115 gathered for a late-night, national-television showcase of the land's top two teams.

"You couldn't believe how much red there was in the stands," said Don Fischer, now in his 28th year as the radio voice of IU. "There were 19,000 in the stands and I say about 14,000 were Indiana fans."

The charged-up Hoosiers made a convincing statement with an 84-64 victory over the Bruins.

"Although Wooden had retired (and replaced by Gene Bartow), most of their guys were back from that national championship team," said May, who had a game-high 33 points. "We had something to prove to them, and I think we did prove something to them."

"It was a big, big game because it was the era of UCLA," Benson said.

The Hoosiers didn't need to prove anything to Knight.

"We went 31-1 the year before. What more of a statement do you need?" UCLA's Washington wasn't so convinced.

"I think we will see them again," he said of a possible post-season rematch. "And then I'm pretty sure the outcome will be different."

The 20-point win over UCLA solidified Indiana's lead in the polls, but it also had its down side.

"It underscored the fact that we had a huge target on our backs," said Abernethy. "Every team came out and gave us their best shot, and those shots almost knocked us down."

Some close calls were soon to follow. The Hoosiers needed two free throws by Buckner with

11 seconds left to hold off a strong Notre Dame team led by Adrian Dantley, 63-60. That was a breather compared to the next game.

Miracle No. 1

Up next was Kentucky at Louisville's Freedom Hall. The Hoosiers were primed for revenge, only to find themselves on the ropes to another upset-minded Kentucky team. Indiana trailed by two heading into the final 10 seconds. A point-blank shot by Abernethy was blocked hard off the glass. Five feet away was Benson, with a defender between him and the basket. The Indiana center took a swat at the rebound. The ball went directly into the basket, a most unlikely putback.

"It wasn't even a tip," Benson said. "I couldn't get the rebound and Coach always told us, 'If you can't get the rebound, get in position to get a hand on the ball and put it back on the board.' In the process of flipping the ball up, I erred in my accuracy. It didn't even hit the backboard. The ball went about 10 feet up in the air and straight down into the basket. There was no skill to that, other than the fact that we practiced getting the ball up on the board."

"I was shocked the ball went in because it wasn't a shot," Fischer recalled.

Given new life, the Hoosiers outscored the Wildcats 13-4 in overtime to win, 77-68.

There would be one more close call before the Big Ten season. Indiana was the guest of honor for the 24th Holiday Festival at Madison Square Garden, where the Hoosiers ran into unbeaten St. John's before the largest crowd to ever watch a college game in New York -- 19,694.

The nationally-ranked Redmen rallied from eight points down to tie the score at 65-65, but late baskets by May and Abernethy allowed the Hoosiers to make their escape from New York, 76-69.

If the Hoosiers thought conference play was going to offer them any relief, the league opener at Ohio State showed otherwise. It took a blown lay-up by the Buckeyes and two Benson free throws with 19 seconds left to preserve a 66-64 squeaker.

On January 10, the Hoosiers went to Ann Arbor for what was the first of three meetings with an exceptional Michigan team. Although Michigan was built for speed, it was Indiana bolting out of the gate quickly with a 16-2 start. With Benson scoring 33 points on 16-for-18 shooting, the Hoosiers went on to win, 80-74.

The rematch at Assembly Hall would be much more eventful.

Miracle No. 2

There was no quick Hoosier getaway on this February day. Michigan used its quickness to seize a 39-29 lead at halftime, Indiana's largest halftime deficit in 73 games.

In the middle of a Michigan flurry was Jim Wisman, Indiana's sophomore guard. After throwing the ball away on successive possessions, Knight yanked Wisman off the floor -- literally. When a picture of Knight grabbing Wisman's jersey showed up in newspapers across the land the next morning, there was some public outcry. But Wisman later came to the defense of his coach and still does to this day.

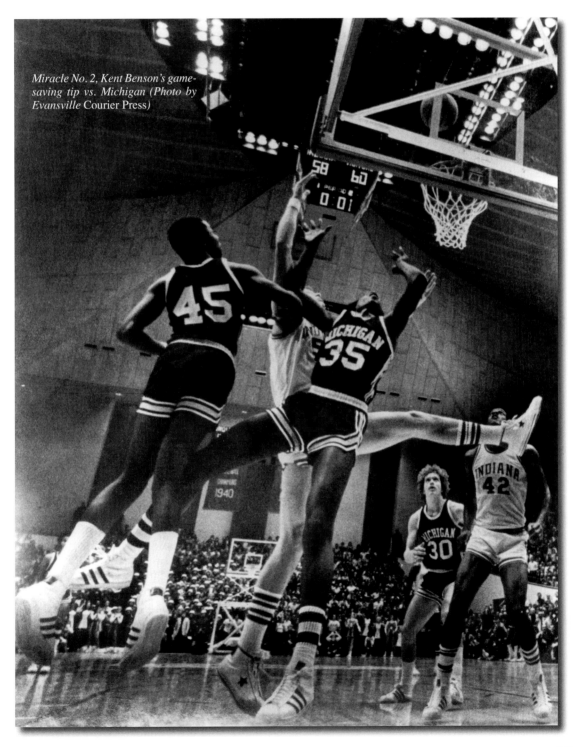

Miracle No. 2, Kent Benson's game-saving tip vs. Michigan (Photo by Evansville *Courier Press)*

"I wasn't prepared," he said from his own business office in Chicago earlier this month. "Michigan's quickness and pressure caught me off guard. That picture made it a lot more dramatic than it was. It was a reaction by Coach when I clearly screwed up. I didn't' take it at the time as a major incident."

With the Hoosiers continuing to struggle on offense, Knight went to his bench for another sophomore guard, Wayne Radford, who averaged four points game. Radford's orders were to score -- not shoot, but score. Shooting was OK with Knight as long as the ball went in more often than not.

As Radford recalled, "It shocked the hell out of me when Coach said, 'We need offense.' I didn't hesitate to do what I had always been able to do, put the ball in the basket."

Radford took 11 shots that day, seven jumpers and four free throws. All of them found the basket except for one field goal attempt. But despite the timely 16 points from Radford, the final minute found Indiana trailing by four and Michigan with the basketball.

With 33 seconds left, Michigan center Phil Hubbard traveled. At 0:22, Buckner rolled in a jumper, his first basket after eight misses. At 0:14, the Wolverines had a one-and-one free throw opportunity for one of their shooters, senior guard Steve Grote. One free throw probably would have ended Indiana's unbeaten season, but Grote missed the front end. May rebounded and the Hoosiers called time with 10 seconds left.

Radford remembers the contingencies discussed by Knight.

"The first option was May and the second was myself because I already had hit five or six shots," Radford said.

The Wolverines were fully prepared for Option No. 1.

"I remember getting the ball at the foul line extended and getting double-teamed," May said. "I passed to Buckner."

Buckner ignored Option No. 2 and took the shot himself from the top of the circle. "Buckner put up a brick," Radford said. "I'm glad we had bullet-proof backboards because it would have gone right through it."

Buckner's shot clanged hard off the rim to the left, where Crews had established position. Crews hurried up a putback that turned out to be a "pass" to Benson, who knew time was about to expire. In mid-jump he redirected the ball toward the basket. The ball caromed off the glass and through the goal as buzzer sounded.

Under the rules at the time, a tip had to be controlled in order to count. After a brief discussion, the officials counted the basket, sending the Indiana crowd into hysterics.

"I had control of it," Benson insists to this day. "I wasn't just slapping at the ball (as he did at Kentucky). There wasn't time to grab the ball, come down and go back up. It was a tip situation. I knew exactly what I was doing. I had only one option. I chose that option and it worked out."

"It was a conglomeration of fantastic happenings," Fischer said. "Jimmy Crews just threw it up toward the basket and Benson tipped it in just ahead of the horn -- bang, bang."

"I can't lie and say it was a pass," Crews said. "It was a shot. I was shooting because I knew there was little time left."

Benson's equalizer saved the Hoosiers from immediate defeat, but there was still work to be done. In the overtime, Michigan once again jumped in front. The Wolverines had a three-point lead and the ball following a Hoosier turnover, but before they could advance up the court, Radford stole it right back and laid it in.

Thirty seconds later, a May jumper gave the Hoosiers their first lead of the day. Two free throws by Benson and Radford in the last minute capped the 72-67 thriller.

"We dodged two bullets that day," Radford said. "The first one was right before the end of regulation. Pulling it out in overtime was the second."

"That was a game where Michigan had control," May said. "If Grote makes the one-and-one, we lose. It was something they didn't do. They didn't handle the pressure."

Cruising to the Finish

Although the Hoosiers would go on to have some anxious moments against Purdue and Minnesota, they encountered no more scares of the Michigan magnitude the rest of the Big Ten campaign. Indiana wrapped up its second straight 18-0 league mark with a 96-67 romp over Ohio State as the Hoosier fans bid farewell to a senior class that would go on to finish with 108 wins, the most by a single class in Big Ten history until the current Michigan State crop passed them.

However, this Spartan class has lost twice as many games. Indiana's Class of '76 lost a mere 12 games. The .900 winning percentage is easily the best of any of the league's four-year groups. And no other Big Ten team has gone unbeaten in a single season, let alone consecutive league campaigns.

Said Buckner, "I'll never forget what Coach Knight said on Senior Day: 'You (fans) take a long look at these people because you will never see another group like them again.' I didn't know how to take it."

By then most of the awards were in. May was named the national player of the year by the *Associated Press*, *United Press International*, the National Association of Basketball Coaches, *The Sporting News* and *Basketball Weekly*. Joining May as a first team All-American was Benson. Benson and May were no-brainers for All-Big Ten first team. Wilkerson was named to the second team.

But despite all the honors, the Hoosiers entered the NCAA Tournament still feeling unfulfilled and with that enormous target still on their back. As May said, "Yeah, I was player of the year, but if we didn't win the title, who cared?"

Stemming the Tide

For all its regular-season success, Indiana's reward was one of the most difficult tournament paths ever traveled by a No. 1 seed. Up first was that same St. John's team IU struggled to beat in New York, a team still ranked in the Top 20. Only this time the game was played on Indiana soil, at South Bend. From a 48-47 lead early in the second half, the Hoosiers pulled away to a 90-70 victory as May scored 33, while Benson and Buckner combined for 35.

The second round sent Indiana to Baton Rouge, La., to face sixth-ranked Alabama, a team as athletic as any the Hoosiers encountered all season. C.M. Newton's Crimson Tide boasted an All-American center, Leon Douglas, a man-child who totally manhandled North Carolina in the first round.

Although the Hoosiers enjoyed several double-digit leads, Alabama inched ahead with four minutes left, 69-68. After Douglas stuffed a May shot with 3 1/2 minutes to go, 'Bama had the ball back and time on its side. The Tide ran off a minute before Douglas drew a two-shot foul. Douglas missed both shots but got his own rebound and missed again.

The Hoosiers were that close to being down three. At the two-minute mark, May sank a guarded 18-footer from the baseline to give Indiana the lead again. After Douglas missed another short jumper, May rebounded. The Hoosiers worked the

clock down to 40 seconds before the Tide fouled Abernethy. A 74 percent free throw shooter, Abernethy stepped to the line with a one-point lead and ... misfired.

"I remember I had a one-and-one and missed," Abernethy said. "They came down and could have gone ahead."

But Indiana's defense, its staple throughout that unbeaten season, came up with the biggest stop of the year. Out of a wild scramble came Abernethy with the ball. A quick foul sent him to the line for another one-and-one. This time Abernethy came through, on both shots, for a three-point lead with 14 seconds left.

"I had a chance to be redeemed," Abernethy said with relief.

One more stop and two free throws by Wilkerson allowed Indiana to play another day, 74-69.

A Hurdle Cleared

The regional final matched Indiana against the nation's No. 2 team, Al McGuire's Marquette Warriors. Such a meeting of top-ranked teams could not happen at the regional level today because the top seeds are more evenly distributed. But in 1976 the seeding was done according to region, and the Midwest Region was loaded with rugged teams.

So there was No. 1 versus No. 2 for the right to go to the Final Four, a barrier Indiana had failed to overcome the year before.

Indiana was off and running against the Warriors until May picked up his third foul in the first half. The Warriors closed an 11-point deficit down to one at the break, 36-35.

The second half saw the return of May and IU's double-digit lead. However, with Earl Tatum scoring repeatedly in the paint, the Warriors drew within 59-56 before McGuire picked up a technical foul, his second of the game. From there Indiana pulled away to a 65-56 victory. Assured of a trip to the Final Four, emotions flowed.

"Even though this team did not show a lot of emotion, that was the most I had seen from them," Fischer said. "A major portion of their goal had been accomplished by just making it to the Final Four."

"Personally, the Marquette game was a high for me because we had not been to the Final Four in three years and this had been a stumbling block the year before," Crews said.

"We could see the light at the end of the tunnel," May said. "It was like, 'Here it is, two more games.' It was right in front of us."

The King is Dead

In America's 200th anniversary year, the Final Four was held in the nation's birthplace, Philadelphia. Awaiting Indiana was UCLA, which breezed through the West Regional. The other semifinal matched a familiar foe, Michigan, the Midwest Regional champ, against unbeaten Rutgers, which came out of the East. It was a unique Final Four, featuring for the first time two unbeatens and two teams from the same conference.

Out of the UCLA camp came comments that Indiana was going to see the real Bruins this time, not the ones Indiana dominated in that November "exhibition." It was in fact a much more polished UCLA team, but the Bruins would have been better off keeping that to themselves.

"David Greenwood remarked that the first game was just and exhibition, that this one was for real," Buckner recalled. "It was bulletin board stuff."

"I remember some smart-aleck comments," Benson said. "That's only going to motivate the team you are talking about. We just had another reason to prove we were better than them."

Early on it looked as though the Bruins were going to walk the walk. With the 6-11 Washington driving on Benson, the Bruins surged to a 7-2 lead as Benson picked up two quick fouls.

"I was guarding Washington way out on the floor," Benson said. "He was so quick."

Even though the game was barely two minutes old, Knight sensed the urgency and called his quickest timeout of the season. He took Benson off Washington and gave the assignment to Abernethy. With Abernethy hounding the Bruin All-American, Washington would not score another basket until midway through the second half.

"When you are guarding a 6-11 guy and you are 6-7, you can only do so much," Abernethy said. "He can always get his shot off, so you've got to hope he's not going to make them. Part of it was hard work and part of it was just hoping."

In addition to his defensive work on Washington, Abernethy also supplied 14 points and six rebounds. Abernethy's numbers might have been greater had he not been forced to sit out the last seven minutes following a scary collision with Washington.

"I was just running up the court and collided knees with somebody," said Abernethy, who feared he might not be able to return for the title game.

"I spent a lot of time in the hotel room that night with an ice pack on while all the guys were at a nice restaurant. I wasn't sure what was going to happen Monday night."

Just as important as the all-around play of Abernethy against UCLA was the board work of Wilkerson, who pulled down 19 rebounds.

"That was unheard of for a guard," May pointed out.

Indiana's 65-51 victory finally convinced the Bruins, although they were still reluctant to admit it. Said Marques Johnson, "Material-wise, I don't think they have as much as we do, but I'd say they are the best team we've played since I have been here."

A Call to Glory

So now it was down to one game, Indiana vs. Michigan.

The Wolverines had made easy work of Rutgers, setting up the first title game between two teams from the same conference. Noting that Michigan had extended Indiana twice in two hard-fought losses, the pundits were pointing to the difficulty of beating a good team three times in one season. It was almost a no-win situation for Indiana.

As Crews recalled, "I'm sitting in the lockerroom thinking, 'We've won all these Big Ten championships, beaten them four times in the last two years. We know we're better and yet we also know they could beat us, big-time.' "

Three minutes into the game, it looked as though fate agreed. On a Michigan fast break, Wilkerson took a crushing elbow to the head and was knocked cold. A pall fell over the Hoosiers.

"There was real concern," Fischer said. "It took them an eternity to get Wilkerson off the floor. He wasn't moving. The longer it took, the more you were scared that it was his neck or spine. It was a very scary scene."

"What was more concerning was when they carried him off the floor unconscious," Benson said. "It definitely affected our concentration, our game plan. In the back of our minds, we were concerned about his health."

When play resumed, Knight's first choice to replace Wilkerson was Radford, the hero of the last Michigan game. Apparently the Hoosier coach wasn't looking for instant offense at that point. Radford took a hasty shot, missed, and was returned to the bench in favor of Crews.

"Unfortunately, I took a shot that didn't drop and got a seat on the bench the rest of the game," Radford said. "I would have played 30 minutes if I had made that shot. Instead, I played 30 seconds."

Crews played a steady first half, but the Indiana offense wasn't clicking. Later, Knight was to say, "When I saw the game films, I saw that Jimmy really did a good job."

Knight's hunch at the time worked out well in the end. Just before halftime, Knight inserted Wisman, the same sophomore guard whose jersey was yanked in front of cameras in the regular season escape against Michigan. This time Wisman would stay on the floor -- for the rest of the first half and all of the second.

In light of Wilkerson's injury and 61 percent shooting by the Wolverines, the Hoosiers were fortunate to be down by just six at halftime, 35-29.

"Indiana played in shock the rest of the half," Fischer said. "They were dazed by it all. There was a feeling of *déjà vu* from the year before, to May's injury."

As May said, "It was like, 'Now what? We got this far and this happens.' It was off my turnover that Wilkerson got hit."

A six-point deficit and the loss of a key player would be cause for much concern in most locker-rooms, but, as Wisman said, "There was no panic by any means."

"If I were a fan, I would have been concerned because we were six points down," Abernethy said. "But as a player I did not have that much concern. We believed in what our coach would say. He instilled that confidence in us at halftime. He had done it all year long. That track record gave us confidence."

Benson clearly recalled Knight's halftime words.

"The first thing Coach said was, 'Boys, Bobby is OK. He's resting comfortably at the hospital. He will be fine. The next 20 minutes are going to go down in history if we just play like we are capable of playing.' "

"It was kind of interesting how Coach handled halftime," May said. "Somebody said he waited two years to say what he said. It was something like, 'If you guys want to make history, you've got 20 minutes to prove it. There is nothing I can write on this board for you. We're not going to make any changes.' Boom, that was it."

Thundering Home

And boom went the Hoosiers.

With Benson and May powering inside, Indiana scored on 21 of 22 possessions over a 12-minute stretch the second half. The only reason that one trip came up empty was because Benson missed a one-and-one.

Five minutes into the second half, Indiana caught up at 39-39. The Hoosiers took the lead at 45-43 and traded baskets until freshman Rich Valavicius came off the bench to supply a jumper that gave Indiana a 55-51 lead with nine minutes to go.

Indiana was a 63-59 leader with six minutes left when May retrieved a missed shot directly underneath the basket. Only May could explain what happened next.

"The ball is going out of bounds. I grab it underneath the basket. I get it, jump back into the defender and throw up some 'b.s.' -- some reverse English on the ball so that it goes straight up and comes straight down into the basket. You should have seen the look on Grote's face. It was a look that said, 'Give me a break.' I knew then that we had them."

May's improbable basket launched an 8-0 spurt that put the Hoosiers in command, 71-59. With no shot clock back then, the Hoosiers went into their spread offense and picked apart the Wolverines for lay-ups and free throws. The final margin was 18 points, 86-68.

It was all Fischer could do to choke out the words as he called the final seconds.

"It's a blur until the final minute of the game," he said. "To me it was the most memorable portion of any basketball game in my memory. I had tears rolling down my cheeks. I can still see Quinn Buckner doing a little jig on the sideline ... Scott May coming out and hugging him.

"Coach Knight had this tough guy attitude, but he melted down, too," Fischer added. "No question, there were tears in his eyes. Watching those kids, they didn't do all the antics you see today, the hot-dogging. They were just so happy and gratified. When I go back and listen to that last minute, I still well up a little bit."

"It was a dream come true," Benson said. "The first thing I did was thank God. The next thing I did was point to Mom and Dad (Bob and Mary Ann Benson)."

Benson was named the tournament's Most Outstanding Player. Joining him on the all-tourney team were May and Abernethy.

"I don't think we could have lost that night," May said. "We were determined. We dominated them."

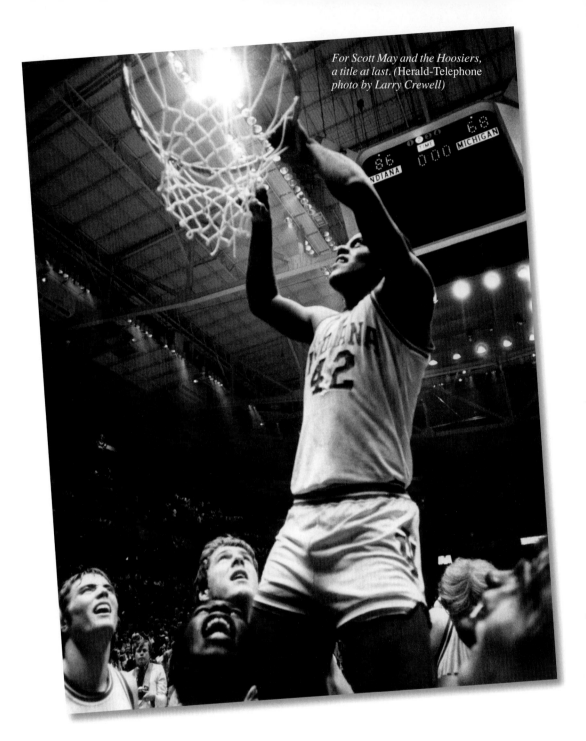

For Scott May and the Hoosiers, a title at last. (Herald-Telephone photo by Larry Crewell)

Perfection Attained

Indiana's perfect season was complete, it's two-year quest achieved. In 32 games, the Hoosiers faced 16 opponents who were ranked at the time. No college team has gone unbeaten since. How long before the next unbeaten comes along? Or will there be a next one?

"It was tough back then," Knight said. "We had some close calls."

It is going to take a team that is very, very mature," said Crews, who as the head coach of Evansville understands how difficult it is to win any basketball game, let alone 32 in a row.

"Part of that maturity is to keep your eye on the important things," Crews said. "Today, it's harder because the kids are exposed to so many things."

"If the right coaching staff has the right mixture of players with the right attitude, it can be done," May said.

"Coach Knight deserves a lion's share of the credit," Abernethy said. "He nurtured us, taught us for four years. We embraced it and tried to carry it out as best we could. It took everybody buying into the system, sacrificing individual pursuits and goals for the betterment of the team."

Abernethy admits to a little scoreboard-watching until the last unbeaten goes down each year.

"In the last 10 years I have watched with interest," he said. "I don't think I've ever talked to a teammate about it, but I'll joke around with my kids."

"Records are made to be broken," Benson said. "Whether this one is or isn't, it is pretty incredible to have held it 25 years. We sure have enjoyed the ride."

This Bucket Battle Was a Riot

Although football games are often foolishly called "wars," this grudge match almost resulted in one. In 1971 I was in the IU student section when the game boiled over. Thirty-five years later, I revisited that day.

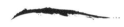

Bloomington Herald-Times
November 17, 2006

There have been some wild and crazy Old Oaken Bucket games over the years, but the 1971 contest at Bloomington put the "wack" in "wacky."

You think last month's brawl between Miami and Florida International was scary? The '71 IU-Purdue game not only had Hoosiers and Boilermakers scuffling all over the field, it also involved fans, coaches and band members.

It was a sight to behold, let me tell you. I observed it from the student section at Memorial Stadium and wondered, 35 years later, just exactly what I witnessed on that raw, overcast afternoon of November 20, 1971.

To set the stage, Indiana was floundering along with a record of 2-7. The Rose Bowl season of 1967 was a distant memory for coach John Pont, whose last winning season at IU was 1968. Having been trounced by Purdue the year before, 40-0, Pont was in no mood for another humiliation.

"Pont was hopped up all week long," recalled Carl Barzilauskas, a sophomore defensive tackle at the time. "Practice was balls to the walls."

"That was the most spirited week of practice we ever had," linebacker Jerry Johnson said. "The electricity spilled over into the game."

Upset in the Making

Purdue brought a team stocked with potential NFL players such as running back Otis Armstrong, quarterback Gary Danielson, tackle Dave Butz and wide receiver Darryl Stingley (whose NFL career was cut short by a paralyzing hit from Jack Tatum).

Who would have thought an overmatched Indiana team would lead from start to finish -- by as many as 21 points?

The upset started unfolding on the game's third play when Barzilauskas, who went on to carve out a pretty good pro career for himself, got one of his big paws on a Danielson pass and tipped it to linebacker Rob Spicer, who intercepted and returned it for a touchdown.

Later in the first quarter, Rick Sayers, Purdue's All-Big Ten tight end, hit the turf after catching a short pass. Trailing the play was IU defensive end Joe Pawlitsch. Sayers popped up off the ground just as Pawlitsch was trying to hurdle him. Pawlitsch's foot caught Sayers square in the head and knocked him cold. From a Purdue perspective, it was an intentional kick. From a Hoosier perspective, it was an accident.

"I'm sure Joe didn't mean it," Barzilauskas said. "He wasn't like that."

Frustrations Mount

At any rate, the bad blood started flowing right there. Adding to Purdue's frustration was that every bounce seemed to be going Indiana's way. The Boilermakers thought they had recovered a second-half fumble, but the officials ruled the play dead.

Then, with Indiana leading 31-17 in the fourth quarter, Hoosier running back Ken St. Pierre fumbled at the Purdue seven, only to have the ball bounce right into the hands of Steve Mastin. The Hoosier tight end gladly took it to the end zone for what turned out to be the decisive score.

"We were playing our ass off, beating a team with NFL players on it, and they were ready to take it out on us," said Johnson, now a public defender in Owensboro, Ky.

The 'Boiling' Point

As time was running out on the Boilermakers, Danielson skidded out of bounds into the Hoosier bench -- into the tempest, it turned out.

This is where the extreme differences of opinion occurred. Danielson alleged he was kicked by an Indiana player.

"Danielson got kicked and Pont did nothing about it," Butz told reporters after the game. The Hoosiers contended that Danielson started it all by throwing the ball at Pont.

"Danielson got up and threw the ball right in Pont's face," recalled IU linebacker Dan Grossman, now a Bloomington eye surgeon and the father of Bears quarterback Rex Grossman.

"I was right there," Grossman said. "About four or five of us jumped on Danielson. Purdue players came running over and then both benches emptied."

Mob Nentality

Now the real battle was on -- Hoosiers and Boilermakers tangling all over the field. Compounding the problem was the fact that IU students were gathering near the field to celebrate the victory. When the benches cleared, many students chased the players onto the field. The scuffling went on for a good 10 minutes before security could restore order.

But as soon as the game ended, the mayhem started all over again. Everybody was fair game, it seemed, including the Purdue mascot, Purdue Pete. A fan wrestled away Pete's hammer and was using it on the helpless fellow.

"A fan was down there in the end zone knocking the crap out of Purdue Pete," Grossman said. "He hit him so hard the paper-mache was flying off him."

"I have never seen another fight like that one," Johnson said. "There were piles of people. I remember Pont jumping on top of a pile trying to break it up. Everyone was involved -- players, coaches, fans. Today, there would have been multiple suspensions."

Barzilauskas tried to play peacemaker but gave up.

"I might have pushed a few people around, but that was it," he said. "I've been in some nasty fights before, but nothing to that extent."

In the midst of the pandemonium, Barzilauskas saw IU defensive end Marshall McCullough calmly gather up Purdue helmets, stick them under his all-weather parka and sneak them off the field. "We were admiring those helmets later," Barzilauskas laughed.

Another Boilermaker helmet was last seen making its way up the stands, handed off from fan to fan.

Strike up the Band

Then the Purdue band had the bad idea of going ahead with its post-game show. Talk about sitting ducks. I still have a vivid memory of those band members using the tips of the flag poles to fend off IU fans in medieval jousting fashion.

The fans did pause long enough to hoist Pont on their shoulders and gleefully escort him to the lockerroom.

Meanwhile, Purdue coach Bob DeMoss fumed. In his post-game press conference he warned the Hoosiers had better "buckle their chin straps and be ready" when they visited West Lafayette the following year.

Midnight Madness

Emptying Memorial Stadium didn't result in a cease fire, either. The hostilities spilled over to the parking lot and continued long into the Bloomington night.

"Coming out of the lockerroom 40 minutes later, guys were chasing guys all over the parking lot," Barzilauskas said. "People were busting windows. I went out later that night and people were still getting into it in the bars."

Keep in mind that student unrest was at an all-time high. The Vietnam War was still raging and Kent State was only a year removed. So the sight of a student revolt didn't seem all that shocking then. In hindsight, however, it turned out to be a disturbing chapter in the IU-Purdue rivalry.

"I was watching a college game several years later and Danielson (a TV analyst following his pro career), was still talking about that day," Barzilauskas said.

By the way, Purdue did get its revenge in convincing manner the following year, 42-7. It was the final nail in Pont's coaching coffin and the first of five straight Bucket victories for Purdue, a harsh payback for one hellacious day in Memorial Stadium.

IU Returns To Glory Days

In the aftermath of NCAA sanctions imposed on the Indiana University basketball program in 2008, it was if a massive cold front moved in and stayed for almost three years. And then, with the flick of a shooter's wrist, the clouds lifted. Since then, IU athletics have been on a welcomed upswing. Indiana University Alumni Magazine lured me out of retirement to write about the resurgence, and I gladly accepted. Here is the piece in its entirety.

IU Alumni Magazine
September, 2013

The human pyramid that sprung up near the pitcher's mound on June 9 said it all.

This collection of limbs and torsos, a spontaneous cream and crimson mosh pit, belonged to the IU baseball team, which had just punched a ticket to Omaha for the College World Series after sweeping favored Florida State in Tallahassee.

We're talking Indiana BASEBALL – not men's basketball, not men's soccer, not the usual Hoosier banner makers, although those two programs had their own reasons to celebrate earlier in the past year.

It was a tremendous year. Men's soccer added another star to the Indiana jersey; men's basketball team won its first undisputed Big Ten title in 20 years; high jumper Derek Drouin won both indoor and outdoor NCAA titles; baseball coach Tracy Smith was national Coach of the Year after leading the Hoosiers to that College World Series appearance. It was a year that saw IU tie for second place for the men's Capital One Cup, the national all-sports championship trophy. Among the women's teams, water polo coach Barry King was Coach of the Year in the Collegiate Water Polo Association Western Division and the team finished in the top 20. Other women's teams with solid seasons included tennis, swimming and diving.

Welcome back, Hoosiers.

Prior to this resurgence of IU athletics, an entire generation of alumni endured a period of mediocrity. You couldn't blame them for rolling their eyes every time they heard their parents or grandparents talk about a "Golden Age" of athletics.

From Doc Counsilman's first of six men's swimming championship in 1968 to Bill Mallory's last of six bowl games in 1993, Indiana was winning NCAA championships, Big Ten championships and going to bowl games with regularity. In addition to Counsilman and Mallory, the coaching staff boasted other future Hall of Famers -- basketball coach Bob Knight, soccer coach Jerry Yeagley, track coach Sam Bell and diving coach Hobie Billingsley.

However, as those coaches retired or left the university, the success rates gradually dropped off.

Knight's last Big Ten champion was 1993. His last Final Four team was 1992. Although the Hoosiers had a surprising dash to the Final Four under Mike Davis in 2002, there wasn't another Sweet Sixteen appearance from 1995 to 2012, and only one conference title, a shared one at that.

After Mallory guided the football team to six bowl games from 1987-94, the Hoosiers went bowling only one time after his firing in 1996.

Swimming, diving and track had winning moments but could not match the high number of champions churned out by Counsilman, Billingsley and Bell.

Even men's soccer, arguably the IU's most consistent sport, flattened out despite the best efforts of Mike Freitag, who followed Yeagley with a championship run his first year (2004) but couldn't sustain it after that.

And when Kelvin Sampson's improprieties dragged the men's basketball program into a deep quagmire in 2008, the program suffered under NCAA sanctions into 2011.

Out of those dark times came the promise of a grand new era of IU athletics, beginning with a single, swift stroke. In December, 2011, a basketball splashed through the net, unleashing three years of pent-up frustration as Hoosiers fans swarmed Branch McCracken Court. It was an emotional, shared feeling that told the rest of the collegiate world, "Indiana University is back."

The 'Shot' II

For IU fans, there was "The Shot," Keith Smart's jumper the jumper that vaulted the Hoosiers over Syracuse in the 1987 NCAA title game. But a quarter of a century is a long time to live in the past.

In the wake of Sampson's missteps, and the three dismal basketball seasons that followed, the IU fan base was starved for a signature moment. And when it came, it ignited a tidal wave of emotion …

> December 10, 2011: Top-ranked Kentucky invades the den of upstart Indiana, winner of its first eight games. Still reeling from three straight losing seasons, Indiana has much to prove in order to convince the skeptics that it is for real. And who better than mighty Kentucky

*Christian Watford's game-winner vs. Kentucky was a shot in the arm for the entire Hoosier nation. (*Herald-Times *photo by Chris Howell)*

INDIANA
UNIVERSITY

NCAA

BASKETBALL
CHAMPIONS

to provide a measuring stick? For most of the game, Indiana is equal to the challenge, even opening up a 10-point lead with eight minutes to go. However, Kentucky chips away and ultimately takes a two-point lead with a mere 5.6 seconds to go. A gallant Indiana effort, but not quite enough, it seems. But those last few seconds are now cemented into Hoosier lore. Verdell Jones weaves down the court past a Cody Zeller screen, spins and shuffles a pass to Christian Watford, anxiously waiting at the 3-point line. Watford rises up and fires over a leaping Kentucky defender. As the clock strikes zero, the ball plunges through the net, lifting the Hoosiers to a stunning 73-72 upset and lifting the fans out of their seats and onto Branch McCracken Court in a celebration unmatched in the history of the Assembly Hall. It is played and replayed again and again on ESPN, You tube, you name it. It winds up winning an Espy as ESPN's most dramatic sports moment of the year.

One of those rushing the court was Casey Smith, a Hoosier baseball player.

"It was the shot heard 'round the world," Smith recalled on the eve of leaving for the College World Series. "I honestly think that shot turned around every program at IU. It put us all on the map. Until the day I die, I will thank Christian Watford for what he did on the basketball court. It made me, as a baseball player, think, "It's our turn.' Then soccer goes out and wins a national championship, and now we are doing this."

All the President's Men

In the 2012-13 academic year, athletics kept IU President Michael McRobbie on the go. In August, 2012, he was sending off seven qualifiers to the Summer Olympics. In December, 2012, he was presenting the NCAA championship trophy to the men's soccer team. In March, 2013, he was presenting the Big Ten championship trophy to the men's basketball team, which won its first outright title in 20 years. In April, 2013, he was dedicating the new baseball and softball fields. In between, he made it a point to watch in person all 24 sports.

"Not many college presidents go to see water polo and such things," noted IU trustee Phil Eskew, Jr.

And to think that for the better part of his first year, 2007-08, McRobbie was busy for more unpleasant reasons.

"I was devoting maybe half my time during the week to the whole Sampson business," McRobbie said. "It was in many ways an unfortunate example of how problems in athletics can affect a whole institution."

"This was not Indiana University. We played by the rules," said Eskew, Jr., who began his term as a trustee in 2006. "We were the pride of the Big Ten. It was so embarrassing."

As much as the Sampson fallout damaged the university's squeaky clean image, there was an even deeper, more painful reason the university was hurting. In the summer of 2007, brain cancer claimed the life of football coach Terry Hoeppner, who had the program on the rise and the fan base excited about it. Just when it looked like IU had found its perfect fit, it was tragically taken away, and a devoted husband and father with it. Between that and the ensuing Sampson debacle, IU athletics felt cursed.

In the fall of 2008, the Sampson debacle claimed another casualty when then Athletics Director Rick Greenspan announced his resignation amidst "failure to monitor" charges from the NCAA. To right the Hoosier ship, McRobbie knew he needed a man who understood the importance of doing things right, someone who bled Hoosier crimson.

No Glass Half-Filled

On January 1, 2009, Fred Glass officially became IU's fifth athletics director in eight years. One of the first things he did was bring the department closer to the athletes. He took the first step toward fixing that by eliminating eight upper-level administrative jobs and hiring nutritionists, academic advisors, trainers.

"Instead of people two or three levels above the student athletes, we moved them down to people who literally tape the ankles and work them out," Glass said.

When McRobbie asked Glass to consider being IU's next AD in the fall of 2008, Glass was shocked at what he heard when he started asking around.

"The thing that was most sobering for me was that more than one coach asked me why I would take this job," he said. "That broke my heart. Bloomington is the quintessential college town, has the most beautiful campus in the country, has such great tradition in athletics. To think people so involved it had come to believe it was no longer a good place to be … (the challenge) became personal."

Glass considers himself lucky to have been an undergraduate student at IU during a high time for athletics, "even though you don't know you are in a Golden Age at the time," he told an audience at the Bloomington Press Club in April, 2013. "Think about this: Sam Bell, Jerry Yeagley, Hobie Billingsley, Bob Knight. The list of iconic coaches goes on. I want to be a part of a new Golden Age."

With a law degree from IU and a highly successful practice going for him in Indianapolis, Glass understood the importance of following the law to its letter, even the vast and complicated laws of the NCAA. He accepted McRobbie's offer, but on the condition that the president shared his vision.

"I felt I could come here and keep the pots from boiling over, but that doesn't do it for me," Glass said. "I want to be part of something excellent. (McRobbie) said, 'absolutely,' that athletics are a very big component of Indiana University. He has been very true to his word."

It was a matter of reaffirming priorities, and Glass has his "Big Four:"

Playing by the rules;

Achieving academically;

Excelling athletically;

Integrating with the university.

"Anybody in our athletic department can recite these because I am shameless about hammering them in," Glass said.

To prevent future missteps, Glass reshaped the compliance department. He hired Kris Fowler as associate athletic director of compliance and Julie Cromer as senior associate athletic director for administration and compliance. He instituted regular meetings for the compliance department and monthly meetings with the coaches. On November 24, 2011, IU went off probation. Sixteen days later, Watford made IU basketball relevant again. From there the Hoosiers went on to win 27 games and reach the first Sweet Sixteen for the first time in 10 years.

Back in Black

What makes Glass proud is that the athletics department has not been a financial drain on the university. In fact, it is self-supporting. The budget is not funded by student fees, tax dollars or university subsidies. To be in the "black" all four years of Glass's tenure is saying a lot for a department that isn't largely funded by a filled-to-capacity football stadium.

"Michigan, Ohio State and Penn State each make more money on one home game than we do in an entire seven-game home schedule," Glass pointed out.

Helping IU meet ends is the revenue from the Big Ten Network, which provides each conference school with about $19 million a year.

"That $19 million impacts IU a lot more than Ohio State because their budget is twice as big as ours," Glass said. "Their budget ($126 million) is twice as big as ours."

When Glass came on board he noted that each of the 24 facilities needed an upgrade of some sort.

"It felt like Rip Van Winkle, like we had fallen asleep in 1973 and hadn't done anything facility-wise in 30 years," Glass said.

The Big Ten Network money as helped in that regard. If you haven't visited the Bloomington campus in the last five years, take a spin around the athletic complex.

Take in the north end of Memorial Stadium and its majestic, limestone towers, giving it a classic facelift in 2009. It houses a 25,000-square foot weight room, one of the largest in the country.

Look at the sparkling new softball diamond, Andy Mohr Field, and the spacious new baseball stadium, Bart Kaufman Field, christened by the first ranked baseball team in IU history, and now the first College World Series qualifier in Indiana history.

On the south end of the complex, feast your eyes on Cook Hall. Opened in 2010, it is multi-purpose practice facility for the men's and women's basketball teams. From 17th street at night, you can see the IU insignia gleaming through the atrium glass.

And then there is the south end of Memorial Stadium, bearing a message you can't miss. In huge, bold, letters it proclaims: "The Spirit of Indiana … 24 sports … one team."

And while Glass gets a lot of credit for the facilities upgrade, Greenspan also laid some of the groundwork. It was Greenspan who supported construction of the new baseball field, Cook Hall and the expansion of the football stadium. And it was Greenspan who made some critical hires, including Hoeppner, basketball coach Tom Crean and baseball coach Tracy Smith.

Greenspan's son, Ben Greenspan, a former IU baseball player and now an assistant under Smith, hopes IU supporters do not forget his dad's role in this resurgence.

"I think it has lots to do with the efforts of my dad and also the current administration," Ben said. "Both had a hand in its current success. Dad is very proud of the things he accomplished in Bloomington, very proud of the coaches he hired. He's proud of where the program is."

Ahead of the Curve

Although it is unlikely IU probably will become a football factory, it is excelling on its main mission, educating its student athletes. Since 2009, IU has placed 24 players on the Big Ten All-Academic Team. IU athletes have a cumulative GPA of 3.07. Sixteen of the 24 teams have posted perfect one-year APR scores (progress toward graduation), including men's basketball, an eyesore under Sampson. All 24 sports currently exceed NCAA standards. By attending all 24 sports, McRobbie is making a statement that all of them matter.

"That was something my wife (Laurie) and I decided to do a year ago," he said. "My wife is very supportive of women's athletics and Title IX. She can speak with good conviction on how it has impacted women's sports."

The McRobbies' commitment has not gone unnoticed. Women's tennis coach Lin Loring, whose tenure goes all the way back to 1978, surely understands it. In 10 of the last 11 semesters, Loring's program has won the Herbert Award for the highest team GPA, which means a dinner with the university president.

"How many tennis teams in the country can say they've had dinner with the president of the university?" Loring said. "Our seniors have had dinner with him four years now."

"Some teams never had a sitting president at their games before," McRobbie said, "so we wanted to show our support for athletics across the board, not just the marquee sports. One of the beauties of visiting all the sports is that you are able to put venues and faces and names with the reports you see."

The coaches also feel Glass has their back – as long as they play by the rules. Todd Yeagley is one who appreciates the patience the administration showed as he was restoring the tradition his father started. He rewarded them with the school's eighth NCAA title, putting that coveted "star" on the front of the soccer jersey.

"Fred doesn't make rash decisions when it comes to results," Yeagley said. "He can look past a down year or two. What you love about him as an AD is that he gives you a framework of trust, that if you stay on course, work hard and things are stable, he will stay with you 100 percent."

The athletes feel it, too. Ashley Benson, who led the IU volleyball team to the Sweet Sixteen in 2010, talked about the support Glass has showed for the lower-revenue sports.

"The way he treated us and all the programs pushed us all to be better, to take our individual programs to a higher level," said Benson, daughter of All-American basketball player Kent Benson and an All-American in her own right. "Before that it felt like we were lost. There was a cloud, and as soon as Sampson was gone, the light started shining through."

Passing the Torch

Not only is the Hoosier Nation back on board again, so is the nation itself. When *Sports Illustrated* came out with its pre-season college basketball edition in November, 2012, the cover featured IU sophomore Cody Zeller, a.k.a, The Big Handsome, posing in front of the Sample Gates in his Hoosier warm-ups, pin-striped pants and all. The caption read, "Best Player … Best Team … Best Pants."

After all Indiana University had been through, it was once again cool to be a Hoosier.

"I've got striped pants now," 15-year-old Dalton O'Boyle said on a visit to Kaufman Field this past summer. "When I first got them a couple of years ago, I didn't know the significance."

Dalton's father, Casey O'Boyle, attended IU in the late 1980s and early '90s, back when the Hoosiers were still in their heyday.

"In those days you got spoiled as an IU fan," Casey said. "It seemed IU sports were on top of the mountain. But somewhere toward the end of Bob Knight's career, things tailspinned. Indiana football went down drastically, and IU basketball was mediocre. It got to the point my 15-year-old son had no idea what IU basketball was about."

Casey would argue that the Watford shot is right up there with Smart's shot for the impact it made on the perception of Indiana athletics.

"Let's face it: The Smart shot was for a championship, and it will always hold a special place in Indiana hearts," he said. "But the Watford shot was the signature moment that put IU back on the map. And that's important for young people, not old guys like me. It's for my son, his buddies, for future IU fans. Until that point, everything they heard was just history, something they read in a book."

More on the Way?

So has a new "Golden Age" arrived? It will be hard to match the 2012-13 year, but the program appears to be on solid footing.

"I feel these things are fluid," former IU running great Bob Kennedy said. "It all starts with people. Fred Glass did a great job of keeping the right people in place and continuing to give them the tools to make them successful."

As an officer in the IU Varsity Club, Kennedy knows the importance of improved facilities.

"Facilities are super important," he said. "Recruiting is a big part, and when I was 17, that stuff impressed me. It says this university is committed to doing the things necessary to give kids success."

If nothing else, the current administration has put the disturbing, recent past behind them. As Glass reflected, "We had been through a pretty tough decade. I was the fifth AD in eight years. There was the tragic death of a football coach we felt was going to lead us to the Promised Land. And then the horrific sanctions that came out of the Kelvin Sampson situation.

"My goal is to have another Golden Age at Indiana," Glass added. "We want to show that the last 10 years were abnormal. We are going to establish a new normal. One by one, we are removing the obstacles and are seeing excellence across the board."

Chapter 11
Going Pro

If you are one of the fortunate ones, you get to cover the occasional professional sporting event. With Indianapolis just up the road from Bloomington, I was afforded my share of opportunities to cover the pros. Looking back, I now realize how lucky I was to cross paths with the likes of Mickey Mantle, Larry Bird, Peyton Manning, Reggie Miller, Michael Jordan, Pete Sampras and many other legends. My encounters with Mantle were covered in Chapter 2. Here are some others.

Not Just Another Day in French Lick

August 18, 1992, was a sad day in Hoosierland. It was the day Hoosier legend Larry Bird announced his retirement from professional basketball. The editors suggested taking the 60-mile drive to Larry's home town, French Lick, for a man-on-the-street story. Making the trip with me was a Herald-Times *colleague, Casey O'Boyle. We stopped in at the usual gas stations and restaurants in French Lick and the adjacent town, West Baden. In the end, however, our best material came from the regulars at some of Bird's old watering holes. Hey, it was a dirty job, but somebody had to do it. This article was co-authored with Casey.*

Bloomington Herald-Times
August 19, 1992

FRENCH LICK, INDIANA

It looked like just another day in French Lick. A kid was spinning his bicycle around the Shell station in West Baden on French Lick's northern edge. People were relishing the fried chicken at the Villager Restaurant. The gang at the Jubil Pub was nursing a cold beer on a hot August day.

But this was not just any day in French Lick-West Baden. This was August 18, 1992, the day native son Larry Bird announced his retirement from the Boston Celtics.

There was a mixture of sadness and expectation on the part of the locals.

"Larry's put in a lot of good years," said Donnie Fullen, the attendant at the West Baden Shell station. "I'd rather see him go out this way than go on with injury."

"I knew it was coming," said Larry Kalb, who operates a limousine service. Thinking back to the four years Bird starred at Indiana State, Kalb added, "He put in a great 17 years. He should go out while he can. If you look at the last few years, he didn't play that much. I think everybody knew he was going to retire. I'll be glad to see him back around here. I give him a year and he'll be coaching Springs Valley High School."

That's where Bird prepped.

"We used to play on the school grounds together," said Frankie Andrews, wearing a Celtics' shirt.

"He's had a wonderful career," said Dave Emmons. "He should enjoy the rest of his life. I'm happy for him. I'm sure he's got a lot of other interests. I'll be glad to see Larry come home."

"He would jog around town all the time," said Kalb. "It was no big deal. It wasn't like people were pulling up and saying, 'Hey, Larry, give me your autograph.' "

From a pump at the Shell station, Kalb motioned to the Jubil Pub next door.

"It was nothing for him to go in there and slap $200, $300 down on the bar and buy drinks for the house," he said.

Not true, said Trish Drake.

"Larry would just come in here like anybody else," she said. "He doesn't flash his money around or act like a big shot. Larry is just Larry. He doesn't want to be treated any differently."

"He would do nothing special," said bartender Larry Seybold. "He'd order drinks and there would be no big deal."

Entire walls are not dedicated to the average patron, however. The north wall of the Jubil is plastered with posters autographed by Bird.

"People around here wouldn't really consider Larry a celebrity, although he's accomplished a lot for a small-town boy," Drake said.

"It's unbelievable to have a friend that great," Andrews said. "When he comes around here, he's just one of the guys."

A man with a speech and hearing impairment came over to express his feelings. He motioned with his hands, a movement similar to the patented Bird shooting stroke.

"Him and Larry used to shoot baskets together," said Gary "Goose" Allen, translating for the impaired man, who nodded and made an elbow-bending motion. "I guess they used to drink a few beers together, too."

"Larry would come in here and play the juke box, any country music song that was popular at the time," said Drake. "One time he brought in Bill Walton and they played pool. It's kind of a sad day because basketball won't be the same here. When the Celtics were playing, people would pile in here to watch Larry. How many small towns in the whole U.S. can say they have an Olympic gold medalist and one of the greatest basketball players ever? As far as I'm concerned, thanks for the memories, Larry."

Bird Comes Home to Roost

Five years later, Bird came out of retirement to coach the Indiana Pacers.

Bloomington Herald-Times
May 13, 1997

INDIANAPOLIS, INDIANA

From a Hoosier perspective, all was right with the world Monday. Larry Bird was back.

It was if he had merely been on loan to the Boston Celtics the last 18 years. Indiana was where he belonged, with the Pacers -- if not as a player, then at least as a coach.

With the introduction of Bird as the Pacers' new head coach, the whole state of Indiana took notice, not to mention the NBA. In one swift move, the professional basketball team that calls Indianapolis its home truly became the Indiana Pacers. Larry Bird not only belongs in Indiana, he belongs to all of Indiana.

From his boyhood days in French Lick to his college days in Terre Haute, Indiana has forever been home to Bird.

"I always knew I'd make it back here some way or another," he said at Monday's press conference at Market Square Arena. "French Lick and West Baden have always been my home. They are my type of people."

From a public relations standpoint, the hiring of Bird is a stroke of genius. The Pacers are competing against the Colts for the entertainment dollar and also are campaigning for a new arena to replace MSA, which wouldn't ruffle Bird's feathers at all.

"I never could shoot in this arena," he said.

From a coaching standpoint, the jury will be out on Bird for at least a year or two. However, all you have to do is tell Bird he will fail.

"Growing up, I was always told I wasn't good enough because I wasn't going up against the best players in Indiana," he said. "I went to Indiana State and was told the same thing. I wasn't there long before I knew I could compete."

After five years of retirement, the thrill of competition is what drove Bird back into the game. As he told Bob Ryan of the *Boston Globe*, there was no competition on the golf course playing against all those "fat bellies." A front office job with the Celtics under new head coach Rick Pitino wasn't going to be good enough, either.

In conversations with former Celtic teammate Kevin McHale, now the general manager of the Minnesota Timberwolves, Bird said, "(McHale) would talk about the fish he caught and the golf he was playing, but that's not what I wanted. I didn't want to be sitting there behind (Pitino). I wanted to be involved, to be competitive."

Bird realizes there is the risk of failure, but he does not view this as a mid-life crisis.

"I know I'm taking a chance, but this is something I wanted to do. My heart was in it to coach. I wanted to be the Pacers' coach in the worst way."

So far, the players have been highly receptive.

"His enthusiasm is great," said Pacer guard Fred Hoiberg. "He will have great respect from the fans and even greater respect from the players. The whole thing now is about respect."

From Bird's days as a player, the Pacers know he will keep long hours. Even Bird himself said, "There's not a player here who will beat me to practice or be the last one out the door. Players will have to work as hard, not necessarily hang around for an hour to shoot, but to work on their weaknesses."

Citing as an example the poor free throw shooting of Dale Davis, Bird said, "Dale Davis

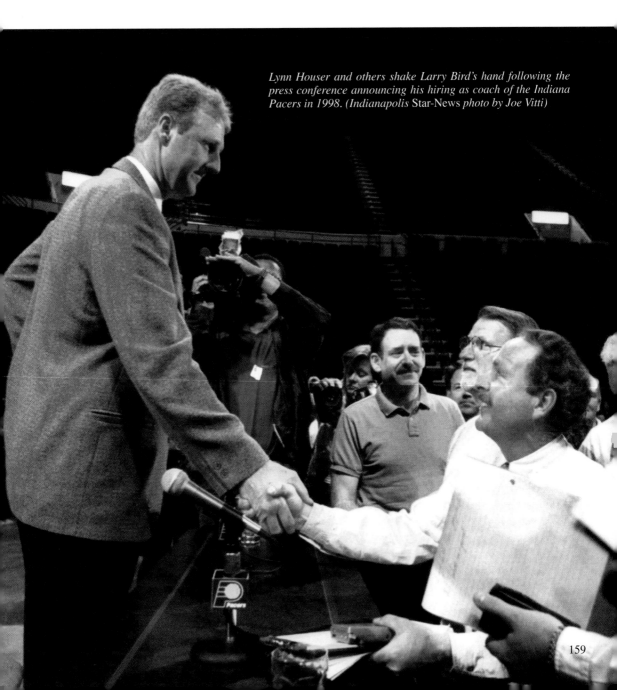

Lynn Houser and others shake Larry Bird's hand following the press conference announcing his hiring as coach of the Indiana Pacers in 1998. (Indianapolis Star-News *photo by Joe Vitti)*

will have to shoot 100 to 150 free throws a day. There are things I will tell the others. I hope they listen because that will make them better basketball players."

A perfectionist throughout his career, Bird will now have to exercise some patience.

"I have two young children," he said. "My patience wears thin. These are grown men. I don't expect them to play like Larry Bird. I've got to play to their strengths."

Bird kept referring to his future players as "our kids." His goal is to make them the best conditioned team in the NBA so they can play a faster game. He knows the Pacers have board strength in Dale and Antonio Davis, and he also knows the Reggie Miller is a much better shooter in the open court.

"My philosophy is to get the ball off the board, up the court and in the hole as quickly as possible. The game is simple. It's not hard to play if you are playing together. I'll probably make mistakes. I just hope when we're drawing up a play in the final seconds, I don't put myself in."

Bird exhibited that dry Hoosier humor throughout the hour-long interview in front of about 200 members of the media. When asked if this made him bigger than Bob Knight, he replied, "I hope I win more games than Bobby Knight -- 30 to 35 won't do it."

And the preferred method of conditioning is nothing like McHale's, whose idea of getting into shape according to Bird is "switching from Miller to Miller Lite."

Bird also was asked if he would ever seeks the opinions of former teammate Danny Ainge, now the head coach at Phoenix.

"I would never consult Danny Ainge on anything except to do something on the court so his man wouldn't double-team me," Bird quipped.

Having added some polish over the years, Bird is evolved into something more than "The Hick From French Lick." It's as if he's been groomed his whole life for this job. And although you won't catch him in an Armani suit, he is just as smooth as Pitino himself, in a Hoosier sort of way. Monday, he said all the right things, and said them honestly and succinctly.

There is no timetable for Bird in this coaching venture, but his contract has a provision for graduating into the front office when he's ready.

"If everybody is happy, I'll go on," he said.

Right now, everybody is happy in Hoosierland. The Bird has landed.

Pacers Leave Bulls Pawing in the Dirt

Reggie Miller provided a lot of dramatic moments over his 18-year career, especially when he shot down the Bulls in Game 4 of the 1998 Eastern Conference finals. And the Bulls provided additional column fodder with their persistent whining. Even though the Bulls had the final say, winning the series in seven games, it was fun while it lasted for this Pacers' beat writer.

Bloomington Herald-Times
May 26, 1998

INDIANAPOLIS, INDIANA

Had it all the way.

Was there any doubt when Reggie Miller caught the ball with time to square up that the shot would not go down?

So what if it was Game 4 of their Eastern Conference finals against the five-time champion Chicago Bulls.

So what if the Pacers were down a point with only 2.9 seconds left.

So what if Miller had played 42 rather ordinary minutes on a bad ankle.

When it comes to theatrics, Reggie is right up there with Chicago's Michael Jordan, who almost had the last laugh. There were some 16,000 Hoosiers with binding underwear as Jordan's desperation shot had a cup of coffee on the rim before falling off, giving the Pacers a 96-94 win.

Ain't life great when you're 2-2 with the mighty Bulls? So what if the Bulls take out their frustrations on the Pacers the next two games. For one deliriously wonderful weekend, the "Hicks" from Indiana upstaged the NBA's darlings. And what makes it even sweeter is the fact that the Bulls were reduced to whining like a bunch of adolescents who had their phone privileges cut off.

Check out Chicago coach Phil Jackson: "I don't know if I can watch the last 10 minutes of the basketball game without calling Rod Thorn (NBA Vice President of Operations)."

Wah, wah, wah.

Jackson ranted on about the officiating of Ronnie Nunn, Hugh Evans and Bill Oakes, calling it "Munich '72 revisited."

Wah, wah, wah.

Jackson was referring to the controversial Gold Medal basketball game of the 1972 Olympics at Munich, Germany. It was the game where the Soviets were given multiple chances in the final seconds to beat the Americans before finally doing so, 51-50.

Granted, there were some calls that were, say, questionable -- as if the Bulls never received any of the kind in their five championship years.

"Them of all people should not be bitching about holding, hitting and punching," Miller said. "They get all the benefit-of-the-doubt calls."

"It's us against the world -- you saw that in the fourth quarter," said Jordan, who thought the officials were influenced by some lobbying by Indiana coach Larry Bird after Games 1 and 2 in Chicago. "Give some credit to Larry Bird. After the first couple games, he fought for more awareness of our defense. It's all a matter of jostling for position."

Maybe the officials did forget that any Bulls game is unofficially thought of around the league as the Michael Jordan Worship Hour. They dared to call four fouls on His Airness, two shy of disqualification, of course.

Admittedly, the Pacers did get some breaks. When was the last time an offensive foul was called on a member of the Bulls in the final minute of a one-point game? It happened to Dennis Rodman, the master of disguising the cheap shot.

And when was the last time with the game on the line that a jump ball call was reversed, giving possession to the Bulls' opposition? It happened with 2.9 seconds left, awarding the Pacers and Miller their final opportunity.

And when was the last time an opponent flew into the Chicago bench, said "hello" with his elbows and was not excused for the duration? Miller did with 4.7 seconds left after a takedown by Chicago's Ron Harper. It appeared there was more pushing and shoving than punches thrown, although you will never get the Bulls to agree on that.

"Everybody saw Reggie as the aggressor," Jordan said. "In the midst of that whole melee, nobody got thrown (ejected)."

"I didn't throw any punches," Miller said. "I'm not dumb enough to throw a punch in a playoff game. I was just trying to push my way out before I got hit. I was trying to get out of the ruckus."

The only real punches thrown were of the verbal variety -- during and after the game. Jackson said the officials acted "scared" and virtually gave Indiana an "eight-man defense."

"We've got to roll with the punches," Jordan said. "I'm not going to look at my teammates and point any fingers. We are all in this together."

Reggie wouldn't buy that.

"Knowing the competitor Michael is, he is cussing out everybody on that plane."

"I'm not going to worry about what people think of us," Jordan said. "Whether it's Utah or Indiana, they still have to come through Chicago."

And beginning with Game 5 Wednesday, the world will get back to normal in Chicago, where the Bulls will once again get the calls and the Pacers will get to whine about the officials.

Until then, allow the humble subjects to enjoy watching the good king squirm.

Sun Setting on Aging Bulls

After the Bulls had to reach down deep to beat the Pacers in Game 7 of the 1998 Eastern Conference finals, you sensed their great run was nearing an end. As history would show, it was indeed the last title for the Bulls in the Michael Jordan era.

Bloomington Herald-Times
June 1, 1998

CHICAGO, ILLINOIS

As the sun was sinking into Lake Michigan on a spectacular Chicago twilight, you had to wonder if the sun also wasn't setting on the pride of the Windy City, the Chicago Bulls.

Not only had their legs started to show their age, you had to wonder if the fires of desire were starting to flame out.

Here were the five-time NBA champs, locked in a life-and-death struggle with the Indiana Pacers, a team which had dared to make them go to a seventh game before earning the right to defend their championship against the Utah Jazz.

These were unfrequented waters for the Bulls, not used to having to go the distance against an Eastern Conference rival. Unlike the more recent vintages of conference fodder, this Indiana team was more persevering, more gritty, more worthy.

This was a Pacer team playing its third conference final in five years and determined to get it right after losing Game 7 to New York in 1994 and Orlando in '95. Would the third time be the charm for Indiana, or would it be three strikes and yer out?

Like Chicago, this was an Indiana team also realizing the curtain was about to come down. The Pacers went into the game fully aware they weren't getting any younger, either.

Those were the stakes as the two rivals squared off at Chicago's United Center, where the Bulls lose about every stock market crash. In fact, rumor has it that a Bulls' loss sends the stock market spiraling downward. The Dow-Jones is Bullish on Chicago, you know.

You might want to buy some stock this minute. The Bulls have lived to fight another day, thanks to a gritty 88-83 win.

After all the excuses, finger-pointing and whining that went on beforehand, these two teams walked off the court filled with mutual respect. The winners won with class and the losers lost with dignity.

"This was one of the toughest series in my whole career," said Scottie Pippen, Chicago's all-purpose forward. "They gave us everything we could ask for. It was a very enjoyable series compared to some of the others we had, like the Knicks. I can't say the best team won. We just came out on top. I have a lot of respect for Indiana."

"Indiana gave us one heck of a series," said Chicago coach Phil Jackson, who is imminently on his way out of Chicago after this season. "This was two teams testing each other out, trying to find areas they could exploit."

Despite being named NBA Coach of the Year in his rookie season, Indiana's Larry Bird in so many words said he felt like a failure.

"I didn't get them to where I wanted to take them," he said. "I feel bad for them."

"He was truly Coach of the Year," Indiana guard Mark Jackson said. "He did a brilliant job. He made the game fun for us. It's disappointing we didn't win it all."

"We knew we would be right there at the end," Bird said. "It was just a matter of making plays. Chicago made the plays."

Bird couldn't resist one parting shot at the officials, who in the first half allowed Chicago to play aggressive, especially on the boards, while calling it tight on the Pacers. After a Chicago reporter complimented Bird for being "a breath of fresh air," Bird thanked the man and added, "The refs still stink."

When the calls weren't going so well for the Bulls, they reverted to their old whining ways, costing them a technical foul. Michael Jordan wasn't going to hear any more of that and told his teammates in no uncertain words at halftime.

"I told them to leave the refs alone," he said afterward. "Every time we mouth off, we give up free points. I told 'em to shut up and play."

Asked if the Bulls are showing some chinks in the armor, Jordan replied, "People are going to say, 'The Bulls lost their swagger in this series.' Well, probably, but nobody has taken anything from us yet."

If this in fact the end of a dynasty, the end of a reign, all you can do is tip your hat to the Bulls and say, "Long live the king."

Jordan's Worst Nightmare: Dan Dakich?

Former IU basketball player Dan Dakich never enjoyed a pro career, but he is forever linked to Michael Jordan, maybe the greatest pro of them all. The 25th anniversary of one of the most stunning upsets in NCAA history recalled the night Dakich and IU shocked Jordan and the North Carolina Tar Heels.

Bloomington Herald-Times
March 22, 2009

When the score flashed across your television screen late the March night, it had to be a mistake, you thought.

No way could No. 1 North Carolina lose to an Indiana that had lost eight games.

But there's that score again: Indiana 72, North Carolina 68.

Oh, come on now. Who does Indiana have to keep Michael Jordan from dunking them into oblivion?

Who is going to keep Sam Perkins from scoring at will inside? And how could Indiana possibly handle North Carolina's trapping defense?

Somebody call the network. That score ain't right.

But it was. Look it up: March 22, 1984 — 25 years ago today.

It really happened because Dan Dakich was there. He was the Hoosier guard credited with making Jordan look like a mere mortal.

Legend has it that when Dakich learned of this impossible defensive assignment, he went back to his room and puked. It's true, he now says, but for other reasons.

"I had been sick as a dog all week," he said over a salad last week.

Dakich was more than happy to talk about perhaps the greatest upset in IU history, although at the time the Hoosiers didn't think of it that way, either out of hubris or naivete.

"You got to understand, at Indiana you kind of expected to win," Dakich said of the attitude cultivated by coach Bob Knight. "It wasn't that anybody was going to awe you. You were expected to play at that level."

Radical Game Plan

Dakich recalled the first team meeting of the week leading up to the Thursday night date with North Carolina in Atlanta.

"I will never forget it. Knight walks in, and the first thing he says is, 'Anybody who doesn't think we are going to kick North Carolina's ass, get out of here.'"

Nobody left, of course. Then Knight unveiled a game plan that essentially scrapped some of the things he holds dear: the four-pass minimum on offense, the screens on the defenders, the up-close-and-personal defense.

The way North Carolina trapped on defense, setting screens only would have drawn more defenders to the ball, Knight believed. He wanted to maintain as much spacing as possible so when the Tar Heels did trap, a Hoosier was going to be open. The marching orders then were to shoot.

"There wasn't going to be any screening," Dakich said. "We wanted to spread things out. I would be willing to bet we didn't score a single point off a screen."

Getting the green light to shoot was all Steve Alford and Stew Robinson needed to hear. They made the Tar Heels pay dearly. Alford, a freshman then, leaped into the national spotlight with a 27-point game, including a 25-footer that gave the Hoosiers a four-point halftime lead.

"Alford was making everything," Dakich said.

Robinson made some huge shots the second half and finished with 14. The Hoosiers also got a solid 16 points from junior center Uwe Blab.

Taking the Air out of Jordan

But the game was really won on the defensive end. Although Jordan was the national Player of the Year, the Hoosiers were more concerned about stopping Perkins inside.

"This might sound crazy," Dakich said, "but our priority was to take away the inside, basically allow nothing at the basket."

If the Hoosiers shut off the inside, Jordan wouldn't be able to go over them for dunks. The plan called for the Hoosiers to sag off of him, take away his lanes to the basket. While backing off an offensive player was foreign to most Hoosier defenders, Dakich saw the logic in it.

"I don't want to dispel the myth, but Jordan wasn't a 30-point scorer back then," he pointed out. "He was about a 19. We were supposed to give up ground so he couldn't get past you. Under no circumstances were we to give him an offensive rebound or a back cut."

It was genius. Jordan picked up two early fouls, one of them a charge drawn by Dakich, and had to sit the last 10 minutes of the half.

"I remember looking over at Coach Knight and seeing how happy he was about that play," Dakich said.

Wherever Jordan went, Dakich went. It was all Jordan could do to score 14 points.

"If they were shooting a free throw and Jordan was down at the other end, I would stand right next to him the whole time," Dakich said. "I'm looking at him this one time, seeing those wide shoulders and thinking, 'Oh my God!'"

Trying to shut down Perkins was another thing, however. The Tar Heel center scored 26 points.

"We failed miserably," Dakich said of that goal.

Nothing Could Be Finer

But the offensive game plan also worked as Knight said it would. Indiana made 24 of 37 shots, 65 percent.

With 5 1/2 minutes to go, Alford scored on a breakaway to give Indiana 59-47 lead. With no shot clock to hurry the offenses back then, all the Hoosiers had to do was hit their free throws at that point. But they missed four straight one-and-ones, allowing the Tar Heels to close the deficit to two in just two minutes.

Finally, Alford ended the free throw drought, and the Hoosiers went up by four.

"I can still vividly, vividly feel this," Dakich said. "A four-point lead in that game seemed like a lot."

Still, it took two free throws by Blab at 0:19, and two more by sophomore Mike Giomi at 0:05 for the Hoosiers to hang on.

Then it was bedlam. The photo on the front of the *Herald-Telephone* sports page showed Dakich leaping into Blab's arms. Moments later, he found himself talking to Billy Packer of CBS.

"We are running off the floor and some girl from CBS grabs Alford and me," Dakich said. "I had no idea why I was there. Then they ask me, 'How did you stop Michael Jordan?' I didn't know what to say."

Once they got back to their hotel, the celebration was rather subdued, though.

"We knew we had beaten the No. 1 team, but it was odd," Dakich said. "I'm mean, we're Indiana. We are supposed to beat No. 1 teams."

History The Judge

The passage of time has helped Dakich appreciate it more.

"I was at an Olympics practice the next year and Jimmy Crews (the former Hoosier) comes over and says, 'You know, everybody is going to remember you shutting down the greatest player ever.' I didn't believe him. Greatest player ever? At the time I thought Sam Perkins was the guy."

Now Dakich is known as "The Guy Who Shut Down Michael Jordan." Whether totally accurate or not, Dakich is reminded of it almost daily.

"I do a lot of radio shows, and they often use it as a form of introduction," he said.

Dakich now has his own radio show on 1070 The Fan in Indianapolis. In 1993, he crossed paths with Jordan in a golf tournament.

"Jordan told me we got lucky, that it would never happen again," he said. "Well, it doesn't have to happen again."

It just had to happen once.

Feel the Magic?
Bird Would Rather Not

At the end of a 2009 Pacers' press conference, GM Larry Bird recalled – with much prodding – the storied meeting between his Indiana State Sycamores and Magic Johnson's Michigan State Spartans in the 1979 NCAA title game.

Bloomington Herald-Times
March 27, 2009

It is a game Larry Bird would like to forget, but the media won't let him. As every fifth anniversary rolls around, he is forced to talk about it.

You know the game, the 1979 NCAA final between Indiana State and Michigan State. It wasn't just David vs. Goliath. It was better than that. It was Bird vs. Magic.

Even as collegians, they already were households words — Larry Bird, the blue collar Hick from French Lick, and Earvin Johnson, the Magic Man who drove Michigan State's high-powered offense.

Almost one in four homes tuned in March 26, 1979. Its 24.1 share of the ratings is the still highest of any NCAA final. Although the game itself was almost anticlimactic — Michigan State won rather easily, 75-64 — it is credited for ushering in the modern era of college basketball. The following year, March Madness was splashed all over a new network, ESPN.

The NBA also got a big boost from the game when Bird and Johnson took their act to the pro ranks the following year and reignited the league's most compelling rivalry, Celtics vs. Lakers. Bird would gain a measure of revenge when the Celtics beat the Lakers in the 1984 finals, but Magic got the last say when the Lakers beat the Celtics in '87.

But even that loss in '87 pales in comparison to the painful ending of Bird's college career. The lasting memory for television viewers that March night was seeing Bird with his head buried in a towel, trying to hide the tears.

"It hurts just as much today as it did back then," he said before a room full of reporters at Conseco Fieldhouse, where he took a few minutes off from his job as Pacers president to revisit that epic game.

"There have been a lot of great champions and a lot of great finals since then," he said, "but every five years they want to bring this up."

Although Bird did not shoot well in that final (7-for-21), he still finished with 19 points, 13 rebounds and five steals. Johnson had 24 points and seven rebounds.

Had the Sycamores beaten the Spartans that night, they would have been college basketball's most recent unbeaten champions, not the 1976 Indiana Hoosiers. And to think that Bird was briefly an Indiana Hoosier before leaving Bloomington in September 1974.

"That was a tough time in my life," he said. "Even before I went to IU, I thought about staying out a year and just working, but they might not have wanted me then. I knew it was going to be a struggle financially. I was busted, broke, didn't have anything. It was just not a good situation for a kid like myself coming out of a small town. I watched IU play, knew they had a great team. Even when I was up there I looked around and wondered who I could beat out to get a couple of minutes a game."

It is old history now. Bird left IU, rode a garbage truck in Terre Haute for a year, enrolled at Indiana State in 1975 and went on to lead the Sycamores to the four greatest years in the history of the program. As Bird's senior year rolled around, he agreed to appear on the cover of *Sports Illustrated* — an error in judgement he says now.

"I wish I hadn't done that," he said. "Everything changed overnight. It changed our team. I went from a pretty quiet 30 points a game, doing what I did, to doing a lot of requests, a lot of photos. It just took away what I was comfortable with. I guess the country just couldn't imagine a kid coming from a small town, dropping out of IU, going to work and coming through all the tragedies I went through, then taking a small school to the next level."

The biggest of those tragedies was losing his father, Joe, who took his own life in 1975. Although Bird's family was dirt poor, he passed up early entry into the NBA, even after the Celtics drafted him after his junior year.

"I had the best times of my life in college," he said. "Playing basketball and going to school, you can't beat that. Talk about having the opportunity to make money, that meant nothing to me. The only thing that meant something was to stay there and get an education. That's what I promised my mother."

If only Bird could have capped it off with a national championship.

"To win 33 games in a row and get all the way to the last game was a heck of a ride, but we didn't get it done," he said. "It broke my heart not to bring a championship back to the city of Terre Haute and to the Indiana State Sycamores."

The Sacking of the Cleveland Browns

To this day in Cleveland, there is no bigger villain than Art Modell, the former owner who packed up the city's beloved Browns and shipped them to Baltimore. You didn't have to be a Browns fan to feel Cleveland's pain. As a Cleveland fol-

lower from my youth, the thought of Cleveland without the beloved "Brownies" chilled my bones like an icy gale off Lake Erie.

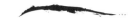

Bloomington Herald-Times
November 8, 1995

The Baltimore Browns? You must be kidding. The Browns playing anywhere but Cleveland is unthinkable.

It has gone beyond the thinking stage, however. Browns' owner Art Modell already has signed on the dotted line.

The Browns are going to Baltimore.

One week Cleveland is losing the World Series to Atlanta and the next it is losing the Browns to Baltimore. That big splash you heard was the many Cleveland natives jumping into Lake Erie.

If you take the Browns out of Cleveland, you might as well take the Yankees and send them to Birmingham. Take the Celtics, too, and move them to Las Vegas. Take the Canadiens and move them to Honolulu.

Cleveland and the Browns are one of sport's perfect marriages -- like Green Bay and the Packers, Pittsburgh and the Steelers, New York and the Yankees, Boston and the Celtics, Montreal and the Canadiens. The Browns reflect their city – rough and brawny. Their fans are blue-collar types who love it when the gales blow off Erie and into the musty old stadium they affectionately call "The Mistake By The Lake."

For almost 50 years, neither rain, sleet nor gloom of defeat has kept the fans of Cleveland from their appointed dates. They kept coming when the weather was the kind only an Alaskan seal could like. They kept coming after Otto Graham and Jim Brown went off to early retirements. They kept coming after Bobby Mitchell and Paul Warfield were traded away. They kept coming after a trio of devastating setbacks in the 1980s, to wit:

* The Interception (1980) - Brian Sipe's ill-advised pass with the Browns in range for a game-winning field goal in the playoffs is intercepted by Oakland.

* The Drive (1987) - With a 20-13 lead and a 98-yard cushion between them and a first-ever trip to the Super Bowl, the

Browns let John Elway and the Denver Broncos go the length of the field to send the game into overtime and ultimately beat them, 23-20.

* The Fumble (1988) - With another Super Bowl beckoning, Cleveland's Earnest Byner fumbles on the way to a game-tying touchdown at Denver.

But the fans kept coming back, in legions of 70,000-plus for home games, an attendance figure that annually puts them among the NFL leaders. Apparently, that isn't enough for Modell, who wants luxury boxes. He wants those corporate dollars. The fans' hard-earned, blue-collar dollars are pocket change to him.

Where's the loyalty, Art? When the Browns were laboring through those losing seasons in the 1970s and '80s, the fans stuck by you. Is this how you repay them?

"I'm going to do what I have to do to protect my family, my franchise and my employees," he said.

Did we miss something? Is somebody holding his family hostage? Modell is like the guy who lets his wife put him through college, then dumps her for some bimbo.

The aftershocks are being felt by Browns fans all over the country, including those in Bloomington. Bloomington has its own Browns Backers Association, one of the hundreds of chapters that make up the largest fans' organization in the world. Every week for the past four years, the local Browns Backers have gathered to watch the games at Yogi's Grill and Bar, owned by Jim Karl, a Browns fan from way back.

The Browns Backers who came to Yogi's for Sunday's game against the Oilers were almost in a state of shock, Karl said.

"It was like somebody took the life out of them," he said.

"It was like a death in the family, or getting divorced," said Craig Moore, president of the local Browns chapter. "It was a combination of shock and sadness."

Moore and Karl have Ohio roots, which makes the move even harder to take.

"I don't have a clue who I'm going to root for now," Karl said.

"I have a hard time thinking of any sports team with as much of a tie as Cleveland has for the Browns," said Moore. "If that can be broken, then any of them can be broken."

Also smarting is John McCluskey, who spent six years in Cleveland before coming to Indiana University to teach Afro-American studies.

"The Browns are so important to the city," he said. "I'm not thinking of the players or the won-lost record, but what they mean to the city. The Browns not only give the fans something to do, they are a source of pride."

If the Browns are allowed to leave Cleveland, no city is safe. We will have entered a new era of franchise free agency, where any city with a stadium and a deep wallet can bid for a team.

"It's the ultimate in free agency," Moore said. "Not only can players go where they want; so can the owners."

Will it be long before we have a yearly auction? Can't you see it: "Who wants the Dallas Cowboys this year? Tampa says $1 billion. Do I hear $1.5 billion, Seattle? Los Angeles bids $1.5 billion. Going once, going twice ..."

Brace yourself. The Browns are only the beginning.

Sampras Too Good or Too Nice?

An annual summer assignment was covering the RCA Tennis Championships in Indianapolis. The draws were great in the 1980s and 1990s, attracting such top names as Jimmy Connors, John McEnroe, Andre Agassi, Boris Becker and a noble superstar, Pete Sampras. For all of his achievements, Sampras seemed underappreciated, something I could never figure out.

Bloomington Herald-Times
August 15, 1997

INDIANAPOLIS, INDIANA

It never ceases to amaze me how indifferent the American sports fan is to Pete Sampras.

As he walked off the court at Indianapolis Thursday, a three-set loser to Sweden's Magnus Larsson, Sampras departed to a mere smattering of applause. Larsson, on the other hand, was cheered wildly.

It's OK to root for the underdog, but I find it hard to root against Pete Sampras under any circumstance. It isn't just because he is an American. Tennis has a way of cutting across international lines. Sampras I'm sure has his foreign admirers, too, but the puzzling question is, why he doesn't have more American fans?

What's not to like?

He's personable, humble, approachable and a gentleman at all times. He doesn't complain and he doesn't make excuses. In another time he would be the classic American hero -- a Lou Gehrig, a John Wayne, a Neil Armstrong.

But it is Sampras's misfortune to have landed in the middle of the MTV generation, where everything is loud, vulgar and boorish. It is this generation which prefers Dennis Rodman and Andre Agassi over Pete Sampras.

Agassi is clearly the crowd favorite again at Indy, one year after he was excused from the Tennis Center for openly cursing an umpire and drop-kicking a tennis ball into the upper deck. Got to love that whacky Andre, even though he hasn't won a grand slam event since Bill Clinton got re-elected.

All Sampras does is win. Quite often. He already has won the Australian Open and Wimbledon this year and has been ranked No. 1 four years running. He is without question the best player of our time. He has it all -- the groundstrokes, the volleys, the big serve, the big heart. He is so good, so efficient, that he is ... boring, you say?

If that is boring, it is the nature of the beast. It is not Pete's fault that technology has transferred tennis from the finesse game it used to be to the power game it is today. The big, tightly strung racquets have changed tennis dramatically. It's not the same sport when Ken Rosewall and Rod Laver played. It's not even the same sport when Jimmy Connors and John McEnroe played. Even Sampras admitted that "It's always a battle of services on the men's game."

You can't blame that on Sampras, just because he has mastered the serve. As fellow player Wayne Ferreira said, "Sampras is probably the best ever. If somebody can do that at that level, I don't see how tennis can be that bad. We've got a lot of great players -- good, strong, tight competition, great athletes, good shot-makers. I mean, the serve has become very powerful, but guys are starting to overcome that now by being such good returners. So the game changes over the years, but it always evens itself out in different aspects."

Sampras has risen above this pack, like no one since Laver and Rosewall. And like those greats, he just goes about his business. He is not controversial. He is not confrontational. He is not contrary.

Some point to that for his lack of emotional appeal. You want emotion? How about the tears he wept during a match after learning his coach and confidant, Tim Gullickson, was dying from brain cancer.

How about last year's U.S. Open match against Alex Corretja, when Sampras, vomiting from over-exertion, picked himself off the court and won the match in a fifth-set tiebreaker.

You think that would have endeared Sampras to the American public forever, but there he was Thursday at Indianapolis, walking off the court to only polite applause.

One of these days, it's going to dawn on us what a privilege it is to watch a legend in the making -- a legend with no flash, no gimmicks, no nonsense. For the time being, we are not worthy.

For Pete's sake, America, wake up.

In the Wake of 9-11, United We Stand

When the NFL resumed play after the shock of "9-11", the games were dwarfed by larger issues. The feeling in the RCA Dome on that Sunday confirmed that.

Bloomington Herald-Times
September 24, 2001

INDIANAPOLIS, INDIANA

After taking a week off to ponder more profound issues, the show that has become the National Football League went on in stadiums across the land Sunday.

It was another way of saying that life goes on in America, no matter how severe the wounds.

The horrors of September 11, 2001 have certainly left their scars, but the fact that Americans can still gather to celebrate a pastime shows their resiliency.

As some 56,000 Americans gathered Sunday at the RCA Dome to watch the Indianapolis Colts play the Buffalo Bills, you could feel a national bond that had been long forgotten the last time the Colts hosted a football game.

You could feel it when members of the Indianapolis Fire Department and law enforcement agencies were honored before the game -- to genuine, appreciative cheers.

You could feel it when the stadium shook with spontaneous chants of "USA, USA."

You could feel it when 56,000 voices sang "God Bless America," "America the Beautiful" and the "Star Spangled Banner."

The members of the fire department who started the national anthem did not need any help in finishing it. Midway through they turned it over to the fans, who willingly took it from there.

Never has "The Star-Spangled Banner" been sung with such conviction in the RCA Dome.

"It was really neat when the whole crowd started singing it," said Colts safety Chad Cota. "The emotion I got from it was easy to turn over into the game."

How many times in the past have minds wandered off the subject matter when the national anthem has been played? We Americans are good at paying lip service to such phrases as "land of the free" and "home of the brave," but this latest national crisis has forced us to really reflect on their meaning. The thought was not lost on Marcus Pollard, the Colts' tight end.

"I can tell you I cried," he said. "It was particularly emotional for me, thinking about the firemen, the police officers, the volunteers who lost their lives. It could have been me. It made me realize how blessed I am to be able to pay tribute to them."

"It was certainly emotional during the national anthem," quarterback Peyton Manning said. "Even though you are focused on football, you can't help but think about what's going on." "The pre-game ceremonies were pretty emotional, seeing the firefighters, EMT and police officers out there," said Indianapolis tight end Ken Dilger. "The national anthem definitely was more special today. It was tough for me, personally, to keep my emotions in check for a few minutes."

Defensive end Chad Bratzke spent six years in New York playing for the Giants before coming to Indianapolis. Seeing the images of the World Trade Center on the big screen during the pre-game memorial struck an emotional chord.

"New York was home for six years," he said. "I tried to prepare myself, but I didn't do a very good job. I had to hold back a couple times."

How unfortunate that it took a catastrophe to bring it closer to home. To say we have failed to appreciate our freedoms and our privileges is a gross understatement. How long will it be before we once again take them for granted? Hopefully never, now that we have seen how costly the price of freedom is.

But this is not the time for preaching. This is a time for healing. Playing our games again is an appropriate way to start picking up the pieces. At Indianapolis Sunday, you sensed that the healing already had begun when the fans booed the Bills as they made their entrance. We like our villains in athletic uniforms, not in battle gear. And we like them out there for us to take issue with, not slinking away like cowards.

Football is a game of heroes and villains. The Indianapolis-Buffalo game had its fair share of both. Fans cheered the good plays, moaned the bad ones and voiced their displeasure when they felt the home team was wronged. The many scuffles among the players seemed to indicate that Americans are a little testy in the aftermath of September 11.

We Americans will continue to have our differences, but that is business as usual. We are not happy unless we have something to quarrel about. But as a whole we stand united, united as we have not stood for a long, long time.

Reggie Goes Out in a Blaze Of Glory

Reggie Miller's final season as an Indiana Pacer began with much promise but was torpedoed by an ugly brawl in Detroit in November. The end came in the playoffs against the very same Detroit Pistons. Miller still made it a memorable night with a gallant effort in defeat.

Bloomington Herald-Times
May 20, 2005

INDIANAPOLIS, INDIANA

Reggie Miller will not have a championship ring to show for his 18 years in the NBA, but he walked away a champion in the hearts of everybody who participated in the final game of his memorable career Thursday night.

Miller, 39, turned back the clock in a losing effort to the Detroit Pistons, a loss that not only ended the Pacers' season but also ended a career that will surely land Miller in the Hall of Fame.

Miller scored 27 points in 33 minutes and nearly single-handedly kept the Pacers in the game until the Pistons put the final hammer down.

"He went out with guns a blazing," said Detroit coach Larry Brown, who coached Miller for four years in the mid-1990s. "I can't imagine a guy playing his last game in this league, 40 years old, and having a game like that. It's mind boggling. I was convinced he was going to win the game."

Brown did a classy thing by calling timeout with 15.7 seconds left and his Pistons safely ahead, the purpose being to give Miller a chance to take his final bows. He departed to a mixture of cheers and tears. Even the Pistons, those dastardly accomplices of that unsavory night in November, sought out Miller to give him a going-away hug. "I was proud to be a part of Reggie's last game and see him get that ovation," Brown said.

Rip Hamilton, the Detroit guard who is often compared to Miller, exchanged a long embrace before letting Miller ride off into the sunset.

"I just told him 'thanks' for the opportunity to play against him," Hamilton said.

Miller scored his 27 points on just 16 shots. He was 4-for-8 from 3-point range. After struggling throughout the series, Miller decided to relax and enjoy what would be his last pro game.

"I'm just glad I made some shots. Tonight, I just wanted to concentrate on having fun. Instead of my usual pre-game routine, I wanted to look around, look at the fans, absorb this. I wanted to feel their presence, wanted to feel like I was still in high school."

"He played like he was 22," Brown said. "We've got to cherish that."

"We really saw one of the true, vintage, Reggie Miller performances you could ever see in a playoff game," Indiana coach Rick Carlisle said. "It was fitting that our distant memories of him are playing 33 minutes, going 11-for-16 from the floor and scoring 27 points. He goes out in a wave of glory."

Although Miller left the fans wanting more, the decision to retire is final. When asked if he would reconsider, he said, "Did you see Games 3 and 4?" noting the poor performances he had in those pivotal games.

There was a lot of good will on the court for two teams forever linked by the violent incidents of November 19, when the Pacers not only mixed it up with the Pistons, but also their fans. Brown was quick to point out that this series was all about basketball.

"We played three (regular season) games since the fight and six in the playoffs, and you saw guys hugging each other," the coach said. "It shows that kids can just play basketball."

The Pacers definitely got the worst of the fallout from November 19, losing Ron Artest to suspension for the duration of the season and Jermaine O'Neal and Stephen Jackson for extended periods. Mix in the injuries to O'Neal, Jeff Foster, Jamaal Tinsley and Jonathan Bender, and it's a wonder the Pacers even made the playoffs, let alone advance to the second round and throw a scare into the defending champions.

"You hate to lose a playoff series," Carlisle said, "but our guys have to realize they have been one of the unlikeliest stories in the history of professional sports. The reality is, we got beat by a team that's just better."

Miller saw no reason for the Pacers to hang their heads.

"On the one hand, this has been one of the most trying seasons for us, but at the end of the day, it was also one of the most rewarding. It brought our coaches, our players, our fans together. Just to be here now, after winning the Boston series and going six games with the world champions."

Miller was candid about failing to bring a title to Indianapolis.

"We had one common goal, but I wasn't able to deliver a championship here. I didn't get the ultimate prize, but I tried."

As Miller left the court Thursday night to a standing ovation, he patted his heart, right over the word "Indiana" on the No. 31 jersey that will be retired quicker than you can say "Boom, Baby."

"It's bittersweet," he said. "Words can never express what I feel for the city of Indianapolis. When I came here I didn't know anyone. I was 2,000 miles from home. But the first time I trotted out onto the floor at Market Square Arena, I knew I was home. This city has embraced me. We've grown up together. We've celebrated together. Tonight, we cried together."

Artest Dares to Turn His Back on Pacers

After almost single-handedly scuttling the previous season with his part in the brawl in Detroit, Ron Artest had the gall to demand a trade early in the following season. Given all his other misguided episodes, Artest quickly became the source of much outrage throughout Indiana.

How dare you, Ron Artest?

How dare you demand the Indiana Pacers trade you after all you put them through?

This is the team that stood behind you after you:

* *Destroyed a television camera in New York;*

* *Did a drive-by brushing of Miami coach Pat Riley;*

* *Delivered the flagrant foul in Game 6 of the 2004 Eastern Conference finals that ended any chance of the Pacers overtaking the Pistons;*

* *And committed the greatest sin of all, charging mindlessly into the stands in Detroit, taking your teammates and an entire franchise down with you.*

Now you have the audacity to demand a trade?

You didn't even have the decency to first consult coach Rick Carlisle or CEO Donnie Walsh or president Larry Bird. You remember Larry Bird, the guy who kept defending you?

Of all the options for a cover photo for its NBA basketball issue, *Sports Illustrated* chose you and Bird, together. The posed shot had Bird standing firmly behind you with arms folded as if to tell the world, "Stand by your man."

Why can't you be a stand-up guy? Why can't you take your differences behind closed doors instead of airing them out in public?

You say you have problems with Carlisle and your role in his offense while all along leading people to believe you were about winning a championship. Nobody ever doubted your competitiveness. Anybody who plays defense as relentlessly you do is dear to a Hoosier's heart, but the moment you started fancying yourself as a No. 1 option on offense, you obviously forgot about Jermaine O'Neal.

Not that you are a liability on offense, but you are known to force a shot or two. Let's face it. You have never been a great shot-maker. You are shooting 42 percent over your career. Of course you had lots of time to work on your shot last year during your season-ending suspension handed down by commissioner David Stern.

You might be interested to know the Pacers made the playoffs without you, even with all the injuries and other lengthy suspensions handed to O'Neal and Stephen Jackson, two teammates who had your back that night in Detroit. Not only did the Pacers make the playoffs, they made it to the second round before losing to the Pistons again.

You say you are tired of constantly being reminded of your past and that a change of scenery might wipe the slate clean. You mentioned New York. You think the New York media are going to forget your indiscretions? New York hasn't forgiven Major League Baseball for allowing the Dodgers and Giants to move to California.

Then again, New York just might dig a character who asked to wear Dennis Rodman's number last year. That sure worked out well for you, didn't it?

New York might also like a guy who shaved the music label of his CD into the back of his head. Heck, New York has put up with Latrell Sprewell and Stephon Marbury, so what's one more powder keg?

That's assuming somebody out there is willing to take a chance on you. Major shoe companies are scared to death of you, which is why you are pushing a little-known German brand of sportswear, Kix.

The Pacers really have no choice but to let you go now, but what can they get for a guy who might go off at any time, whether it's to promote a CD or pummel a heckler?

Your teammate and friend, O'Neal, already has said, "See you later." That is the prevailing sentiment, Mr. Artest. Take your bad haircut, your bad CD and your bad attitude somewhere else. Close the door behind you and keep on going.

We dare you.

It's a Lonely Ol' Night for Manning

For all the times Peyton Manning had quarterbacked the Colts to victory, he had yet to win The Big One at the time this column was written. After the 2005 season ended in a devastating playoff loss to the Steelers, Manning looked more vulnerable than ever.

Bloomington Herald-Times
January 16, 2006

INDIANAPOLIS, INDIANA

"So sad and lonely," said the elevator operator on the ride up to the press box following the Colts' season-ending loss to Pittsburgh Sunday.

You wouldn't expect such an astute observation from a source who struggled with her English, yet the lady on the elevator nailed it. Having just seen Peyton Manning do some serious soul-searching in front of microphones and cameras, the words stuck in your head.

So sad and lonely, Peyton Manning appeared as he tried to explain another playoff failure.

Manning will once again take the brunt of the criticism as losing quarterbacks usually do, and losing the big games continues to be the knock on him. Don't think for a minute he isn't aware of it.

"I can't argue with the truth, but it's certainly not a lack of effort," he said. "I never step onto the field or walk off the field saying, 'I should have done more to prepare for this game.' I was never more prepared from an off-season standpoint. I can't tell you how much I studied these guys the last two weeks. We expected to play Pittsburgh and I really studied them hard."

Sacked five times, Manning could have leveled some of the blame at his offensive line, but he knows those guys have his back on the vast majority of plays. In trying to explain the breakdowns Sunday, Manning was diplomatic.

"I'm looking for a safe word here, guys. Pittsburgh just did some things that gave us trouble. Let's give them credit for having a good blitz package," he said.

Manning also could have passed the buck on to place kicker Mike Vanderjagt, who shanked a tying field goal in the final seconds.

"One play is not the reason why the Colts didn't win this game," Manning said. "Mike has been so awesome, such a clutch kicker, that people are surprised. It's nothing he has to apologize for because he has made so many clutch kicks."

Those are pretty kind words for a guy Manning once described as "our idiot kicker," but this Indianapolis team is family, a family that might be broken up after this season. Who knows where Edgerrin James, Reggie Wayne and Corey Simon will be next year with the personnel decisions facing the Colts in the off-season.

"It feels like college, like you are losing seniors," Manning said.

All that provided some extra incentive for the Colts, who realized that this might be their best shot. This was the year the Colts had all the pieces in place, the offense, the defense, the home field advantage.

And then they neglected to take advantage.

"You put so much to get into this position," Manning said. "Such a long season -- so many games, so much time studying things, so many third downs. We played so well from September to November, but the last two games, teams have come in here and outplayed us. You want to play your best football in December or January."

The Colts are now inviting comparisons to the Buffalo Bills of the 1990s, but that is unfair to the Bills. At least the Bills made it to the Super Bowl four straight years, something no other team has done. The Colts are more like the Atlanta Braves, a regular-season success story but post-season "disappointment," a word Manning kept throwing out there.

"It's disappointing now and it will be more disappointing tonight and tomorrow," he said. "It takes time to move on from a game like this, time to make your peace with the football gods and get ready for the next season."

It wasn't for a lack of urgency, Manning claimed.

"I've always played with a real sense of urgency. I've never said, 'It's OK, we'll get 'em next year.' It's not OK. You do feel a sense of urgency. Hopefully we will give it another try next year. Obviously, you get tired of saying that, especially after a playoff loss. Pretty soon you run out of years and there won't be a next year. I play every year like this is going to be the last game of my last year."

You know Manning will be taking another long look in the mirror between now and training camp. He said that in so many words Sunday.

"I'm going to keep trying. That's all I'm saying. All I can do is come back and try to be a better player next year, a better quarterback. You just have to keep sawing wood."

As Manning exited the interview area, he lacked the usual swagger, the usual bounce in his step, the usual light in his eyes.

So sad and lonely.

Quarter to Three, Just You and Me

After covering some very bad Indianapolis Colts teams in the 1990s, the 2006 Colts took me to the Promised Land, the Super Bowl. In addition to filing daily updates that week, I also kept a blog. Here's what I blogged after the Colts beat the Bears in Super Bowl, XVI, 29-17.

MIAMI, FLORIDA

It's a quarter to three, and I just returned to the hotel. I'm still trying to grasp what I just saw, a championship. Not just any championship, but a championship for the city of Indianapolis. If ever a city deserved one, it is the capital of Indiana.

Historically speaking, Indy hasn't had that much to hang its hat on, other than the 500, but a Super Bowl victory is about as good as it gets. I feel so privileged to have witnessed this Indianapolis coming-out party.

True, Indianapolis is far removed from the "Nap Town" image of old, but last night's triumph put a great big circle around the city in the old Rand-McNally. It now has joined an elite group of cities than can claim Super Bowl champion. With apologies to baseball, pro football is now the national pastime. Heck, NASCAR has probably gone around baseball.

But to be the toast of professional football at this hour – man, that's big. Indianapolis is the king right now, ladies and gentlemen. Let's give it up for the Circle City!

I suspect there is still some revelry going on around the Circle at this hour, sub-zero temperatures and all. If I were there right now, I'd put on my long-johns, my sock hat and my mittens and frolic right along with them.

You see, that's the downside of my job. While others are out celebrating great victories, I have a job to do. OK, so it's hard to feel sorry for any sports writer – and I would be the first one to admit that – but there are times when I wish I could just pack up my gear right after the game and commence to celebrating.

I thought of that as I watched the post-game celebration on the field at Dolphin Stadium Sunday night. Colts fans around me were basking in the glow of victory and ready to continue on into the night while I had to go back to my laptop and crank out a story (stop the violin music, please). As I was headed down the tunnel to the work room, I could still hear the music blaring from the post-game party. It was Rare Earth's "I Just Want to Celebrate."

It called to mind an emotion I felt on another rainy night almost 20 years ago, the night IU beat Syracuse in the 1987 NCAA title game. By the time I had finished my story, the party was over, the streets empty. I really wanted to share the moment with somebody, but there was nobody to be found. To this day, IU's '87 title hasn't sunken in because I wasn't able to put some closure on it with some back-slapping, high-fiving, beer-guzzling friends.

I hope that doesn't happen with this championship. Having covered the Colts now for over a decade, I feel I am entitled to enjoy this victory. Writers aren't supposed to be fans, but it's hard not to admire this classy Colts' team. They have surely paid their dues to get to this point, and I hope the Bears can get there, too. They are every bit as likeable.

So, if you see me down at Nick's, or Yogi's, the Irish Lion or some other pub, step right up. Let's hoist a glass or two because, as the song says, I just want to celebrate.

Chapter 12
Characters

We all know someone who qualifies as a "character," a colorful person who will not go unnoticed or be forgotten any time soon. "Character" also can describe someone who possesses an unsinkable spirit. You often find these individuals in unexpected places, even at a compost dump as I did in 1997. This chapter also tells the story of Bobby Wampler, a character worth writing about.

Talkin' Trash

The only compost site in Monroe County was operated by Dave Porter, an educated man who took "green" to an extreme. After a few trips to the dump site, I had to find out more. Turned out he made a lot of sense.

Bloomington Herald-Times
July 15, 1997

He sits there amid the filth, the flies and the foul smell of decay. His kingdom consists of mountains of molding wood, castles of dried brush, streams of smelly sludge and meadows of dead grass.

But to Dave Porter, the sight of rotting wood is as brilliant as a summer rainbow. The scent of de-

caying vegetation is a breath of fresh air. A sunken step in the sludge is a tiptoe through the tulips.

To Porter, life is one big compost pile.

Porter's 70 acres on West Vernal Pike is just that, a sprawling compost pile. Yard waste of almost any kind can be found there in some form of decay. Porter himself comes across as one of the half-decayed characters in Stephen King's horror novel, *Pet Sematary*.

You will find Porter in the middle of this natural mountain of waste, sitting under a big shade tree with his two dogs, Rama and Beatrix. You might even catch him playing the fiddle or boiling molasses from the many maple trees brought to him as waste.

To Porter, waste is in the eye of the beholder.

"Yard waste is what the average person thinks of when they no longer want it," he said. "Waste to you may not be waste to someone else."

But this is no standard garbage dump. Porter is only interested in organic waste, the kind nature will break down in its own way and in its own time.

"I want your glass clippings," he said. "I do not want your beer cans."

Porter spends a good portion of his 12-hour day turning away truckloads of inorganic material. Sometimes the public unloads it in spite of him.

"I have to play cop," he said. "I'm here to make people behave themselves better than their children."

It is not uncommon for Porter to arrive at dawn and find a heap of inorganic waste material dumped in front of his gate. People will leave ev-

173

erything from old automobile engines to broken toilets. Sometimes they take something with them. One day he was shocked to discover someone had stolen the large, stainless steel kettle he was using to make maple syrup.

"When crap like that happens," he said, "I want to bulldoze the entrance and say, 'Leave me alone.' "

Porter has been a self-described loner for most of his 48 years.

"What woman in her right mind would want to live with me?" he said.

Porter seems perfectly happy observing life from his spot under that shade tree.

"Step into my office," he says, shooing away one of the mutts from a bucket seat that serves as a chair. Wooden pallets serve as a floor. The decor is a foul-smelling barrel filled with brine of some kind. And for real atmosphere, a pig skull rests on top of a crate, inevitably calling to mind the beast of prey in the novel, "Lord of the Flies."

Porter's working attire is a dirty, long-sleeve shirt, soiled blue jeans, construction boots and a straw hat. A farmer's tan gives his face some color and some hard lines. While sitting there, you have to constantly wave off the flies and endure the odor of garbage. When asked if it always smells that bad, he offers a confession.

"There's some sort of dead animal in that barrel, a squirrel or something. I just haven't had it in me to dig it out yet."

Even Porter has his limits, it appears. Just don't call him "eccentric," he warns. The mere mention of that word launches him into a sermon on the evils of landfills and public dumps.

"Landfills are stupid," he sneered. "Just because you put something in a landfill does not mean you've dealt with the problem. You just put it out of sight. Just because you flush something down the toilet doesn't mean it is gone."

Composting is the only way, Porter says.

"It's the best way to use organic waste. It reduces the volume. The material is a food source for some other organism. That is why it goes away."

If Porter's world were perfect, there would be compost piles in place of all landfills. The idea is to not to stack waste on top of waste, but to spread it all out and let nature takes its course.

"There is no short supply of space in Indiana," he points out with a wave at all the open property around him. "Why are we in such a hurry? We have to quit being so wasteful. If you want to recycle a jar, just wash it and use it again. To smash it up, haul it away and then re-melt it is ludicrous."

Listening to Porter, you realize he is no dummy. He says he has three degrees from Indiana University, including one in biology. He says he has worked as a lab technician, an instructional designer, a photographer, a market gardener and as a humble "gopher" boy. You could see how he wouldn't last long in a job like that. He is much too independent.

He says he has lived in these parts since 1958 and remembers a Bloomington where "the trees made a canopy over the streets. Now all the streets are opened up so that global warming can run its course."

Porter speaks with disgust of bureaucrats and "flatlanders" -- people whose feet never touch the soil. They only touch the sidewalks, the carpets, the tarmacs of the world. Porter also loathes the "sleaziness of capitalism." As he was speaking, two truckers unloaded their trash and then left without paying, as if to underscore his point.

Porter himself is a living contradiction. All the while he is talking about caring for the land, he is abusing his body by chain-smoking. There is probably some sense to it, though. If nothing else, it keeps the flies away.

But in the middle of the squalor and stench and the decay is a slice of life, a garden. On one end is patch of day lilies. Not far away are some rhubarb plants and some herbs, mustard and garlic. Porter harvests his crops and peddles them at Bloomington's Farmers' Market.

"I've been going to Farmers' Market since they started it," he said, picking a batch of rhubarb and handing it to his visitor. "If it can be grown here, I've tried to grow it."

If you like, Porter will give you a tour of his empire. The wood pile is particularly impressive, with tree stumps up to six feet in diameter sprinkled throughout the heap.

"I am dumfounded at all the wood thrown away," he said. "In many places, people would want it for energy. Here, it is a waste. That tells you about our value system. We're too rich."

As you pull away from this smoldering dung heap, you steal a look in your rear view mirror and catch Porter plucking the fiddle. And there he remained, a 20th Century Nero fiddling away as his empire burns around him.

Editor's Note: A few years after this article was published, Dave Porter was taken by cancer.

'Spanky' an Ol' Rascal

One of my summer beats for the H-T was covering the Bloomington City Golf Tournament, a month-long match-play event sponsored by the newspaper since the tournament's inception in 1929. In 1980, a City Tournament Hall of Fame was established. Beginning in 1985, I was charged with writing the biographical sketches on each inductee. One of personal favorites was a character named Steve "Spanky" Stanger.

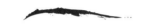

Bloomington Herald-Times
July 25, 1999

Steve "Spanky" Stanger believes in the power of supination, the golf gods, Seamus MacDuff, Ben Hogan, space junk, a good laugh, a cold beer and a strong woman.

But when told he was about to enter the Bloomington City Golf Hall of Fame, Stanger had a heck of time believing that.

"I was a little bit overwhelmed," he said.

Believe it, Spanky.

In ceremonies following the conclusion of the 71st *Herald-Times* City Golf Tournament at Cascades today, Stanger will be the 32nd inductee into the Hall of Fame since its inception in 1980.

"Nobody will appreciate it more," said long-time friend and former co-worker, Larry Behme.

Stanger has played in 25 city golf tournaments dating back to 1973, when he won the Junior Championship Flight that first year. It would be 16 more years before his next title came along. In 1989 he won the men's crown by defeating Steve Hinds, 3 and 2. Over the course of his colorful career, a career still active, Stanger has fashioned a record of 39-18 and has reached the quarterfinal level six times.

Stanger came out of Owen County, where he established a name for himself as a high-scoring guard on the Owen Valley basketball team. In fact, he never saw a shot he didn't like. He lived by the maxim: "If you're hot, shoot it. If you're not, keep shooting 'til you get hot."

As a high school golfer, Stanger was considered average.

"I remember one of my teachers writing in my yearbook, 'To a mediocre golfer.' That put a fire in me," Stanger said.

He became a student of the game, particularly of Ben Hogan's book, *The Modern Fundamentals of the Game*. It was between those pages Stanger that learned all about the technique of "supination," a way to pronate the wrists at impact.

He would practice the technique by the hour with the help of a makeshift "supinator," a stick with a weighty hunk of led on the end. The head was made out of "space junk," Stanger claimed.

As the story goes, he was on his way to California to look for work in the early 1980s. When Stanger's car, an aging Plymouth Barracuda, broke down in the middle of the desert, Stanger hit golf balls while he was awaiting roadside assistance. When he went to retrieve the balls, he stumbled over a heavy object.

"At first I thought it was a cannon ball, but where could it have come from?" Stanger explained. "It could only have come from outer space."

Hence the theory, "space junk."

Believing the object to be magical, Stanger fixed it to the end of a shovel handle and swung it repeatedly to strengthen his wrists. The effect was indeed magical. As drives started booming off his clubs, Stanger's game went to the next level.

In 1984 he reached the finals of the Championship Flight before losing to another future Hall of Famer, Bob Burris, 6 and 4. He made the semifinals in 1985 and '88.

The year 1988 also was good for Stanger's personal life. In October he wedded Donna Jones, a young lady he met on the golf course. It was only fitting that their marriage ceremony was held in the Cascades clubhouse.

And when they had a son in 1992, Spanky was tempted to name him Striker Straight Stanger. Donna would have none of that. They compromised and named him Hogan, after Stanger's idol.

Donna put stability in Stanger's life. Until she came along, he had a tendency to stay out too late. It wasn't unusual for him to show up for the first tee after having slept in his beat-up Chevy station wagon, the successor to the Barracuda.

With bloodshot eyes peeping through wire-rimmed glasses and a toothy smile poking out from under a thick mustache, Stanger resembled the actor Cheech Marin as he staggered up to the first tee. Only Cheech never launched a drive 300 yards.

It was no coincidence that Spanger's first city title came the summer after his October wedding. With his lust for the night life behind him, he was at his very best, beginning with a 20-hole escape in the opening round against an up-and-coming youngster by the name of Troy Gillespie, who was two years away from winning his first city title.

Stanger needed a birdie to match Gillespie on the 19th hole and then outdrove the powerful Gillespie on the 20th, something few other golfers could claim. In fact, Stanger drove the green and won it with another birdie.

The rest of the '89 tournament trail had such formidable foes as Gary Lawson, George Finley, Denny Smith and then Hinds, who was playing in his third final in five years.

Although it remains Stanger's only championship, he continues to be a major hurdle for any Championship Flight qualifier.

His presence also is felt on the golf course in another way. Since 1986 he has been an assistant course superintendent at the Bloomington Country Club. His first boss at the Country Club was Behme, who answers to "Boss" when Stanger addresses him.

Incidentally, the nickname "Spanky" has nothing to do with the Young Rascals, although Stanger certainly has a lot of rascal in him. He inherited that tag when his boyhood baseball coach couldn't come up with the name Stanger. It usually came out "Spanger" or "Spangy."

Stanger is probably one of the most popular characters to ever set foot on Cascades, the Country Club or any other area golf course.

"Spanky has a direct line to the golf gods," Behme said.

If Stanger wasn't a believer in the golf gods before, he is now. On the opening day of this year's Championship Flight qualifying tournament, Stanger was struggling mightily. His second shot on No. 10 went into the big maple tree near the 16th tee. What went up did not come down.

Having already suffered an embarrassing whiff on 10 and now facing a penalty stroke, Stanger climbed up into the tree in search of the missing ball. He didn't stop at the first limb. He methodically worked his way up until he was a good 40 feet off the ground. And still he couldn't find the ball.

He finally abandoned the search and worked his way back down, but not without a scare or two.

When somebody asked him about his round, Stanger said, "Usually, I say, 'I didn't whiff and nobody got hurt.' Well, this time I whiffed and almost got killed climbing a tree."

The story doesn't end there. The next day, the second day of qualifying, Stanger was passing by that same tree when the ball plopped softly by his feet. Stanger was certain he was having a mystical moment right of out Michael Murphy's book, *Golf in the Kingdom.*

"It had to be Seamus MacDuff," claimed Stanger, alluding to the legendary golf ghost of Murphy's classic. "I've got the ball on my mantle now."

Next to it he can place the plaque he will receive today commemorating his induction into the Hall of Fame.

"The city tournament is really exciting," Stanger said. "Everybody wants to play Augusta, but they aren't going to. So you make a tournament where everybody can compete. That's what the city is.

"I knew Phil Talbot. He used to start us off at the State Am -- he and Eddie Lawson and George Poolitsan. They were class people (and all City Hall of Famers). "Walter Sadler taught me the etiquette of golf. He made sure I knew about the game, how great a game it was. "I played a lot of golf with John Gillaspy. We were golf rats. We would play golf all morning at Pine Woods and, if it got too hot, jump in Rattlesnake Creek and look for balls. "I was obsessed with golf, even though it was hard. But you know what? If golf was easy, we would all be on TV." But not up a tree.

Hoep' Still Hip

When Indiana University introduced Terry Hoeppner as its new head coach in December, 2004, some of us needed no introduction. I knew the guy from my days in Kendallville, where he coached the East Noble High School football team. He was a likeable character then and thankfully hadn't changed a quarter of a century later. Sadly, he was taken by brain cancer in 2007, just two years into his career at IU.

Bloomington Herald-Times
December 20, 2004

As Terry Hoeppner addressed the media Friday in his first press conference as the new football coach at Indiana University, I could hardly wipe the smile off my face. In my mind, the university could not have made a better choice.

How did I know that?

Because I spotted the same gleam in Hoeppner's eye that I saw a quarter of a century ago.

Bear with me as I take you back to the fall of 1979. I was about to begin my fourth year of covering East Noble High School football for The *News-Sun*, a small daily in Kendallville, a town of about 15,000 located about 20 miles northeast of Fort Wayne.

At that time East Noble was known as a "basketball school," and rightly so. The football program averaged about two wins a year. The 1979 season promised the usual futility, so I wasn't exactly looking forward to it. That was before I got to know East Noble's new head football coach, 32-year-old Terry Hoeppner.

It didn't take long at all to get to know the man. Hoeppner was one you took an instant liking to, the kind of man most guys wish they could be — tall, handsome, rugged, a bit of a rogue — your basic chick magnet. Hoeppner looked strangers straight in the eye, gave them a firm handshake and usually followed it up by saying something funny or clever.

He could have passed for a college student. He wore his hair over his ears, roamed the sidelines in bell-bottom pants and sang verses from the latest pop music. He was forever crooning the "Pina Colada" song, the Rupert Holmes hit that topped the charts in 1979.

Come on, you know the song. It tells the story of the guy who is losing interest in his lady, so he places a personal ad seeking a woman of adventure, someone who likes pina coladas, walks in the rain, blah, blah, blah. A lady answers his ad and agrees to a rendezvous. Lo and behold she is the man's girlfriend, one and the same.

The point is, Hoeppner is that kind of wishful romantic. He confirmed it at Friday's press conference by offering a bouquet of roses to his blushing wife, Jane.

"Unexpected gifts, guys. It's all about unexpected gifts," Hoeppner said with a wink.

Of course, the East Noble players gravitated to their new coach. He made practices fun. He was one to put in a "Thursday Night Special," a trick play cooked up on the eve of the game. I recall a punt play he coined "Punt, John, Punt," named after John Isenbarger, the halfback-punter on the 1967 IU Rose Bowl team who had the bad habit of thinking "run" first and "punt" second.

His players called him Coach Hoep' for short. Even after defeat, the guy had a way of keeping the game fun for his players. As one player told him, "Coach, I've been playing sports since the sixth grade and this is the first time I ever looked forward to coming in on Saturday."

Not that Hoeppner took defeat lightly, but he had a great way of bouncing back and bringing his players along for the ride. After one of the six games his East Noble team lost by less than a touchdown in '79, Hoeppner said, "On Friday night I swear I'll never coach again, but on Saturday I'm rejuvenated and ready to start all over. Win or lose, every week is a new week. You can't rest on your laurels or dwell on your misfortunes."

Hoeppner will surely have to give himself the same pep talk at IU. That unsinkable attitude was on display Friday.

"I know we can win here — no doubt about it," he said.

In front of him as he spoke was a crystal bowl with a single rose in it. Athletic Director Rick Greenspan was about to remove the display when Hoeppner said, "Leave it up there. I love it. If you play in the Big Ten and don't aspire to going to the Rose Bowl, you are selling yourself short."

Hoeppner talked non-stop for a good 20 minutes without benefit of notes, which didn't surprise me. He was always a good story-teller. And he never ran out of stories, having spent time in the company of coaches such as Bear Bryant and Lou Holtz, having had NFL tryouts with the Packers and Cardinals, having played in the old World Football League. With a background like that, Hoeppner could keep you entertained for hours.

"If you had a party after the game, the first person you wanted to invite was Terry Hoeppner," said the long-time radio voice of East Noble sports, Fred Inniger. "Terry would tell a story as funny as heck, then I would go home and tell my wife the same story and she would go, 'oh.' You just couldn't tell a story like Terry Hoeppner could. The kids loved his stories. He was hip and in touch with the times."

Although Hoeppner is a self-described "player's coach," he knows how to keep his distance. As Inniger said, "Hoeppner has what I call 'channeled discipline.' There is a line the kids are not going to cross. Hoeppner has a way of getting kids to decide what he wants them to decide without being a George Patton."

Even though Hoeppner's East Noble team was headed for a losing season, it was competitive and enjoyable football. You could see the turnaround in progress. The bleachers were filling up on Friday nights. The players were proudly wearing their jerseys around Kendallville. The fans were talking about Hoeppner's latest trick play.

One East Noble player was so inspired by Hoeppner that he penned new verses to the old Chambers Brothers hit, "People Get Ready," and slipped the modified version under Hoeppner's door. One of the verses went, "People get ready, there's a team a coming ... Steady as steel, we're going to take that wheel."

You could see the wheels turning in Hoeppner's head Friday as he talked of ways to get fans excited about IU football again. He talked about bussing players to the game early and having them march through the tailgate areas, "encouraging" the hard core tail-gaters to get their fannies into the stadium. He talked about connecting with the fan base.

"We are going to have fun in the community," he promised. "We are going to cross the street. I love the idea of going out and selling the message of this university and Indiana football."

As Hoeppner continued to speak, you could feel the good vibrations filling the room.

"I think we just hit a home run," said Mark Deal, the former IU football assistant.

Seeing that familiar twinkle in Hoeppner's eyes, hearing the unabashed enthusiasm in his voice, I could see he had not changed a bit in 25 years.

People, get ready.

Getting to Know You, John Daly

Golfer John Daly certainly qualifies as a "character,' and he also has character, an Indiana family will tell you.

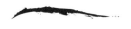

Bloomington Herald-Times
August 14, 2005

It is almost impossible to look at the photograph of Tom Weaver and his daughters and believe that any good could come out of his death.

There he is in that snapshot from 1991, with 8-year-old Karen safely tucked under one arm, grinning back at the camera, while under his other arm is 12-year-old Emily, her head fixed to his shoulder. It wasn't long after that picture was taken that the Weaver girls were fatherless.

On August 8, 1991, Tom was in the gallery at Crooked Stick Golf Club in Carmel during the PGA Championship. Sometime that afternoon, an electrical storm sprung up. Warning horns blared. Fans scurried for cover.

Weaver had hustled back to the parking lot and was only a few feet away from the safety of his car when a lighting bolt struck him square in the chest. Just like that, a 39- year-old man was gone.

What kind of god takes a man in the prime of life, leaving two daughters without their father and a wife without her husband? What possible good can come out of such an inexplicable event?

Those answers were 14 years in coming. It wasn't until this past May, when Karen Weaver received her diploma from Indiana University, that this chapter came to a close.

A Golfer's Success

The 1991 PGA Championship saw a 25-year-old nobody, John Daly, come out of nowhere to claim the season's last major tournament.

In his first season on the PGA Tour, Daly had barely made the radar. He was the ninth alternate for the '91 PGA, and got into the field only when Nick Price withdrew because his wife went into labor. Even then it took three others ahead of Daly to decline the last-minute invitation.

But Crooked Stick, a course noted for its long fairways, was perfectly suited for Daly, a long-knocker from back in his days at the University of Arkansas. From the moment Daly boomed a drive off the first tee, he had the fans in his pocket. He fired a 69 that first day, putting him within two strokes off the lead. Most unheralded golfers would have been positively giddy after that, but Daly's mood was curtailed by the news that a spectator had been killed.

Daly followed with rounds of 67, 69 and 71 to win the tournament by three strokes. The $230,000 payoff, his first big paycheck, could not have come at a better time. He still owed $175,000 on his house and about $25,000 on his car.

Daly figured he could pay off those debts and have enough money left for something special. He knew just the place for it.

A Child's Uneasy Feeling

Even an 8-year-old knows when something isn't right.

Upon returning from a friend's house on that August day, Karen Weaver wondered why there were so many cars in front of her home, a home that was unusually crowded for a Thursday afternoon. As soon as she looked into the eyes of her mother, Dee, Karen felt fear.

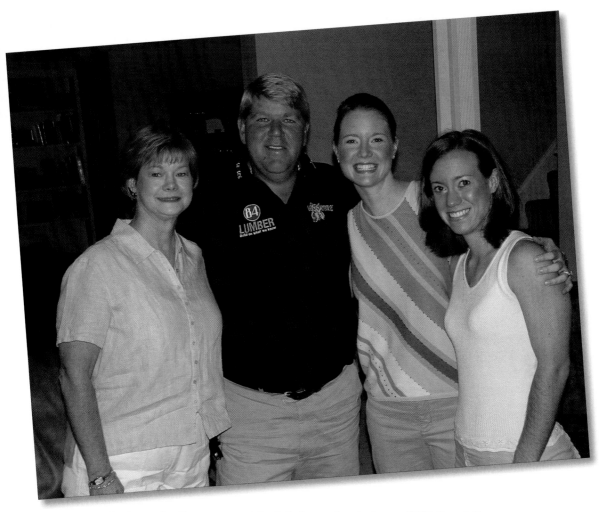

The Weaver family got to meet John Daly face-to-face in August, 2005. From left are Dee Fisher (mother), Daly, and sisters Emily Weaver and Karen Weaver. (Courtesy photo)

"As I walked into the house, something came over me," Karen recalled. "I felt something wasn't right, that something bad was going to happen. Then I saw Mom's face. The look reaffirmed my feelings. "I don't really remember much after that," Karen continued. "My sister, Emily, was away at camp. Mom said I didn't start crying until Emily came home. I'm not really sure why. I was probably waiting to make sure Emily was okay. Once she was there, then it was okay for me to cry."

To this day, Emily has not picked up a golf club. At the time of Tom's death, she had just started playing golf -- with his full blessing.

"It was our father-daughter time," Emily said by phone from her home in Oswego, Ill. "I would get tired after the fourth hole and then he would play both our balls while I drove the cart. My husband (Curtis Edmondson) plays now, but it's hard for me to let him go, especially when the weather is bad."

About a week after Tom's death, the family received notification that a trust had been established for the children, earmarked for their education. The amount: $30,000. The donor: John Daly.

The Other Side

Anyone who has followed the career of Daly will know about his battles with alcohol, gambling and women. One of his wives had a brush with the law. Daly himself has incurred the wrath of the PGA Tour for some unsportsmanlike behavior on the course. His nickname is Wild Thing.

But Daly also has a gentle side. He is active in more than a dozen charities, one of which he kept to himself, the donation he made to the Weavers in 1991. That gift came with one catch, that it be used for the education of the Weaver children. Daly didn't even know their names. He just wanted to make sure their future wasn't compromised by tragedy.

As Daly said in this month's issue of Golf Digest, "I just felt it was the thing to do, and it felt good. I won a major, but we lost a human being while I was doing it. I almost felt a part of his death."

Full Circle

Fourteen years later, it was Daly receiving a phone call from out of the blue. That $30,000 helped Emily, now 25, become a respiratory therapist. It also helped put Karen, 22, through Indiana University. The chapter was closed on May 7, when Karen received her degree.

The whole family was there at commencement. Karen felt Tom was there in spirit but wished had been there in person.

"When everything was over and I was back at my apartment, I was sad," Karen said. "This was something Dad wasn't able to experience."

Emily and Dee also have their moments of sadness.

"Yesterday (Monday) was the anniversary of Dad's death," Emily said. "It has gotten a little easier, but in the beginning it was a very hard day."

"I still think about Tom on a regular basis," said Dee, who remarried in 2000. "Little things the girls do remind me of him. They are strong, independent women now, and I have moved on, too. I married a wonderful man."

It was Dee's second husband, Steve Fisher of Noblesville, who tracked down Daly, a surprised Daly at that.

"I never followed up on it because I felt if I did get in touch with them, it might bring up memories of that day when their dad got killed," Daly told Golf Digest. "So now, 14 years later, I got a message that one of the girls is graduating and that they want to get a hold of me."

'Could I get to know you?'

Monday, the three of them -- Karen, Emily and Dee -- will have a chance to thank Daly in person. He is participating in Fuzzy Zoeller's Wolf Challenge at Covered Bridge Golf Club in Sellersburg and they have been invited. The girls already have given thought to what they will say to Daly.

Said Emily: "I will say, 'Thank you for your selfless gift. It was at a time when I was not aware of the impact. But now that I'm done with school and am married, I have a much greater appreciation of the sacrifice you made.' "

As for Karen, who hopes to go on to medical school, she will tell Daly, "Thank you for your generosity and, if it's all right with you, could I get to know you?"

Editor's Note: Karen, Emily and Dee did have their day with Daly, and it was an emotional moment for all of them. Karen went on to become a doctor and is now practicing family medicine. Emily did get qualified as respiratory therapist but is presently a stay-at-home mother of three. Dee is still happily married to Steve Fisher and continues to work for a school corporation in the Indianapolis area.

You Can't Keep a Good Girl Down: The Fall and Rise of Jenny Hollars

Just a remarkable story of perseverance.

Bloomington Herald-Times
August 13, 2008

Despite the demands of being a wife, mother, athletic director and cross country coach, Jennifer Hollars still makes time to run five days a week. She can't help herself. It's in her blood. From the time she was a little girl, she preferred running shoes over roller skates.

But while running one day last June, Hollars felt a "stabbing" pain.

"It was on my right side, so I knew it wasn't a heart attack," she said. "But I felt this rattle in my lung, like there was a bubble there."

When the symptoms returned in future runs, it was time to seek a medical answer. After a series of tests, her condition was diagnosed as "Spontaneous Pneumothorax," a small rupture of the lung. It wasn't life-threatening, but it was serious enough to require some delicate surgery, a procedure that took place last week. The recovery kept Hollars in the hospital for three nights and forced her to miss cross country camp for the first time in her 11 seasons as the Bloomington North girls' coach. She rejoined the team this week.

For Hollars, it is just another reminder that, while her body generally is an efficient machine, like all machines it does break down on occasion. Still vivid in her memory are two most untimely breakdowns, the cross country state finals of 1988 and '89.

So Close, Yet So Far

In 1988 she was known as Jennifer Warthan, the up-and-coming sophomore daughter of Charlie Warthan, coach of the North boys' cross country team. Jennifer already had established herself as a state-caliber runner and was running a strong fourth at the state meet when, with the finish line in sight, she collapsed. Although she was able to get back on her feet, it forced her to settle for sixth.

Running out of gas is not uncommon in big meets, when runners are pushed beyond their normal limits. So Warthan wasn't too worried about it when she returned to the state meet in '89, a favorite for the title along with rival Jill Schuler of Floyd Central.

For most of the race, Warthan and Schuler set a pace far ahead of the pack, waging a fierce battle for first. With about a half-mile to go, Warthan suddenly broke away. Entering the home stretch, she had put almost 150 yards between herself and Schuler.

"I was feeling great," Hollars recalled. "I remember pulling away and just being out there in nature, exerting myself, pushing myself and feeling wonderful."

Engine Failure

However, just 50 yards from the finish, her body began to shut down. First, she started to veer off course. Then she started to stagger. Watching closely from the sidelines, her father sensed the warning signals.

"About 80 yards out I noticed she was starting to lose speed and looking incoherent," Charlie said. "I was yelling at her, but she wasn't picking up my signals."

Said Hollars, "I remember hearing my dad's voice loud and clear and almost in slow motion, 'Where are you going? You're going the wrong way.' Then I remember thinking, 'Oh God, please don't let this be happening again. I'm so close.' Then I remember my legs going numb."

Hollars went down in a heap. As her supporters looked on in disbelief, Hollars tried to get up but fell. She made another attempt and fell again. By this time Schuler had caught up to her. In desperation Hollars tried to crawl. One by one, more runners went by her. It was agonizing to watch.

"I was thinking, 'Crawl, just crawl,'" Hollars said. "I was too dizzy to count the runners going by me, but it was heartbreaking each time."

Even for the few moments she was able to get to her feet, she was wobbly and disoriented. After falling for the last time, she wound up crawling the last 10 yards, coming in a devastating 14th. Her coach at the time, Ralph Sieboldt, was stunned to learn of the sudden turn of events.

"I was standing out on the course a quarter-mile from the finish, and Jenny goes by at least 100 yards ahead," he recalls. "I was elated. Then I get to the finish line, see all these people around her and come to find out she went down."

Nineteen years later, it is still a blur to Hollars.

"I kind of remember hearing someone near the chute say, 'Don't touch her. She can't finish.' Then I remember being across the finish line and people helping me up. I was really out of it then. I can't remember crawling. It was very surreal, like a bad dream. It felt like an eternity. I fall, and the next thing I remember is getting to the line. I don't remember getting up and falling again."

When asked to revisit his daughter's painful collapse again last week, Charlie asked for a moment to compose himself.

"It was pretty horrible," he said in a voice choked with emotion. "It was horrifying to know she had the talent and the heart to do it. On the other hand, I was able to take strength in the fact that she was able to push herself to a limit most athletes cannot commit themselves to. Most will never find out how good they are. She was able to find that out."

The Long Road Back

That particular night was a long one at the Warthan household.

"My legs were heavy and sore," Jennifer said. "I could hardly move. And then I was totally depressed. I had built up to that moment, had that dream, and was so excited to cross that line in front of everyone else, knowing what I had achieved. I had that vision since I was a small child. I had always insisted I go with my dad to all the meets, even the away ones. The realization that I had only one more shot at it was really scary."

The depression did not go away any time soon.

"I moped around the house, was quiet at school," said Hollars, a model student throughout her high school career. Wondering if there was something physically wrong with her, the family sought the advice of a physician. They found out it was equal parts mental and physical.

"The theory was that I just ran to a level where my body shut down, Jenny said. "I was stressing out at the beginning of races, running too hard. It was more about picking my pace."

Girl on a Mission

Like young athletes are wont to do, Hollars eventually got over it and came back her senior more determined than ever.

"She handled it a lot better than some of the people around her," Sieboldt said. "Spiritually, she is really a strong, young lady."

When Hollars returned to state for the last go at it, she had a better game plan. She decided to hang back the first half-mile, conserve her energy, then gradually turn it on. She also vowed to stay relaxed.

Her plan worked like a precision instrument.

"At the half-mile mark I was 15th or 20th," she said. "But once we made the turn, I started picking girls off. I had this pre-visualized point where I would kick it and go, where I would break my competition. That's exactly what happened."

As Hollars broke to another big lead entering the last 100 yards, the only question was whether her body would hold up. As Rex Kirts wrote for the *Herald-Times*, "With Warthan bearing down on the finish line far in front, breaths were being held, silent prayers being said."

This time, thankfully, there was plenty left in the tank.

"I just tried to remain strong and wasn't uptight," Hollars said. "I knew once I got through that first half-mile, I wasn't going to let it happen again. I knew I had not exerted everything, that if I needed another gear, I had it. I wasn't going for time. I was just going for a state championship."

Light at the End of the Tunnel

And this time she was not to be denied. Hollars crossed the finish line standing up and well ahead of her old nemisis, Schuler. Within seconds she was engulfed by family and friends and even strangers, many of whom had witnessed her agonizing finish the year before.

"It felt so good to cross that line, Hollars said. "It was such an exciting, thrilling moment for me. I remember seeing the line on the ground, stepping over it and feeling this complete sense of peace. It was, 'Wow, it's finally real, this goal I have been dreaming about.' "

Not only did she walk away with the gold medal that day, she also received the Charles Maas Award for mental attitude.

The ordeal of her junior year, followed by a triumphant redemption, is something Hollars still draws strength from today in her duties as a devoted mother of two, a coach of many and the girls' athletic director at a school with a proud athletic tradition thanks to inspiring stories like hers. Sieboldt, now retired, still marvels at her three-year high school quest.

"I always tell people, in my 30 years of coaching, it was the highlight and low light of my career," he said. "I was lucky enough to coach several state champions, but her winning that title her senior year was just a great accomplishment."

Hollars looks back on it now and believes she is the better for it, that she set an example for anyone who thinks they cannot take another step.

"I want to be remembered for putting it all out there in whatever I do," said. "Now it is being channeled into being a mom and a wife, into being a good A.D. and being a good role model for all my girls and all my sports teams."

Then, with her eyes tearing up and her voice wavering the way her legs did on that haunting day in 1989, Hollars concluded, "It's about the journey — all the work and effort. Going through that makes you think about the bigger picture. If I hadn't gone through that, I don't know if I would be the same. Sometimes you need experiences like that to make you grow.

"Looking back, the state championship means a lot, but the race that means the most to me was my junior year, when I fell down, because that was some effort. I'm really proud I was able to do that, even though it didn't turn out the way I wanted at the time. I didn't get the glory or the medal, but I know how hard I tried."

Editor's Note: Hollars and her North girls' team advanced to the 2008 state finals, finishing 21st. She would take a total of seven teams to state before retiring from coaching in 2012. She now is a full-time mother and teacher and goes by the last name "Hester."

Lebron Would Be Wise to Follow Damon's Lead

Talk about pressure! Damon Bailey dealt with it from his junior high days, when Bob Knight started bragging about him. It never really let up until Bailey hung up his jersey after a brief pro career. In this piece Bailey talked about handling all those expectations.

Bloomington Herald-Times
February 23, 2003

Even though high school basketball phenomenon Lebron James is about to make his millions in the NBA, you want to feel sorry for him.

And how do you feel sorry for a future millionaire who already has been showered with gifts, including a Hummer vehicle valued at $50,000?

Would it help to know that James, from this point on, may never have a life he can call his own? How about the enormous burden of living up to the expectations of a "can't miss" prospect? How about the possibility of being subjected to never-ending scrutiny?

James, a senior at St. Vincent's-St. Mary's high in Akron, Ohio, has had a taste of all this ever since his picture appeared on a 2002 cover of *Sports Illustrated*, hailing him as the best high school player in the country and destined to go straight to the NBA out of high school.

Ever since then James has been in the national spotlight. Television could not wait to make money on him. Several of his high school games have been aired on pay-per-view. If James can maintain some semblance of normalcy through all that, he is gifted in ways beyond the basketball court. If the day comes when he feels overwhelmed by it all, it would behoove him to consult a young man who walked in his shoes 15 years ago, Damon Bailey.

If anybody understands what James is going through, it is Bailey, an Indiana legend in his own time — and well before a youngster's time.

With Bailey it started in 1985 when Indiana coach Bob Knight attended his Shawswick Junior High games. Then Knight was quoted in John Feinstein's *Season on the Brink* saying Bailey was better than any guard on the IU team.

Before Bailey ever played a minute of high school basketball at Bedford North Lawrence,

Sports Illustrated named him the country's top ninth grader — ninth grade, for the love of sanity.

From that moment on, Bailey would play in front of packed houses, home and away. The most fans to ever watch a high school game in Indiana turned out for Bailey's last — the 1990 state championship game. Even with the game aired on state and national television, a crowd in excess of 40,000 filled the RCA Dome in Indianapolis and watched as Bailey rallied BNL to a 63-60 victory over Concord.

Over his four-year high school career, an estimated 800,000 fans watched him play in person. Bailey was exposed to the spotlight early and often. Post-game questions from reporters were routine his freshman year of high school. By his senior year the madness had evolved into full-scale press conferences. And although he was at ease in front of cameras and microphones, he did not always welcome them. There were times he just wanted to be a kid.

While attending a recent IU practice, Bailey talked at length about those days under the microscope. Asked if he enjoyed all the attention, he said, "I had fun because I didn't know any better. The limelight in my case was something I grew up with. Having Coach Knight coming to watch and being in the book was really just a part of my life, so I didn't know any different."

There was a downside, Bailey added: "It forces you to grow up defensive. You definitely miss out on some things that other high school kids can enjoy. There is good and bad to everything, and that is part of it. If you are going to reap the benefits of being a Lebron James, there are going to be some negatives to go along with it."

Earlier this month, James lost his high school eligibility for accepting some throwback jerseys worth $800. He took it to court and was reinstated. Bailey understands that fans can be all too generous and that it takes a strong will to resist the hand-outs.

"I understand there are rules, but there is a fine line with some of that," he said.

Bailey had the benefit of strong guidance from his parents, Wendell and Beverly, and many other members of the community also looking out for his well-being. One of them was his high school coach, Dan Bush.

"Everything that could have been thrown at Damon was thrown at him at that time," Bush said. "We tried to keep as much of it away as we could. We tried to be fair with everybody, but we wanted to be most fair to Damon. We wanted him to be a kid.

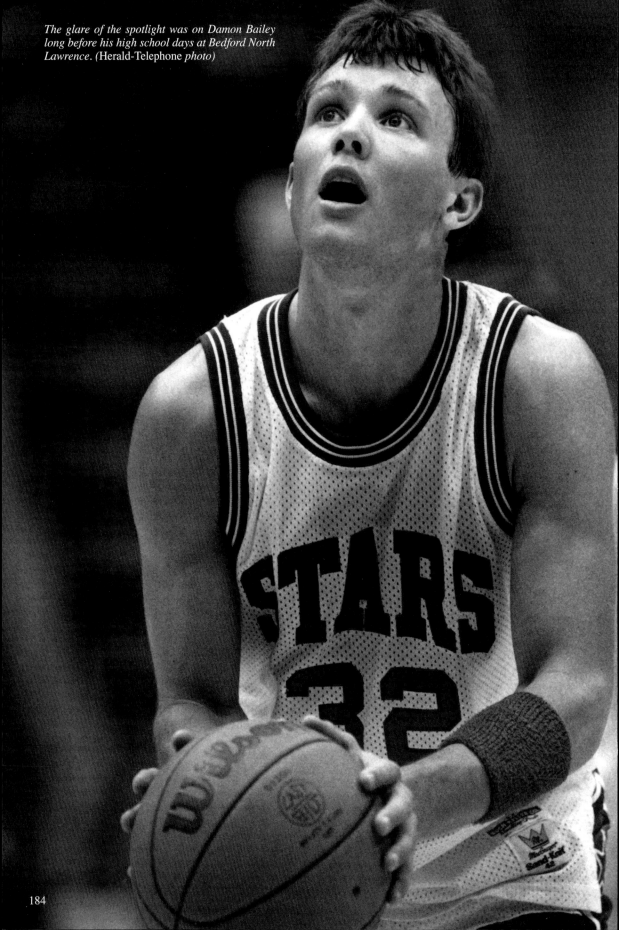

*The glare of the spotlight was on Damon Bailey long before his high school days at Bedford North Lawrence. (*Herald-Telephone *photo)*

"Damon was mature beyond his age," Bush went on. "You have to give his mom and dad a lot of credit. They never let him get too full of himself. Most kids with that kind of success would have been hard to live around. Most kids can't handle it. Not many adults can handle it.

"I remember telling Damon, 'If you don't want to do this stuff, just tell me.' Damon was never a kid who needed a lot of attention. He didn't crave it. He just wanted to play and go home."

Bailey certainly didn't help the cause of privacy by choosing a college close to home and playing for a coach as high-profile and demanding as Knight. Would the spotlight have been less intense had he gone elsewhere than IU?

"Looking back, maybe," he said. "It is something every player is going to question. I made a decision, a commitment, to go here and I tried to make the most of it."

Rumor had it that Bailey had his bags packed on more than one occasion at Indiana. Was there any truth to that?

"I can't say they were ever packed. I may have had the suitcases out a time or two, but nothing was in them," he replied. "To play under Coach Knight magnifies that quite a bit. There are times you wake up in the night wondering, 'What am I doing here? Why am I not someplace else?' But I was happy with the way things turned out."

Bailey doesn't waste his time dwelling on past expectations.

"I think expectations are something you have to set for yourself. Outsiders setting expectations for you I never worried about. What I wanted to accomplish, I knew. I never put a lot of stock in it. I never worried about what people thought."

That doesn't mean Bailey at age 31 wouldn't take a mulligan or two if he had the chance.

"I would love to have the talent and the ability I had then, knowing what I know now," he said. "Just the youth and maturity of getting into the real world gives you a greater appreciation of what goes on."

The fish bowl didn't end with college for Bailey, who was drafted by the Indiana Pacers, spent a year on the injured reserve, then finished up his professional career in the CBA with the Fort Wayne Fury. After almost two decades in the public eye, Bailey is now content to be a husband, father and bread-winner. He co-owns a warehouse in Bedford and lives just outside of town with his wife, Stacy, and three children. To him, this is the good life. There are still times when he is interrupted for an autograph, but he is gracious about it.

"There were times you wish you could do this or that, go out and eat without being bothered, but overall I wouldn't trade anything."

Outside of the summer camps he runs, basketball is no longer in the picture for Bailey.

"I enjoy my business, but when it's 5 o'clock and time to go home, I have three kids I would rather spend time with."

Editor's Note: In 2005, Bailey took over as head coach of the Bedford North Lawrence boys basketball team. After two uneventful seasons, he stepped down. In 2012-13, he became an assistant coach for the BNL girls' team. With his daughter Alexa playing a key role, the BNL girls won the Class 4A state champion. As the head coach the following season, 2013-14, Damon guided the Lady Stars to a second straight 4A championship, giving him the distinction of playing on an Indiana state champion and coaching an Indiana state champion.

Bobby Wampler: Living Life to Its Fullest

And now I give you Bobby Wampler, a character worthy of place in the book title along with Bob Knight. Remember an autistic youth by the name of Jason McElwain? He made national headlines in 2006 when he entered a high school basketball game and hit a string of 3-pointers. Well, a year before that feel-good story, there was another that took place in Ellettsville, Indiana, where Bobby Wampler served as team manager for the Edgewood Mustangs. His story is a two-parter. Part I was a feature on the young man who became an unofficial member of the boys' basketball team, overcoming his many handicaps. In Part II, written six weeks later, Bobby Wampler entered a junior varsity game and cemented his place in local lore.

Bloomington Herald-Times
January 20, 2005

Out of a lifetime of setbacks lives the smile, the ever-present smile of 18-year-old Bobby Wampler.

Wampler's official title is "team manager" for the Edgewood boys' basketball team, but, unofficially, he qualifies as "team character."

And what a character he is -- all five feet and 80 pounds of him. From the moment he walks into Jeff Carmichael's classroom door in the morning to the time he puts the last basketball away for Coach Jay Brown at night, Wampler can hardly stop smiling -- or chattering.

Need some ideas for your basketball team, Coach Brown? Bobby will gladly draw up a play for you.

Need some help with your JV team, Coach Kyle Swafford? Bobby is right beside you.

Need a date for the prom, senior Amber Pedersen? Bobby is there for you.

There is irony in all this. For a young man who seems to be there for everybody else, there was a long, long time when it seemed he wasn't going to be there at all.

In 1986, two months into his life, an infection nearly ended it. A severe reaction to some medication resulted in the shutdown of his vital organs -- heart, liver, lungs, kidneys. As Bobby was being rushed to Riley Children's Hospital in Indianapolis, his parents were informed his that chances of survival were slim.

"On the way up we were told to think about some funeral arrangements," said Bobby's mother, Debbie Mulvihill.

For the next nine months, Bobby was on life-support.

"It was day-to-day for a long time," said his father, Bob Wampler, a custodian at Edgewood.

For almost 36 months, little Bobby was in need of feeding and breathing tubes. It wasn't until the age of three that he uttered his first word and took his first step. He was in and out of hospitals his entire childhood until. At age 14, he had to have a kidney transplant.

And that wasn't the end of it. Just last month he was hospitalized with bleeding ulcers.

The kid is a walking medicine cabinet, requiring a dozen medications daily and vaccinations weekly. You might expect an adolescent facing such a daily ordeal to be withdrawn or bitter, but Wampler is unsinkable -- at least his spirit is. The cheerful way he goes about his business in the classroom and at practice, you would think he was the luckiest person in Ellettsville.

"For our basketball team, Bobby is somebody who brightens our day," Coach Brown said. "He is such a positive person in our gym. I tell our boys all the time, 'If you think you are having a bad day, then you need reconsider and think about what Bobby has to go through just to be here.' Sometimes we mope around after missing a shot or making a bad play when we should be thankful we have the opportunity to just play this game. That's the biggest thing Bobby has taught me. It is a life lesson to see somebody battle through the things he has and come through with a positive attitude."

Carmichael, the Special Education teacher and former volleyball coach, looks forward to seeing Wampler come through his door on the days when the lad's health permits

"I've had some mornings of gloom and despair after a volleyball match and Bobby would come through the door all smiles and high-fives after having blood drawn," Carmichael said. "The thing about him is his will. He just won't stay down. He's kind of like Forrest Gump. He is the poster child for doing the best you can with what you have. I've probably gotten more out of him than he's gotten out of me."

"Mr. Carmichael is like a second father to me," said Wampler, who is on pace to graduate this spring.

"I do expect to graduate from Edgewood High School one day," he added. "That means a lot to me. My sister (Jenny Chandler) graduated from Edgewood and my father works for Edgewood. This my last year and I really want to make it good."

Thanks to his upbeat personality and optimistic outlook, Wampler is a popular presence at Edgewood. Last spring he had the good fortune to escort not one, but three young ladies to the junior-senior prom. Assistant softball coach Jeff Farmer fixed him up with softball players Mandy Kot, Sammy Kot and Pedersen. Wampler still carries a prom picture in his wallet.

"Bobby was king for a night," Farmer said.

"Bobby got off-subject a little bit, but that's how he is," Pedersen said. "He kept talking about all his other girls instead of us."

Probably the closest person outside of family to Wampler is Swafford, the 26-year-old junior varsity coach. Swafford was coaching the Edgewood eighth grade team in 2000 when Wampler entered his life.

"We list him in the program as a manager, but I've always called him my assistant," Swafford said.

Wampler continues to take a seat next to Swafford and looks for any opportunity to help.

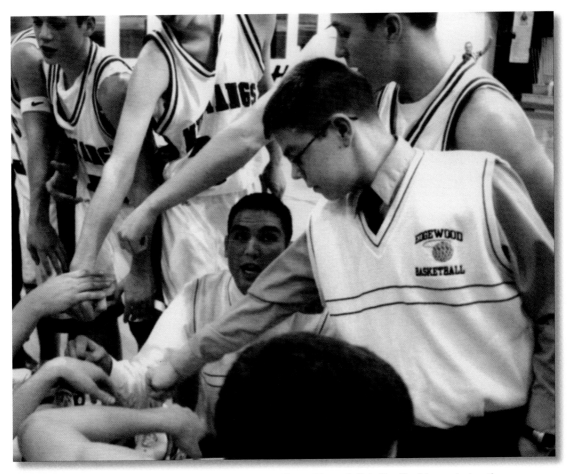

Bobby Wampler listens in on an Edgewood huddle as JV coach Kyle Swafford issues instructions.
(Herald-Times photo by Monty Howell)

"I remember one game where I picked up a technical foul," Swafford said. "One more and I would have been ejected. After the game Bobby came up to me and said, as serious as he's ever been, 'Coach, you could have picked up the second technical because I would have brought the team home for you.'"

It was Swafford's first year of coaching that Wampler needed the kidney transplant. On his first visit to Riley Children's Hospital, Swafford wasn't quite sure what to expect as he entered Wampler's room.

"As soon as I turned the corner, Bobby's response was, 'I'll be ready to go next year, Coach.' That's the kind of kid he is. What he goes through in one day I might not have to go through in my whole life. The small things most people look past are things Bobby cherish the most, just being able to go to practice, play a little one-on-one."

Wampler's transplant was a celebrated success. The donor was none other than his cousin, Gwen Green.

"It was an easy decision to make," Green said. "When it's family, how do you tell a child 'no?' He is so inspiring."

Wampler's willpower has helped Green persevere in her darkest hours. In her words, she is a "recovering drug addict."

"Even though Bobby doesn't know it, he has helped me in a lot of ways," she said. "I have a 10-inch scar on my abdomen that reminds me, 'If Bobby can keep going, I can, too.' He is such a little fighter. He doesn't just fight for his life. He fights to have a life."

The community took notice. Members of the Indianapolis Colts visited him in the hospital. Indiana University invited Wampler to a private gathering of IU basketball greats when it named its All-Century Team. There he got to meet the likes of

Calbert Cheaney, Jimmy Rayl, George McGinnis, Bobby Leonard, Damon Bailey, Archie Dees, Kent Benson and others.

"Kent Benson offered to let me try on his championship ring, but it was too big," said Wampler, who keeps a lot of his sports memorabilia at the house of his grandmother, Dorothy Wampler. Look around and you will see a pair of sneakers that once belonged to former IU star Brian Evans. You will see framed letters from coaches Bob Knight and Mike Davis and scrapbooks full of pictures of Wampler with celebrities.

Having made the best of his situation, Wampler is quick to offer words of encouragement to those who also face hurdles that appear insurmountable.

"I would tell kids, 'It will be OK. You will get through it, but you have to have a positive attitude on life.' " he said. "If you don't have a positive attitude, life is not going to bring you anything.' Some kids tell me to shut up and leave them alone, but I just say, 'One day life is going to hit you in the butt and you are going to wish you had listened to Bobby.' "

"Bobby is what he is," his mother said. "I just wish everybody was blessed to have a Bobby Wampler in their life."

'Little Bobby' Lives His Dream

Disney couldn't have scripted this epilogue any better.

Bloomington Herald-Times
March 3, 2005

A hush sweeps over the crowd as the undersized player toes the free throw line in the waning seconds of a junior varsity basketball game. Even though the game is no longer in doubt, it seems like the air has been sucked out of the gym.

Eying the two most important free throws of his life -- the only free throws of his life - is little Bobby Wampler.

Wampler, a 5-foot, 80-pound senior, isn't even an official member of the team, yet there he is, center stage in one of the most memorable moments in the 40-year history of Edgewood High School basketball.

Who is this Bobby Wampler, and what is he doing on that free throw line?

Wampler is an 18-year-old student manager for the Edgewood basketball team who has had to overcome a lifetime of health issues.

The first years of his life, he was hooked up to tubes. He was 3 years old before he could walk or talk. He might not have lived past the age of 14 had not his cousin, Gwen Green, donated a kidney to him.

So thanks to medical science and a family that extends all the way to coaches and teachers, Bobby is a happy, functioning teenager. He was never happier than he was this past Friday night, the night he actually suited up for the Edgewood Mustangs.

In the week leading up to Edgewood's Senior Night game against South Putnam, the coaches promised Bobby he could warm up with the team. They even practiced warm-up drills so he could get the feel of the routine.

"We had concerns Bobby might try to do too much," said junior varsity coach Kyle Swafford, who has been close to Wampler ever since the lad volunteered as a student manager for the Edgewood eighth grade team five years ago.

Knowing he was going to actually be on the court with the team, Bobby was counting the minutes.

"I remember waking up at 2 o'clock in the morning and not being able to get back to sleep," he said. "I kept thinking, 'Wow! I get to be one of the big boys.' "

Had they put Bobby on the official roster that night, they would have listed him at 5-0, 100 pounds, which would have been a stretch. For the occasion, Bobby wore No. 13, the same number worn by Ollie McPike, the player-manager for the fictional Hickory Huskers of *Hoosiers* movie fame.

"He looked like Ollie out there, about half the size of everybody else," noted Wampler's Special Education teacher, Jeff Carmichael. "I told Bobby before the game not to clink the bottom of the rim like Ollie did."

From the moment Bobby first warmed up with the junior varsity team, he belonged.

"He was a natural out there," Swafford said.

After completing his lay-ups, Bobby stepped behind the 3-point line. When, after three or four tries, one of those 20-footers plunged through the basket, the student section applauded. And then he made another, and another and another. The clamor grew with each make -- and this was just the junior varsity warm-ups.

"Bobby was just working the crowd," said Swafford, who had a surprise cooked up.

Before the game, Swafford approached South Putnam JV coach Matt "Oggie" Brewer with a plan: If the score gets lopsided, Bobby is going in. Brewer was more than happy to oblige. Sure enough, Swafford's 14-5 JV team broke out to a 20-point lead late in the fourth quarter. With 40 seconds to play, Swafford looked down the bench at Wampler and said, "Bobby, get in there."

The words had barely left Swafford's lips when Bobby was tearing off his warm-up suit and sprinting to the scorer's table. A roar rose from the crowd, which was much larger by then as the varsity tip-off was only a few minutes away.

Swafford instructed his players to get the ball to Bobby, then cast a look toward the South Putnam bench. Brewer responded with a nod. When play resumed, Wampler caught a pass near the Edgewood bench. As two South Putnam defenders converged on him, his eyes were bulging out from behind his wire rim glasses.

It wasn't much of a foul. It was more of an intentional, friendly tap. Everybody in the gymnasium knew what it meant.

> Bobby Wampler, student manager, a real-life Ollie McPike, is going to the free throw line.
>
> Wampler looks like he has been there before. He does not shoot underhanded as Ollie did, but his first shot is much truer than McPike's first free throw in *Hoosiers*.
>
> Nothing but net.
>
> Pandemonium.
>
> Fans are hugging, high-fiving, laughing, crying.
>
> And amid all the bedlam, Bobby drains the second free throw to show them the first was no fluke.

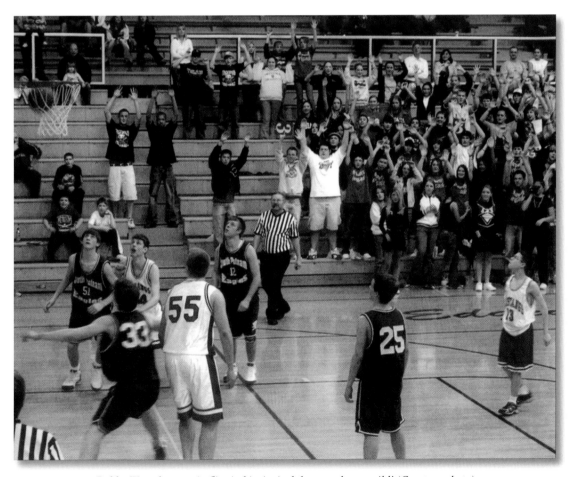

Bobby Wampler eyes it, flies it, hits it. And the crowd goes wild! (Courtesy photo)

"It was so loud I couldn't hear myself think," Carmichael said. "How many people in that gym could have stepped up to the line in that situation and hit two free throws?"

"I knew I could make 'em," Bobby unabashedly said later.

Emotions flowed freely.

"I couldn't keep it in," Carmichael said. "That's the most I've cried in a long time. I didn't think I had that kind of emotion. This just shows that you can't judge a book by its cover."

You have to know Jeff Carmichael to appreciate the sentiment. As a former college athlete and high school volleyball coach, Carmichael is as intense as they come.

"Give me 10 minutes on the volleyball court, and I can be a jerk again," he says with a bit of pride.

But kids like Wampler have a way of softening up even the grumpiest of old men. After making the free throws, Wampler went for greater glory. In the remaining 30 seconds, he hoisted two uncontested 3-pointers. It was probably a good thing neither found its mark. School officials might have had to cancel the varsity game for being anticlimactic.

"That would have been big -- even in (IU's) Assembly Hall," Wampler said.

"The roof would have come off," said Swafford, a former Edgewood player who remembers watching Damon Bailey play in the Mustang Corral when Bedford North Lawrence visited in the late 1980s. Bobby Wampler's moment in the spotlight was more meaningful, he said.

"It was cool seeing Damon Bailey play here, but what Bobby did the other night might have been the most special thing that ever happened in this gym."

Wampler still went through his paces with the varsity, basking in the chant, "Bobby, Bobby, Bobby." When introduced during Senior Night festivities, he received a standing ovation.

"You and I will have other things to remember, but this will be Bobby's marquee moment," Carmichael said. "If Dicky V (Vitale) had been there, he would have been screaming."

"One day I will hopefully marry a cheerleader and have kids," Wampler said. "And when they ask me, 'Dad, did you really do that?' I'm just going to smile and say, 'yep.' "

Editor's Note: Bobby Wampler continues to defy the odds and still sits on the bench at Edgewood basketball games.

Chapter 13
Good-Bye, So Long, Farewell

Over the course of a 36 year-career, a lot of people, places and entities dear to you pass out of your life. One of the most difficult challenges for any writer is to pen a proper good-bye. Here are some fare-wells from the heart.

White Sox Have Heavenly Connection

Anyone who called Kendallville home in the 1970s knew Dick Stonebraker, owner of a gas station on the north side of town. If you were in a hurry, you didn't stop for gas at Stonebraker's. Ol' Dick was quite the talker, especially about his Chicago White Sox. When Dick passed away in 1983, Kendallville lost one of its more cherished citizens.

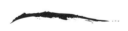

Kendallville News-Sun
October 1983

The other night I had a weird dream. I dreamed I was late for an appointment and nearly ran out of gas. I remember pulling into a Mobil station off a busy highway and waiting almost a full minute before a pot-bellied man in his mid-50s came lumbering out.

"Fill 'er up?' he asked in a cheerful tone.

"Just give me $5 bucks worth and make it quick," I ordered.

"Want your windshield cleaned?"

"That won't be necessary," I replied.

"How's your oil?"

"It's OK."

The man raised the hood anyway and pulled the oil stick. He was a rather curious looking fellow with a rosey face, pudgy nose and white, bushy hair on the sides. He had little, if any, hair on top, which made him look like an aging Ronald McDonald.

"You are about a quart low," he informed me.

As we waited for the pump to register $5, the man hit me with, "How about them Sox!"

"Yeah, how about them," I said, faking my enthusiasm. "Don't forget – just $5 bucks."

"Do you follow baseball at all?"

"Yeah, I'm a Braves fan."

"Too bad about those guys. I follow the Braves on cable TV and I wanted them to beat those Dodgers the other night. The Braves sure had their share of bad fortune this year."

"Can you speed it up a little," I snapped, trying to change a sore subject. By this time, the gas pump already had passed the $5 mark.

"Yep, I've been a Sox fan for almost 40 years. I can remember betting a dollar a game on them against some friends who followed the White Sox and Indians. I used to call this Indians fan, Cleon, in the middle of the night and let him know he owed me a buck," laughed the man warmly.

"You can cut 'er off any time now," I said impatiently as the meter showed $6. Too late, he was already cleaning my windshield.

"You know, I think the Sox are going to win it all, the way Hoyt and Dotson have been pitching. And Bannister is going to come around."

"How much do I owe you?" I interrupted, trying to cut him off.

"And did you see the home run Luzinski hit on the roof at Comiskey?"

I ignored the question, tapping my steering wheel nervously. The pump already was approaching $8 and I had only a 10-spot in my wallet.

"And how about that Kittle kid. Ain't he something! He was working in a steel mill in Gary until the Sox discovered him. And Carlton Fisk should get the MVP award, I think."

I kept checking my watch to give him the message, but he was cleaning the back window by now. The pump was up to $10 and counting.

"I hope I got some spare change to cover the difference," I mumbled.

"Did you say check the tires?" he asked.

"No, I'm in a hurry."

Too late; he already had his tire gauge out.

"Yeah, I've got this friend named Fred who likes the Cardinals. I also won a few dollars off him. Lost quite a few, too, especially when the Cardinals had their good teams in the '60s. Course, it was all in fun.

"I remember taking a group of kids up to Comiskey back when the Sox lost all the time, but we still had a ball. We even got some foul balls!

"This year has been the most fun, though. I'm glad Chicago has something to cheer about after all the bad years the Sox, Cubs and Bears have had. The last time the Sox went to the Series was in '59, you know."

"Yeah, I know," I answered abruptly. "Now what do I owe you?"

"That will be $11.50."

Counting my change, I could come up with only $10.82.

"Aw, that's close enough," he said.

Surprised by this unexpected generosity, I promised to come back and make up the difference.

"Don't worry about it," he scoffed.

I thanked him and started to pull out when it dawned on me who this fellow was. But the kindly man was fading away.

"Dick … Dick Stonebraker, come back!" I cried.

"Dick, don't go! I didn't recognize you at first. I know it has only been a couple of months since your death, but believe me, we still remember you. All those years you waited for the Sox to do something, and the very day you leave us, they take off like a beautiful winged bird. Come back, Dick."

But it was too late. Dick had faded away. I woke up in a panic, looking around my room as if Dick might be there somewhere. All of a sudden I felt terribly lonely. Unable to sleep after that, I got up and did some research.

On the day Dick Stonebraker died, July 20, the White Sox were loping along in the American League West with a 46-43 record. They were a mere game ahead of second-place Texas. Floyd Bannister had a 5-9 pitching record.

From that point on, the Sox played .737 baseball, posted a 56-20 record and won the division by a whopping 20 games! Bannister won 11 of his 12 decisions. It was if Stonebraker had taken the White Sox' losing ways with him.

I remember hearing somebody say that Stonebraker made God a White Sox fan.

It is really kind of sad to know he cannot be here now as the White Sox approach their moment of glory, but I truly believe he is up there enjoying every minute of it. After all, he has the best seat in the house.

A Gates Way into Our Homes

For almost 50 years, Hilliard Gates was the voice of high school basketball, college basketball and college football in my home town, Fort Wayne. His passing in 1996 even prompted some words from Bob Knight. I got to know Gates in my Kendallville years. Even though I was just a cub reporter, he always treated me as an equal.

Bloomington Herald-Times
November 22, 1996

In the press conference following Wednesday night's Indiana-Princeton game, the first thing on Bob Knight's mind was not the scare Princeton had thrown into his Hoosiers. It was the passing of legendary sports announcer Hilliard Gates, who died Wednesday at the age of 80.

"We are obviously pleased to win the basketball game, but it becomes a very, very sad day for basketball people in the state of Indiana and me personally to learn of Hilliard Gates passing away," Knight said.

Knight was introduced to Gates early in his Indiana coaching career when Gates used to call the Hoosier games over television. Gates already had been broadcasting in one medium or another for 30 years by the time Knight met him.

"He was a basketball institution, long before anybody today was actively involved in the game of basketball," Knight pointed out in his press conference.

To this future sports writer growing up in Fort Wayne, there were three radio voices that used to keep me awake at nights listening to the transistor radio under the covers. There was Len Davis, the voice of high school football; Bob Chase, the voice of Fort Wayne Komets hockey; and Hilliard Gates, the voice of high school basketball.

Davis has long since passed but Chase is still calling Komets' games on radio station WOWO. And until 1993, Gates was still calling high school basketball. Over the course of his busy career, Gates also did Zollner Pistons basketball, two Rose Bowls and the first NBA All-Star game in 1950. His nightly television segment on WKJG, "Gates Way To Sports," was a model for the sportscasts you see today.

But radio was where Gates was at his best.

"I probably kept score of a thousand games of Hilliard's over the years," said Bob Hammel, the recently retired H-T Sports Editor. "Without question, Hilliard was my first teacher in the whole field. My first ambition was to be a broadcaster. Then my voice changed (into its present raspy form). He was such a great communicator on the scene. There were a lot of players I never saw play -- players of the '40s and '50s -- but I visualized them. I felt I had seen them, knew how they played. Hilliard's descriptions were so alive."

Gates coined such phrases as "halfcourt shot," a bomb from deep in the corner. A "quarter-court" shot was somewhere in between.

It was fitting that Gates should be inducted into the Indiana Basketball Hall of Fame in the twilight of his career. Through it all, he remained a humble man.

During my days as the sports editor for the *Kendallville News-Sun*, I would cross paths with Gates on many occasions. I was deeply impressed by the fact that he knew my name and was willing to talk "shop" with a relative nobody like me.

"I'm not sure I've used the word 'wonderful' before," said Knight, "but (Gates) was a wonderful man, someone we will all miss. He was a really, really good friend. He was a guy who really enjoyed

sports, really worked at making sports enjoyable. I would bet that all across northern Indiana, outside of personal loss, that this be met with so many people feeling sad, the hearing of his passing."

Gates was at the microphone when Milan toppled mighty Muncie Central in 1954. When that triumph was recreated in the 1986 movie, *Hoosiers*, Gates was asked to recapture the final magic on film.

Bloomington's Don Stratigos, who helped choreograph the penultimate scene, tells a story that reveals how much high school basketball meant to Gates. As actor Maris Valainis, a.k.a. Jimmy Chitwood, was practicing for the epic, Bobby Plump-like shot, he couldn't locate the basket.

"Maris was out there practicing from the top of the key and clanking them off the backboard and rim," Stratigos began. "Gene Hackman (a.k.a. coach Norman Dale) came over and said, 'Get the kid to move in or we'll be here all night.' Keep it in mind that all the kids and fans had to act like he made it anyway -- go nuts, run out onto the floor ... So every time we had to re-shoot, it cost about a thousand dollars. (Director) David Anspaugh decided to give him two more tries and then move him closer.

"Because of the drama of the moment -- how important it was to see the ball leave his hands and see in the frame the ball going in the basket -- you could feel the tension in the entire Hinkle Fieldhouse. It was a surreal feeling.

"He launched the shot ... nothing but net. Everybody in front of the camera reacted as beautifully as they were supposed to. Behind the camera, Hilliard and I were hugging each other and twirling each other around as if we'd won the state championship. Here was this 70-year-old man throwing me around like a doll. Fiction and reality became one. It was beautiful, spontaneous."

Beautiful, spontaneous. That was the way Hilliard Gates delivered sports into our homes for all those years.

He was more than a voice. He was a companion.

The Day Tradition Died

On an April day in 1996, there was a passing of another kind, the end of single-class basketball in Indiana. To a traditionalist like me, it felt like a death in the family.

Bloomington Herald-Times
April 30, 1996

INDIANAPOLIS, INDIANA

It was the end of a tradition. It was history in the making. It was democracy at work. It was the day Indiana high school basketball, as we know it, changed forever.

Mark it down: Monday, April 29, 1996.

On this momentous occasion, the Indiana High School Athletic Association Board of Directors, those watchdogs of Hoosier athletics, voted in favor of class basketball. And it wasn't even close, 12-5 the vote went, brushing aside 86 years of single-class tradition.

In the end it was the only vote, if you believe in democracy. The board members were merely listening to their constituents, the member schools, who when surveyed, approved class basketball by a shocking 233-151 margin.

"We live in a democracy," said Jim Russell, sports information director for the IHSAA. "(The board members) were elected by the membership to represent their intentions and they have spoken. From the association's standpoint, the system works. It was done in a public way. We surveyed the member schools, and we surveyed the student athletes. The fans had a chance to voice their opinions, and the media certainly did."

The IHSAA brass should not be cast as the villains in this matter. Their hands were tied from the beginning. In 1993 a committee representing the interests of small schools produced a petition expressing a desire for class basketball, signed by almost 70 percent of all schools.

The IHSAA spent the next 27 months researching the idea and surveying each and every school. When the survey showed that 60.6 percent of the member schools approved of the idea, the forces of change were put into action.

"We wanted to go in as open-minded as possible and without any sense of direction," said IHSAA commissioner Bob Gardner. "We certainly haven't been hush-hush about it. It has had a fair hearing in the media."

The IHSAA headquarters in Indianapolis was overflowing Monday with members of the media to hear first-hand this historical decision.

"Indiana is always going to be unique," said Gardner. "The gathering here today proves that."

"We've never had an open meeting here before," Russell pointed out, "but Bob Gardner's philosophy is that we have nothing to hide here. Everything has been above the board."

Gardner is prepared for the inevitable backlash for allowing class basketball to arrive on his watch.

"Somebody has to fill that role," he said. "If that's my task, I'll fill it. I'm pleased we have a decision and a direction to go. The length of time involved and the uncertainty made it difficult to deal with."

The issue obviously was not taken lightly.

"Speaking for myself, each board member waited as long as possible before coming to a decision," said Phil Gardner, the principal at Wes-Del who presides over the IHSAA Board of Directors. "I was not totally surprised by the strong vote," he added. "I was on the subcommittee that did the 27-month study."

Having handed out the medals to all five champions and runners-up in last year's state football finals, Gardner had a different perspective.

"The thing I came back to was having had the privilege of handing out medals to 10 groups of players, 10 groups of coaches, and seeing the influence it had on them," he said.

"I didn't really sleep that well last night," said board member Mike Blackburn, the athletic director at Northwestern. "I have an interest in history (as a former teacher), and I'm somewhat of a traditionalist. There were so many things to evaluate. We did the right thing, based on what our schools wanted us to do. I certainly don't think we did something wrong. It was inevitable. If it wasn't passed this year, it would have kept coming up."

It is not a totally done deal. The opposition has 90 days to get signatures from 20 members in each of the five districts asking for a statewide vote of member schools. But, as Russell pointed out, "We've already had a referendum, the survey."

The good news for the opposition is that the first two years of class basketball are put on a trial basis. The new tournament will go into effect in the 1997-98 school year and be re-evaluated in 1999.

"Nothing is set in concrete," Bob Gardner promised. "The bottom line is what's best for the athlete. We are an educational institution. We make decisions based on the best interests of the young people we serve. We do not want to change the image of Hoosier Hysteria. The tradition of Indiana high school basketball will continue, and we have a safeguard (the re-evaluation) if it doesn't."

As Russell concluded, "Indiana is always going to be a basketball state. The essence of the experience will not change."

The publisher of *Hoosier Basketball Magazine*, Garry Donna, isn't so sure.

"This reminds me of when Coca-Cola came out with 'New Coke.' They already had the No. 1 product and then they changed it," Donna said.

Editor's Note: Class basketball survived its two-year trial period and is still the format used in Indiana today.

Doris Seward Gets the Grand Prize

If you read the piece on George William Thompson ("Mystery Man", Chapter 10), you might recall it was Doris Seward who sent the photo that launched me on that treasure hunt. In many ways, Doris was linked to that photo and to that time, a grand generation.

Bloomington Herald-Times
October 4, 1999

"**L**ike some of you ..."
Thus began Doris Seward with each and every personal column she wrote for the *Herald-Times* the last four years, pieces which brought everyday life into our living rooms.

If you knew Doris only through her writings, you might not have realized what a grand lady she was. I got to find out for myself a couple of years ago.

In the spring of 1997, Doris sent the H-T Sports Department a rare photograph. Pictured were four members of the 1906 Indiana University relay team. One of those pictured was Doris's father, Fred. That wasn't her reason for forwarding the photograph, however. What caught her imagination -- and ours -- was the unfamiliar face of a gentleman of color. Doris thought it might be interesting to find out the name and the story behind what had to be one of IU's first black athletes.

The story ended up in my lap. I didn't mind because I was just as intrigued by the unknown as Doris was. My first stop on the trail was Doris herself, figuring she might have a lead on this mysterious figure. Doris was more than willing to help but insisted I come by her house at an appointed time. I knew then that you couldn't just drop in on this lady, 80 years old or not.

And when I did call on her, it was like stepping back into a more civilized time. She was dressed in a manner befitting afternoon company, her hair neatly done and a touch of make-up carefully applied. It was obvious she had gone to a lot of trouble for this interview.

Doris escorted me to her parlor, where a cup of tea and a plate of fresh dates awaited. I couldn't help but feel like the gentleman caller in the Tennessee Williams classic, "The Glass Menagerie."

In the days before my meeting with Doris, I had put a name behind the unknown runner, George William Thompson. The mere mention of that name triggered a whole set of memories, stories Doris's father had shared with her so many years ago.

We spent the better part of the afternoon talking about life at the turn of the century, and what it must have been like to have been a black man in a white man's world.

On Doris's recommendation, I would later interview two more of Bloomington's finest senior citizens, Elizabeth Bridgewaters and Maurice Evans. Sadly, they also have passed on, an enormous loss to our community within the last two years.

It turned out that George William Thompson not only was an outstanding athlete and ambassador for IU, he also was a dynamic community leader. It was Thompson who blazed a trail for blacks in Akron, Ohio -- long before Ohio or the rest of the country ever heard of Martin Luther King. Although Thompson's impact is still felt around Akron, he might have remained a long-forgotten figure at IU had it not been for Doris Seward.

About a week after the story broke, I stopped by Doris's home on High Street to return the picture which had started the pursuit. As always, she was most polite and genteel. After a brief chat over tea, Doris removed an object from one of the shelves in her parlor.

"I would like to you have this, Mr. Houser," she said, handing me a brass cup. On it was the inscription, "St. Louis University Games, 1905, Won by U. of Indiana."

Doris wanted me to have that precious artifact, a reminder of her father and his teammate. She was refreshingly generous that way.

My wife, Pat, once approached her in a public place to tell her how much she enjoyed her columns. Doris thanked her and reached into her bag. She pulled out a bound collection of her works.

"You win the prize," she said. "For being the first person who brightens my day, I give a prize."

Now Doris gets the prize, a bountiful eternity, no doubt. She earned it brightening a lot of our days.

Like some of you ... I'm going to miss her.

This Cat Had Me by the Tail

People aren't the only ones deserving of a proper farewell. The passing of our two precious cats prompted this piece and the next one.

Bloomington Herald-Times
May 7, 2001

It was shortly after Labor Day, 1982. I had just moved from my residence of six years, a little farm house on the property of Charles and Dora LeGras in rural Noble County.

A couple of days later I drove out to check the mailbox at the old homestead, which was abandoned now. Out of the corner of my eye I saw movement. Over in the grass was a black kitten, a farm critter which had been left behind. It paid no attention to me. It was preoccupied with a butterfly.

I drove away rationalizing that this animal was not my responsibility. Later that afternoon, the guilt kicked in. After work I went back to the farm with my dad, Ray, and my stepson, Steve. Our mission: capture the kitten, which already had a keen distrust of people.

Believing the cat was close to starvation and dehydration, it would welcome some milk, I figured. So I stopped at the grocery and picked up some Half-and-Half – the good stuff.

We put the bait in plain view of the cat and took our positions. The plan called for Dad and I to keep the cat's attention while Steve, much swifter afoot, would sneak up from behind and corral the cat with a blanket.

But this cat was on to us.

It helped itself to the Half-and-Half until Steve was within a matter of feet. Just as Steve was about to spring, the cat bolted. The cat was toying with us and loving every minute of it. It was about to disappear into a storm cellar when I made a desperate lunge and got a firm grip on its tail. Scratching and screaming, it went reluctantly into a burlap bag.

For the next two days it holed up in a shed at my new place. On the third day it felt secure enough to venture outside. That night it slept in the garage. One night later, it was a fixture on the bed.

For the next 18 1/2 years my bed really belonged to my faithful companion -- Odessa Marie Houser, I named her. When I would get home at night, no matter what the hour, she would be there to greet me like a worried mother.

Cats aren't known to be the warmest of pets. The saying goes that dogs treat people like family while cats treat them as staff. I must confess that "Odie" had me steppin' and fetchin'.

Even though I was in my 30s, I had never called a pet my own, a pet who claimed me as its champion. Odie did.

Maybe her devotion grew out of gratitude for being rescued, but I was hers and hers alone. She was openly jealous of the other people in my life, especially my wife, Pat. If Pat and I tried to snuggle up on the couch, Odie would wedge herself between us.

Odie did not have much use for women in general, but she did warm up to other men. My father once charmed her with music. An accomplished guitarist, Dad was in the kitchen one night strumming a few chords. Odie was totally captivated. She climbed up on the kitchen table, flopped over on her back and shamelessly swooned at the "other" man in her life.

Odie had a certain royalty about her. The other four cats who have shared the Houser household always deferred to her. If Odessa Marie showed up while they were in the midst of a feeding frenzy, they would reluctantly move over. My wife jokingly referred to her as the Queen Bitch.

Odie was not above bitching if we were slow to feed her or make a lap. And she was prone to pout if we went away on vacation and left her in the company of strangers.

Although Odie's nose may have been out of joint, her heart was in the right place. On the night Pat's mother died suddenly in 1983, Odie consoled the grieving daughter by gently placing a paw on her cheek.

After turning 18 last June, Odie's health went into decline. Her hearing had been gone for some time and her eyes were starting to fail. Odie also was having trouble keeping food down and controlling her bowels. With the quality of her life deteriorating, the time had come to put her down.

The day before she was to meet her Maker, I made it a point to spend as much time with her as I could. I tried to interest her with some string, but she preferred to sleep in the sun on the front deck. I got her to eat a little tuna and crawl up on my lap.

At the very moment she dipped into the Big Sleep, she was cradled in my arms, one of the saddest moments of my life.

In 1982 I captured a cat by the tail. For the better part of 19 years she captured my heart.

We made quite a pair, a boy and his cat.

The One and Only 'Molly the Mooch'

And while Odie was a cat of royalty, "Molly The Mooch" was, well … different.

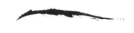

Bloomington Herald-Times
January 23, 2002

Last spring I wrote about Odie Houser, our family cat of almost 19 years. Now I give you Molly Houser, also known as The Mooch, a.k.a. The Moose, a.k.a. Psycho Cat.

Odie was special because we rescued her from an abandoned farm and enjoyed her for the better part of two decades. With Molly, well ... where do I begin?

When Odie was four years old we thought it would be nice if she had the companionship of another cat. My wife Pat thought an all-white cat would make a neat complement to Odie, who was all black. So, for Pat's birthday in 1986, I went shopping for a white cat.

My first stop was the Bloomington animal shelter. I was looking into the various cages when I heard a commotion behind me. I turned and saw a white paw beckoning from the cage. There she was, this ambitious white kitten, shoving two other cats out of the way in order to get my attention. I asked the attendant to let the white one out so I could see it up close and personal.

The audition went well. No sooner had the cat hit the floor when it started bouncing off the walls and making this unusual sound. It was not your ordinary "meow." It was more like a chirp, a most laughable, cheery chirp.

You might say Molly had me at "hello."

The attendant cleaned Molly up, sprayed her for fleas and sent her home with me. My next stop was Pat's office, where I hoped to surprise her. I put a lavender bow around Molly's neck and proudly presented her to Pat. Although the fleas were bailing in all directions, Pat didn't mind a bit as Molly nestled warmly in her arms.

Molly had Pat at first sight.

What a delightful birthday present she was, squirreling around the house making those unique chirping noises. Odie wasn't amused at first but eventually accepted the newest addition to the family. The neighbor cat was another story.

This cat also was all-white and thought it was the baddest thing on the block. Molly didn't buy that. One day the two of them went into a shrub to settle their differences. Leaves and twigs went flying as if a mighty wind had shaken the bush. The neighbor cat came scrambling out and kept on running. Strutting out a few seconds later was Molly, quite pleased that she was the new queen of the hill.

She was one tough cat. About a year later, she took off across the street and into the path of a van. To Pat's horror, Molly disappeared beneath the wheels. That should have used up all nine lives, but Molly came out of it with just a broken hip.

We knew then that this cat was a survivor. She had gotten over rejection by her first own-

Molly "The Mooch" was a picture waiting to happen. (Houser family photo)

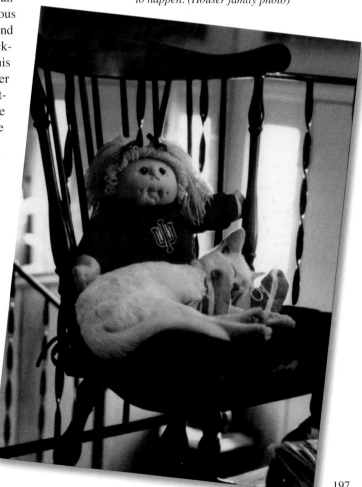

er, had escaped the shelter's Death Row, had weathered Odie's initial disdain, had outlasted the neighbor cat and even had held up under the weight of a big ol' truck.

You think that Molly would have been a little leery of people by then, but she loved company. No party was ever too big or too rowdy for Molly, who would camp right in the middle of it.

No box or basket could keep her from finding a way to wedge her butt into it. And like a poster girl, Molly knew a Kodak moment when she saw one. We have hundreds of pictures of her striking various poses -- climbing trees, hiding on the tops of shelves, peering through windows, sneaking out of boxes. My favorite is one of her curled up on the lap of a doll baby.

"She just goes around making pictures," Pat said.

Molly never saw a meal she didn't like, either. Every morning for 16 years, she would get up with Pat, an early riser, and gleefully lead my wife to the food bowl. Molly knew the precise moment Pat got up because she was sleeping in the same bed -- under the covers and with her head on the pillow, no less. Sometimes Molly would sleep horizontally, leaving me just a sliver to rest on. A girl has to have her space, you know.

Speaking of space, my father once made the mistake of sitting in Molly's favorite chair, the TV room recliner. Molly climbed up on the back and started working her way down until she had muscled Dad completely out of the chair.

I know what you're thinking, that no cat should be allowed such liberties, but Molly had exceptional people skills. Her playful behavior and weird chirping earned her the nickname Psycho Cat, given to her by a family friend.

Pat came up with Molly The Mooch, after Molly's habit of mooching food off you. Our grandson, Alex, interpreted Mooch as Moose, the name that really stuck. All the names fit her well.

The Mooch's favorite time of the year was Christmas, when she could play in all the empty boxes and gnaw at the bows and ribbons. This past Christmas, however, she acted disinterested.

She came out briefly for the first unwrapping and then went back to her nap. She started to sleep away the days and spend less time on our laps. She wasn't even getting up for breakfast and finally stopped eating altogether.

Last week, Molly went to a place we like to call Rainbow Ridge, from a verse about animal

heaven. Molly and Odie are there together in our hearts. After almost 20 years of cats, our house is terribly empty now.

Pat and I are getting through it by recalling all the wonderful, funny, engaging moments those pets gave us. It is our way of surviving the loneliness.

Thanks to Molly The Mooch/Moose, we know a little bit about survival.

When Actions Speak Louder than Words

In the summer of 2011, it was painfully obvious that a great local golfer, Bob Burris, was dying from cancer. At the encouragement of his family, I visited his home to spend some time with him – and feel the love that surrounded him. As you will note, there are not many comments from Burris himself, but those around him had plenty to say. A month after this article was published, Burris passed away.

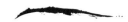

Bloomington Herald-Times
July 19, 2011

What do you say to a dying man?

Sad to say, I've had to write my share of eulogies over the years, but they were always after the fact, after the person had passed on.

But upon the request of the Burris family, I agreed to interview the gravely ill Bob Burris Jr., who is in the last stages of cancer.

For those of you too young to know who Bob Burris is, he is one of the greatest golfers to ever walk the venerable grounds of old Cascades. And I mean walk. He never rode in the cart, always preferring to walk and carry his own clubs.

He was a sight to behold. With long, flowing, reddish-brown locks and a full beard to match, Burris looked like one of those classic holy cards of Jesus. In fact, that was his nickname. The running joke around Cascades was that the real Jesus only wished he could play as well as Bobby Burris.

"We called him 'Jesus,' and believe me, Bobby could back it up," said Steve Hinds, who was in his golfing prime at the same time. What also amazed Hinds was that you rarely saw Burris on the putting green or the driving range. He just showed up and proceeded to pound the course into submission.

"If his tee time was 2 o'clock, Bobby showed up at 1:59," Hinds said. "You thought, 'This guy can't be that good,' but he was."

"Bobby Burris would just get out of his car, walk across the parking lot, step up to the first tee and hit it right down the fairway without even thinking about it," said Ike Martin, another long-time comrade.

And Burris went about it like a silent assassin, hardy saying a word or showing emotion of any kind, just like the rest of the Burris brothers — Ron, Bruce and Mark. For over a half century, the Burris family has been synonymous with the City Golf Tournament. With only a few exceptions, there has been a Burris playing in the tournament since 1947, when Bob Burris Sr. was the first to compete.

When Ron thought about not playing in this year's tournament due to Bobby's declining health, Ronnie's wife, Dee, talked him into it.

"I told Ronnie, 'There has been a Burris playing in this tournament since the '40s. You owe it to Bobby,'" Dee said.

Borrowing Bobby's putter, Ronnie overcame a three-hole deficit with four to play to beat Dave Devitt in the first round, an emotional lift for the entire family.

Over a 20-year period from 1975-94, Bobby won three championships and made it to the finals three other times. He reached the semifinal round eight times. His record over that period was 42-15, a .737 winning percentage during an era bursting with future Hall of Famers.

In 1989, Burris was enshrined in the H-T City Golf Hall of Fame, following in the footsteps of Bob Sr., who was inducted in 1982. Bobby was still winning championships when his father passed away in 1987 at the age of 55. Bobby has had to deal with his own health issues over the years, beginning with a bout of bacterial meningitis that nearly took his life in 1991. Later, it was discovered that Bob Jr. had a hole in his heart, severely limiting what he could do. He played his final city match in 1999.

For the last two years, he has been coping with cancer of the colon. Last April he suffered a stroke, making it difficult to write down his thoughts. In December, after exhausting all forms of treatment, Burris was given six to 12 months to live.

So how do you approach a man who may not see his 55th birthday? I have to admit I was uncomfortable as I sat down in Burris' living room. As always, he remains a man of few words, but he seems to be at peace with the hand he has been dealt. In fact, he continued tending bar at Kenny's Tavern right up through the end of June.

"I had to have something to do," he said.

Confronted with his mortality, Bobby has revealed a different side of himself. He woke up one morning in January and his head was swimming with a song that had come to him. To the surprise of his wife, Debbie, it was about her. He called it, "Blue Eyes."

"Bob has never been a big affectionate guy," she said. "I'm not even sure he knew my eyes were blue."

Helping Bobby put the words to paper was his stepdaughter, Traci Smith.

"Traci has always been the creative one of the family," Debbie said. "She tapped into Bobby's soul somehow."

"I started writing down his thoughts, and it just flowed," Traci said.

The song already has been picked up by Diamond Garden Music in Nashville, Tenn. The verse that really grabs you is the one where Burris refers to the wife he is about to leave behind:

"The pain that scares me most of all
Isn't where, isn't how or when.
I'm afraid that those blue eyes I love,
Will never shine that bright again."

Getting it out there like that has been therapeutic for the whole family.

"If you can find peace in an ordeal this, it is by speaking the words that need to be spoken," Debbie said.

More recently, Bobby has come up with yet another song. With Traci's help once again, the lyrics confront his death and its aftermath. They simply call it, "Bobby's Song."

"One day my pain will go.
My body will be gone.
But your fight will just begin
And you will have to carry on."

What more can you say than that? In the end, it is not what you say to the dying man. It is what the dying man says to you.

Ol' Ray Went Out with a Bang

You would think that your father's passing would be the most difficult farewell of all, but it wasn't. Having lived almost 94 years, "Ol' Ray," as we called him, had a great run. And he had a very good exit strategy, a full military funeral, which turned our hearts of sorrow into hearts of pride.

Bloomington Herald-Times
March 9, 2011

Dad would have been so pleased.

Last Saturday, my father, Ray Houser, was given a proper military funeral in Fort Wayne.

Although Fort Wayne was his lifelong home, Dad's heart was always on the high seas. He served 35 years in the Navy, including World War II, where he sailed on a minesweeper. To the very end of his 93-year run on this Earth, his military career was the thing he was most proud of — outside of family.

He was never prouder of me than when I was in the Navy from 1972-76. Now he has a grandson, Raymond, named after him, who has risen to the rank of master chief petty officer. Dad ascended to the highest rank possible for an enlisted man, chief warrant officer.

I'm sure Dad was beaming from above when Chief Raymond DeMarco showed up in full dress blues for the funeral Saturday. I also dressed for the occasion with a navy blue suit and a star-spangled red, white and blue tie.

Dad had expressed a strong desire for a military funeral, including a 21-gun salute, but with the country still deeply involved in the War on Terrorism, there is a shortage of available military personnel for such occasions. However, friends of the family made phone call after phone call until arriving at a viable alternative, the American Legion. Members from posts around the Fort Wayne area volunteered to accord Dad full military honors. Also stepping up to the plate were the Patriot Guard Riders, the motorcycle "gang" that goes all over the country to see that veterans are not forgotten.

The Patriot Guard planted American flags at the entrance to the funeral home, the church and the cemetery. A group of them stood at attention during the entire Mass said prior to Dad's burial. Greeting us at the cemetery were two representatives of the local Navy Reserve unit. They saw to the playing of "Taps" and the proper folding of the flag that had draped the casket. When they had finished folding the flag, the senior officer inspected it for military precision, and then approached. He dropped to one knee and said, "On behalf of a grateful nation ..."

As the sole surviving son, I was the rightful recipient. And also as a veteran myself, I was allowed to return salute. I must admit now that I often casually saluted when I was on active duty, but this was one time I wanted to get it right. I stood at attention, cocked my right hand crisply against my brow, and then slowly lowered the hand in synch with the Navy representative.

Unbeknownst to me, other members in the congregation behind me were doing the same thing.

I was so moved when I turned around that I could barely choke out a final request, the singing of "America the Beautiful." Right on cue, everyone joined in, including the color guard.

Never in my life was I more proud to be an American, and it gave me a deeper appreciation of those who paid the ultimate price.

Ray Houser was no war hero, but he did devote his life to his country. The military funeral he received Saturday was all he ever wanted in return. Anchors aweigh, my boys.

A Friend Is Somewhere Over the Rainbow

This was the hardest farewell of all. Bob Millican was my tennis partner, fishing buddy, basketball teammate and a guy I admired so much. On June 22, 2004, we were playing tennis. After a changeover, I turned around and ... he was gone, the victim of a massive heart attack. I never had a chance to say good-bye. This personal remembrance was as close as I could get.

Bloomington Herald-Times
June 24, 2004

Bob Millican was a true sportsman in every sense of the word.

When it came to hunting, whether it was quail or mushrooms, Millican had the nose of a bloodhound. When it came to fishing, he knew exactly where to drop the line.

A spectacular double rainbow – just for Bob Millican. (Courtesy photo)

On the basketball court, he was still running with the kids into his 60s. On the tennis court, he tormented opponents with the serve-and-volley.

It was shortly after one of his powerful volleys that Bob took his last breath two days ago. He probably would not have wanted it any other way.

I was with him at the end, and I've got to tell you, I'm hurting right now. More than a tennis partner or a basketball teammate or a fishing buddy, Bob was a great friend.

As good a sportsman as Millican was, he was an even better human being, which is a good thing because he was 6-feet-4 and blessed with strength that was almost scary at times. I saw him single-handedly carry a fishing boat up a steep hill and down the other side. I offered to help, but he said he could handle it easier by himself.

He was nice to everybody, including the less fortunate. Although he ended up in the real estate business, he started out as a teacher in Special Education. That ought to tell you something about the guy.

"Bob was a straightforward, honest guy," said Dr. William Pugh, a friend of Millican's. "He did all the right things. He represented the All-American guy, one of the nicest people you ever wanted to meet."

And what a wonderful family man. He was a devoted husband to wife Kathie and a model dad to daughter Anna and son Jason. Heck, he was even a faithful master to his beloved dog, a Golden Retriever named Oscar.

Underneath that nice-guy exterior, however, was a fierce competitor. Just ask anybody who dared to get too physical with him on the basketball court. A succession of in-your-face hook shots was in their future.

On the fishing pond, we used to wager who would catch the most bluegill. Millican made sure he came out on top by dropping three lines to my one. I didn't mind, because he always volunteered to clean the fish later.

Millican was like the perfect fishing guide. He hooked the boat up to his truck, drove you to the lake, backed the boat into the water, located the precise place where the fish were biting, set your line to the right depth and then watched with pleasure as you reeled them in. Afterward, he would clean the fish for you.

Not only did Bob always catch the most fish, he always found the most mushrooms. If the fish weren't biting on a particular spring day, he would pull the boat ashore and take a hike. He could spot a yellow morel under a fallen tree from 50 yards away.

Millican found a dream house for my wife and me and probably could have made a lot more money in the real estate business. But, as friend Gary Clendening said, "Bob never let making a buck keep him from going fishing."

Sounds to me like Millican really had his priorities right. The closest thing he had to a vice was the occasional pinch of chewing tobacco while waiting for the fish to bite.

"Bob was our hero," said neighbor Brian Werth, who played many a game of basketball and tennis with Millican over the years. "For being a big guy, he was very non-threatening. He is one of the most admirable guys I've ever known."

Did you see that wondrous, double rainbow over Bloomington before dusk Tuesday, just hours after Bob's passing? That had to be Bob saying, "It's all right, fellas. You ought to see the view from up here."

On the night of Bob's death, some of his friends got together for some toasts in his name. I'd like to propose another: Here's to Bob Millican, basketball teammate, tennis partner, fishing buddy and most of all, dear friend. We'll see you over the next rainbow.

Closing One Door, Opening Another

As a way of saying thanks to all the people who got me started, I penned this piece when I left Kendallville in 1984. As you will see, it was not easy leaving that life behind.

Kendallville News-Sun
October 19, 1984

An outdated East Noble High School calendar. A faded picture of the *News-Sun* staff dressed up for Halloween.

A fuzzy, toy replica of Hannah Holstein with a head that once bobbed but now is broken.

A certificate declaring Lynn Houser an honorary member of the "1982 East Noble Championship Baseball Team."

A permanently stained coffee cup with a hand-printed warning: "This is not an ash tray!"

A "Peanuts" cartoon showing Charlie Brown telling Snoopy that "Doing a good job around here is like wetting your pants in a dark suit – it gives you a warm feeling but nobody notices."

Relics. Artifacts. Remnants. Memories of a very special chapter of my life, a chapter that is drawing to a close after eight years. Starting Monday, I begin a new chapter at the *Bloomington Herald-Telephone*.

It all started to hit me the other day as I began emptying out my desk and stripping my bulletin board. I never anticipated staying this long when I first accepted a job as the new courthouse reporter for the *News-Sun* in 1976. A little paper like the *News-Sun* was merely a stepping stone to a glorious career at a metropolitan newspaper, I figured.

Then I learned the sports editor's position was open. I always fancied myself as an expert in the field of sports, so why not give it a try? Covering city councils, school boards and budget meetings was not my cup of tea to begin with.

It turned out to be the best decision I ever made. Within months I was firmly entrenched in a job I would hold for the next eight years. If somebody had told me back in 1976 I would still be at the *News-Sun* in 1984, I would have laughed in their face. But here I am today, only I'm not laughing. I'm torn between the excitement of opening a new chapter in my life and the sadness of closing a satisfying one.

What do you say after eight years anyway? Where do I begin? Where are the words that flowed so easily before?

I have on many occasions written straight from the heart, and that is what I'm going to do now. I will really miss this place, especially the people.

Thinking back over the last eight years, so many faces come to mind. Some of them are no longer with us – Dick Stonebraker, Lee King, Joel Hampshire, Jerry Grocock and Jim Herendeen – people who will be remembered for more than their athletic careers.

As for the living, I think of the many fine coaches I have had the pleasure of working with. Some of the more prominent ones from neighboring schools are West Noble football coach Dutch Raether; Central Noble football coach Mike Tolle; Lakeland basketball coach Bill Leiter; DeKalb basketball coach Roger Hughes; Prairie Heights basketball coach Randy Aalbregtse.

From East Noble, I've enjoyed working with basketball coach Denny Foster; girls' basketball coach Bob Farmer; wrestling coach Don Manger; track and field coach Bob Waterson; football coach Bob Wiant; baseball coach Fred Inniger.

I can honestly say I liked all of the coaches I dealt with. I'll tell you one thing. I wouldn't mind having my kid playing for any one of them.

You know what else I'll miss? The activities I have become accustomed to. I'm talking about noontime basketball at the YMCA; planning projects with the Jaycees; playing Strat-O-Matic Baseball with Jim Pippenger; going to Notre Dame football games with Eugene Poinsatte; belting out a hymn with the Immaculate Conception choir; taking road trips with WAWK's Larry Gilliland; Tuesday night bridge with Ken Napier, Paul Dobler, Dave Kropp and Don Frey; playing tennis with Carl "Doc" Stallman, Larry Blue and Mike "Fleetwood" Cshusta; rockin' and rollin' at the Parlor Lounge; talking sports at The Lockerroom pub; playing softball in the summer; going to The Strand Theater on "budget night;" going for a swim in Bixler Lake; biscuits and gravy at Glen and Nancy's; All-Area banquets at Shook's Lounge; broiled fish at the St. James; dinner theater at East Noble.

Above all, I'll miss my friends, the people who trusted me and let me be myself. If that meant going out and raising a little hell, they understood that writers are human beings, too.

So here's to you my friends: Jives, Hank, Troy, Gregg, "Waffle", Denny, "Biggun' ", John G., Harry, "Skeeter," Frank, Willy, Brannie, "Gigs," Stan, "Sledge," Mick, "Zip," Lance, Kevin, "E-Z," "E.P." and anybody I might have left out.

Last but not least are some extra special friends, my fellow employees at the *News-Sun*. For eight years, they have been more than friends. They have been my family. I only hope the publishers at the *Herald-Telephone* in Bloomington are as kind to me as publishers George and Lee Witwer have been. I hope my immediate superiors are as patient with me as John Peirce, Jim Kroemer, Terry Housholder and Dave Kurtz.

I also hope my fellow workers in Bloomington will be as fun to be around as Troy, Gregg, Kerry, Jan, Jill, Margaret, Mary, Carol E., Carol K., Cleon, Marcia, Sandy, Trudy, Lorraine, Donna, Ron, David, Tom, Wayne, Chris, Imo Jewel, Rita, Wendell, Norm, Bob, Mary I., Ingrid, Barb and all the girls in composing, all the folks in the mail room and all the guys in the press room.

Thanks to all of you for putting up with my loud voice, my lockerroom jokes and my occasional tantrums.

And now it's time for the ol' Armchair Coach to head south. In closing, I want to leave you with these words of wisdom offered by my good buddy, Steven Hankins: "It's not the miles I've traveled. It's the stops I've made."

So long, everybody. See you in the sports pages.

I Love(d) My Job

And then, 29 years later, I penned my farewell column to my Herald-Times *readers, published the day after I retired."*

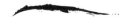

Bloomington Herald-Times
March 7, 2012

When I walked out the Assembly Hall doors following the IU-Purdue game Sunday night, it hit me: I was no longer "Lynn Houser, sports writer."

It is an identity crisis I have been wrestling with ever since last summer, when I made the decision to take an early retirement.

Since then, many of my peers have asked, "Houser, are you nuts?"

A fair question, it is.

Given the present state of our economy, why would a guy who grew up in Indiana, went to Indiana University, lived in Bloomington 30 years and worked in the state's best damn sports department want to walk away from a dream job while he is still of sound mind?

At this moment you are probably questioning the "sound mind" part, but, hey, all good things must end.

For me, it is a matter of moving onto something else while I'm still young enough to take on a new challenge. I have no idea what lies ahead. I do know it is time to do something different.

After 36 years in one career I have become a creature of habit. I've noticed the last couple of years that covering the same events over and over has a way of losing its freshness. That can only lead to staleness, and I would never want to burden my readers with unimaginative writing.

More than that, I have grandchildren who barely know me. I aim to fix that before I miss another birthday, another baptism, another recital, another Little League game.

There were no grandchildren in the picture when I came to Bloomington in 1984. Having spent the previous eight years at the small northern Indiana daily, the *Kendallville News-Sun*, I was thrilled to get hired by what was then the *Herald-Telephone*. To me it was the opportunity of a lifetime.

Bob Knight had Indiana basketball in its heyday, and there was an air of confidence that Bill Mallory would have IU football on the rise in no time at all. IU soccer, swimming and track were national players because of coaches Jerry Yeagley, Doc Counsilman and Sam Bell. Bloomington high school sports teams were no strangers on the state level, either.

And what a sports team I was joining, beginning with sports editor Bob Hammel, who already was a legend when I came on board. To this day, Bob Hammel is the most prolific sports writer I have even seen. How many others could say they wrote a quality cover story and column every day? Hammel did, and he made it look easy. You name a Hall of Fame, and he's in it.

On the desk was John Harrell, in my opinion still the best slot man to ever turn out a page. He personally invented computerized shortcuts to help us formulate agate for our sports pages, while also editing copy and laying out the pages. You can thank him for the website that has all the latest on Indiana boys and girls high school basketball results.

Also on board at the time were Rex Kirts and Andy Graham. Hammel, Harrell and Kirts are all in the Indiana Sportswriters and Sportscasters Hall of Fame, and I'm convinced Graham's time is coming. For a paper of that size, I would even now put that sports department against anybody's — in any state, in any era.

After Hammel retired in 1996, Gary McCann replaced him as sports editor. McCann is now in the College Basketball Hall of Fame. He eventually was replaced by Stan Sutton, a 2004 inductee into the Indiana Sportswriters and Sportscasters Hall of Fame.

So you can see that I've been nurtured by some pretty good mentors over the years. I also was fortunate to have a beat that was broad and varied. I got to cover my share of IU events as well as high school events. I got to cover community events such as city golf and city tennis, and I also got to cover the Colts and Pacers. I am amazed at the historical things I witnessed firsthand:

* Bob Knight throwing the chair (1985);

* Keith Smart hitting "The Shot" (1987);

* The Hoosier football faithful making such a ruckus that Michigan's Bo Schembechler complained about crowd noise (1987);

* The crowning of Indiana's last, single-class, high school basketball champ, Bloomington North (1997);

* Reggie Miller sticking a playoff game-winner in Michael Jordan's face (1999);

* A.J. Moye and IU stuffing No. 1 Duke in the Sweet 16 (2002);

* The Colts punching their ticket to the Super Bowl by finally slaying the Patriots (2007);

* The Colts then winning the Super Bowl by conquering the Bears (bittersweet because the Bears were quarterbacked by Bloomington's own Rex Grossman);

* Austin Starr winning one for Coach Hep' with a last-minute field goal over Purdue (2007);

* And Bloomington South capping off of a perfect season with a state title (2009).

How could I have been so blessed? How could I have ended up at this job, in this great sports department, at this point in Bloomington's glorious sports history? It truly was the work of a higher power.

No wonder I looked forward to almost every assignment. It rarely felt like work. But now it does, mainly because my biological clock is ticking and I yearn to spend more time with my family. The death of my father a year ago this week continues to remind me of that.

Before going, though, I want to thank the H-T for giving me the opportunity to be a part of all this, and for providing a forum for me to write about it.

And thank you, readers, for all the feedback over the years. I can't tell how much a simple compliment could brighten my day. And for those who disagreed with my message, thanks for not killing the messenger.

No matter where I land after this, I will look back on my years in Bloomington and realize, "Houser, you had it made."

Index